Principles of Ear Acupuncture

Microsystem of the Auricle

Second Edition

Axel Rubach, MD
Private Practice
Munich, Germany

132 illustrations

Thieme
Stuttgart · New York · Delhi · Rio de Janeiro

Library of Congress Cataloging-in-Publication Data is available from the publisher.

This book is an authorized translation of the 3rd German edition published and copyrighted 2009 by Hippokrates Verlag, Stuttgart. Title of the German edition: Propädeutik der Ohrakupunktur

Original translation by Ursula Vielkind, PhD, Dundas, Canada; new text parts translated by Ruth Gutberlet, Hofbieber, Germany

Ear illustrations: © Axel Rubach; adaptations by Mathias Wosczyna, Wandlitz, Germany

© 2017 Georg Thieme Verlag KG

Thieme Publishers Stuttgart
Rüdigerstrasse 14, 70469 Stuttgart, Germany
+49 [0]711 8931 421, customerservice@thieme.de

Thieme Publishers New York
333 Seventh Avenue, New York, NY 10001, USA
+1-800-782-3488, customerservice@thieme.com

Thieme Publishers Delhi
A-12, Second Floor, Sector-2, Noida-201301
Uttar Pradesh, India
+91 120 45 566 00, customerservice@thieme.in

Thieme Publishers Rio, Thieme Publicações Ltda.
Edifício Rodolpho de Paoli, 25º andar
Av. Nilo Peçanha, 50 – Sala 2508
Rio de Janeiro 20020-906 Brasil
+55 21 3172 2297 / +55 21 3172 1896

Cover design: Thieme Publishing Group
Typesetting by Thomson Digital, India

Printed in India by Manipal Technologies Ltd., Karnataka

5 4 3 2 1

ISBN 978-3-13-125252-4

Also available as an e-book:
eISBN 978-3-13-169412-6

Important note: Medicine is an ever-changing science undergoing continual development. Research and clinical experience are continually expanding our knowledge, in particular our knowledge of proper treatment and drug therapy. Insofar as this book mentions any dosage or application, readers may rest assured that the authors, editors, and publishers have made every effort to ensure that such references are in accordance with **the state of knowledge at the time of production of the book**.

Nevertheless, this does not involve, imply, or express any guarantee or responsibility on the part of the publishers in respect to any dosage instructions and forms of applications stated in the book. **Every user is requested to examine carefully** the manufacturers' leaflets accompanying each drug and to check, if necessary in consultation with a physician or specialist, whether the dosage schedules mentioned therein or the contraindications stated by the manufacturers differ from the statements made in the present book. Such examination is particularly important with drugs that are either rarely used or have been newly released on the market. Every dosage schedule or every form of application used is entirely at the user's own risk and responsibility. The authors and publishers request every user to report to the publishers any discrepancies or inaccuracies noticed. If errors in this work are found after publication, errata will be posted at www.thieme.com on the product description page.

Foreword

In my foreword to the first edition, I expressed the wish that Axel Rubach's *Principles of Ear Acupuncture* would be widely distributed and accepted. This wish has been realized. It is considered the best textbook in this specialty area and has also become a standard reference in the English-speaking world.

Ear acupuncture has been established in Germany for over 50 years. This began in January 1951 when the German medical society for acupuncture DÄGfA (Deutsche Ärztegesellschaft für Akupunktur) invited the inaugurator of auriculotherapy, Paul Nogier, to teach classes in Munich and thereafter included the method as a permanent feature of its training program.

Later, experiences from Chinese medicine were added and imparted through the DÄGfA lecturers Ingrid Wancura and Georg König. The coexistence of the two schools had a fruitful effect. Both systems have proved to be equally feasible and complement each other, providing patients with great benefits. Ear acupuncture is still the most effective and, in daily practice, the most common form of Western acupuncture.

The complete system of ear points has not only created new opportunities for diagnostics and therapy, but also directed attention to the phenomenon of microsystems in general, and to the existence of somatotopic representations of the entire organism in circumscribed areas. Sufficient scientific studies exist to document the effectiveness of microsystemic acupuncture.

In physics, complex nonlinear systems and the fractal phenomenon, as well as the view of the universe as holographic (described by David Bohm), have been recognized. From this, it is obvious that not only the aspect of self-reflection, but also systemic correlations between the whole and its parts, play a role within microsystems.

Those practicing ear acupuncture must be well acquainted with anatomy, point topography, and the particular indications for treatment. Axel Rubach introduces these topics illustratively and with practical orientation to the anatomy and morphology of the ear, the acupuncture points and their locations, and the specific indications of this method. The easiest way has proved to be the best: avoid complicated treatment procedures burdened with a number of therapeutic obstacles, but rather work out and communicate unambiguous point constellations (pools), knowledge of those points, and the resulting safety in their use.

This newly revised edition contains additional therapeutic examples and improved artwork. For many therapists, this second edition will provide helpful guidance in learning the method of practice, as well as serving as a reference text for those who are more experienced.

Jochen Gleditsch, MD
Otorhinolaryngology, Dentist
Honorary President of DÄGfA
Lecturer in Acupuncture,
University of Munich, Germany

Preface

This book resulted from an idea to create a fundamental work and textbook on the systematics of ear acupuncture. With this in mind, I would like to offer my utmost respect to all those who, since Nogier's ingenious insight, have paved the way for this method with their work and publications. They also laid the groundwork for this book. Additionally, the condensed knowledge and experience of many lecturers from the German medical society of acupuncture, DÄGfA (Deutsche Ärztegesellschaft für Akupunktur), have contributed considerably to the success of this work.

I would like to express my gratitude to my teacher and friend, Dr. Jochen Gleditsch, to whom I owe my knowledge of this procedure and my enthusiasm for acupuncture in general. He initiated the idea for this book and was always on hand with help and advice. His book *Maps Mikroakupunktsysteme*, published in 2002,

offers comprehensive and detailed insights into the essential microsystems of acupuncture and joins the phenomena of the individual microsystems into one concept.

Thanks also to my friend Tom Ots for his input concerning the treatment of addictions and psychiatric disorders.

In this updated edition, our aim was to make the information as accessible as possible to readers and to allow them to secure a path to expertise by testing themselves with the provided templates. We have revised the entire text and the illustrations, adding many new therapeutic examples and making it easier for readers to become familiar with the topic of ear acupuncture. We also improved the book's potential as a reference work.

Axel Rubach, MD
Hans-Juergen Weise, DDS
Claus Schulte-Uebbing, MD

Contributors

Axel Rubach, MD
Private Practice
Munich, Germany

Claus Schulte-Uebbing, MD
Physician in Private Practice
Munich, Germany

Hans-Juergen Weise, DDS
Dentist in Private Practice
Rheinfelden, Germany

Contents

Basics/Theory

1 Introduction

1.1 History

Origins. Contrary to common belief, ear acupuncture is not a more recent form of therapy than body acupuncture. As early as the *Huang Di Nei Jing,* the 2,100-year-old book of Chinese medicine, we find evidence of reflex relationships between the outer ear and individual regions of the body. Records show that these relationships were also therapeutically being used in Persia, Egypt, and Greece about 2,000 years ago. It remains a mystery which culture these reflex relationships were first discovered in, mainly because we have only a few medical records up to the 17th century. As a result, certain elements of this method of treatment (e.g., cauterization in the upper auricular region for the treatment of sciatic pain) owe their survival predominantly to oral transmission from generation to generation in the Middle East and parts of Africa.

In the 17th century, there are indications both in the arts and in medical treatises that the auricle's reflex relationships were also well known in Europe. The first and foremost example is the famous painting by Hieronymus Bosch (1450–1516) called *The Garden of Earthly Delights.* The right wing of this altar triptych shows a symbolic illustration of Hell and—among other things—an auricle on which certain relationships between the ear and the rest of the body are depicted in great detail. The area in the upper auricle, which is pierced by one of the two spears seen, is identical to the zone of cauterization mentioned for sciatic pain. In a case description from the year 1637, the Portuguese physician Zaratus Lusitanus reported on sciatic pain treatment by ear cauterization, and in 1717 Valsalva described in his book *De Aura Humana Tractatus* an auricular area that had been cauterized for toothache.

Also from the 19th century, interesting medical records exist on auricular cauterization for sciatic pain syndrome, such as that of the physician Luciano of Bastia, as well as the documented observations by the surgeon Valette at the Charité in Paris in the year 1850.

The French/Western School. The different localizations of cauterization zones on the auricular helix, which were described in these documents, demonstrate that a systematic approach to ear reflexology did not yet exist at that time. It was not until the 1950s that the French physician Paul Nogier—to whom we also owe the "rediscovery" of the above-mentioned documents from medical history—developed the systematic fundamentals of ear acupuncture on the basis of incidental observations during years of meticulous research. In some of his patients, he had noticed scars in the upper part of the auricle stemming from therapeutic cauterization to relieve the symptoms of the sciatic pain syndrome. All of these patients had found relief—some in Africa, some through a lay healer in Marseilles—after Western medical art had proved to be unsuccessful. The lay healer had learned this form of healing from her father, who had been a physician in Indochina for many years. Nogier first presented his work, under the title *Auriculotherapy,* at a conference on acupuncture in Marseilles in 1956. Hence, he is the undisputed founder of today's ear acupuncture. This very first lecture—translated into German by Bachmann and subsequently published in the *Deutsche Zeitschrift für Akupunktur* (DZA, *German Journal of Acupuncture*; Nogier 1957)—prepared the ground for this method of treatment.

The Chinese School. Nogier's knowledge also reached China, where his publications caused a reconsideration of Chinese traditions that went back thousands of years, thus stimulating extensive and intensive research. Chinese findings up to that date confirmed and complemented his work to a great extent but also produced some contradictions. Nevertheless, Nogier is widely acknowledged as the discoverer of today's ear acupuncture, even in China. The Chinese school of ear acupuncture gained international recognition through the Austrian physicians Georg König and Ingrid Wancura, and because of its good results with acupuncture-induced analgesia.

Both forms—the so-called Chinese ear acupuncture and the auriculotherapy of Nogier—have much in common, although on occasion the localization of points may differ. The sensible objective is to integrate any confirmed knowledge from both schools under one roof and to use it to benefit patients.

Competing research activities of various schools and mutual verification of their findings guarantee some control and reliability of the studies and keep the discussion going. As early as the 1970s, Russian researchers also contributed

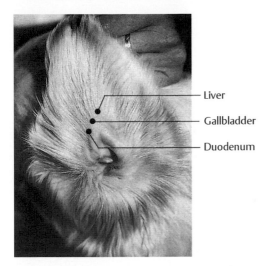

Fig. 1.1 Example of organ projections on the ear of a dog.

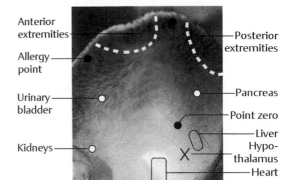

Fig. 1.2 Example of organ projections on the ear of a rabbit (according to Portnov 1979).

significantly to this field, with Durinjan, Portnov, and Velchover the leading authors. Although their research took place mainly in the area of veterinary medicine, their results were comparable to those described in human medicine (**Figs. 1.1** and **1.2**).

Over the past 15 years, positive findings from international research teams, e.g., in the area of perioperative medicine and the treatment of addictions, have added to the insights into the effectiveness of ear acupuncture and encouraged further research.

In perioperative medicine, for example, the literature survey from Usichenko et al (2007) shows that an increasing number of randomized, controlled trials have contributed to the acceptance of ear acupuncture in combination with pharmacotherapy as being an effective mode of treatment as part of integrative patient care. The data from this survey reveal the most frequent perioperative indications for ear acupuncture to be premedication, reduced use of anesthetics during general anesthesia, and postoperative pain therapy.

According to this study, ear acupuncture seems to be an effective complementary treatment for preoperative anxiolysis and to reduce the use of postoperative analgesics.

Examples of recent research work by Usichenko et al, Li and Wang, Vorobiev and Dymniko are described below. Vorobiev and Dymnikov's (2000)

blinded study on postoperative pain therapy shows a reduction in pain intensity and use of analgesics following outpatient surgery. A double-blind study by Li and Wang (2006) indicates a significant reduction in the use of opioids within the first 5 days after liver surgery when applying ear acupuncture. Usichenko et al (2005a) examined the impact on the use of postoperative analgesics in patients who received a hip replacement in combination with the application of ear acupuncture to the "hip joint," "*shen men*," "lung," and "thalamus" points versus ear acupuncture to the "sham" points. Usichenko's randomized, controlled trial on preoperative anxiolysis through ear acupuncture shows that ear acupuncture has the same anxiolytic effect as 10 mg diazepam.

1.2 The Term *Microsystem*

The term *microsystem* refers to the phenomenon of defined body areas that reflect the entire organism in the form of functional interrelationships. Through these body areas, it is possible to utilize well-defined reflex relationships with external or internal regions of the body to provide diagnostic clues or enable therapeutic measures. Synonyms are *zones of representation* and *somatotopy* (from Greek: *soma*, body; *topos*, place); the latter term is mainly used in neurology and neuroanatomy, where it applies to those cortical fields that correspond in terms of nerves and function to certain motor or sensory areas of the body.

The microsystems are not, as one might expect, microprojections of the body drawn to scale, but rather fields of representation, each primarily representing the characteristic reflex relationships with the organism that match the corresponding area. There are different microsystems in the body that are interconnected, each one representing an independently functioning system of individual inherent laws with its own characteristics and special diagnostic and therapeutic possibilities. According to Gleditsch (2005), the overlapping of different microsystems is reminiscent of several sports fields painted on top of each other on a gymnasium floor: depending on the markings, one sport or another will be played. In this sense, the functional coexistence and interaction of the reflex zones of the tongue, mouth, nose, hand, sole of the foot, or auricle can be understood within the overall picture of the human body or the system of body acupuncture (**Fig. 1.3**).

Of the above-mentioned synonyms, the term *microsystem* best describes the concentrated form of whole-body projections within the scope of their organized systematic reflex relationships.

1.3   Scientific Findings Concerning Ear Acupuncture

During the 1980s and 1990s, two experimentally well-founded theories of acupuncture research crystallized from the various explanatory models. With their functional cross-linking and interaction, these form the foundation of today's scientific knowledge on this subject: one theory represents the neurophysiological, or nervous plane, and the other theory the neurohumoral plane.

However, the research results presuppose that the nervous system must be intact if acupuncture is to be effective. They go beyond the hypothesis of "gate control" (Melzack and Wall 1965) by postulating that the major pain-relieving mechanisms are located not only at the spinal cord level, but also in the midbrain region. Here, particularly in the periaqueductal gray matter, an increased secretion of the endorphin enkephalin is triggered by the peripheral stimulus. This results in an inhibition of pain conduction in the descending spinal cord fibers that is mediated by the neurotransmitter serotonin (descending inhibition of pain).

In addition to the sympatholytic effects of needle stimulation, such as the increase in blood flow, the segmental reference of acupuncture is important. This can be verified at the neuroanatomical level. For example, there is significant correspondence between the action characteristics of individual acupuncture points and their corresponding segmental references. Further neurophysiological connections are evident from the frequent correspondence of acupuncture points with the maximum points according to Head (1893) and certain trigger points (Melzack and Wall 1965), as well as from the fact that skin resistance is demonstrably lower at these points.

Ear acupuncture as an independent microsystem can be distinguished from body acupuncture essentially by the fact that the reflex points or zones are only demonstrable when irritated. Ear acupuncture points function like a cybernetic binary system according to the yes/no principle: they are only reactive when the corresponding organ is disturbed or when the corresponding body part is injured or diseased. By comparison, body acupuncture points are part of an energy system that exists in a "steady state," which is why they can be identified at any time.

Presumably, the major scientific theories of interpretation available at present, namely, the neurophysiological and the neurohumoral models, apply to both forms of acupuncture in the same way. On the neurophysiological level, the points of the auricular microsystem exhibit different interactions that can be neuroanatomically understood, i.e., their reflex arcs are connected to higher regions of the central nervous system, such as brain stem and thalamus (Velchover 1967 and Durinjan 1983). This can be explained by the topically close embryological development and by the unusually dense and differentiated innervation of the auricle. The

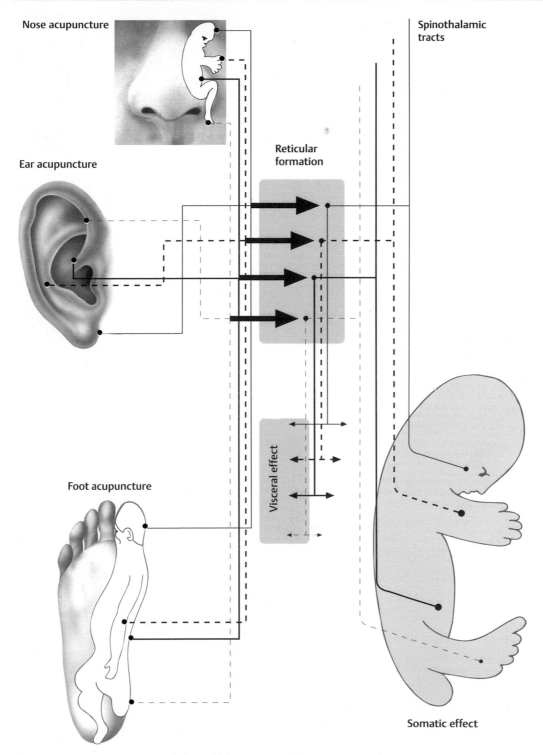

Nose acupuncture

Spinothalamic tracts

Ear acupuncture

Reticular formation

Visceral effect

Foot acupuncture

Somatic effect

Fig. 1.3 Known microsystems (adapted from Bossy 1981).

quick onset of action in acute states of pain can probably be attributed to these relatively short reflex paths (**Fig. 1.4**).

1.4 Ear and Body Acupuncture— A Comparison

Both ear acupuncture and body acupuncture originated in ancient China. However, it only became possible to take advantage of all the therapeutic possibilities of ear acupuncture as a result of Nogier's discoveries and systematic work.

Body acupuncture, on the other hand, has not experienced major changes to its basic principles since the first records were written more than 2,000 years ago. It is based on a system of correspondence, *yin* and *yang,* and on a system of 12 channels—six *yang* and six *yin* channels—which run along anatomically identifiable lines over the surface of the body as defined by acupuncture points. The system of five elements with its five phases of transformation, used as a universal reference system, was added as an essential ingredient to complement these fundamentals of acupuncture.

In contrast, the auricle is endowed with a microsystem that is independent of the modalities of body acupuncture. This microsystem exhibits a direct reflex relationship to the entire body. Ear acupuncture works with a number of systematically arranged reflex points that, when irritated, can be identified in certain anatomically well-defined areas of the outer ear. The image of an inverted embryo described by Nogier (see **Fig. 2.12**) may provide a rough orientation; with its disproportionate representation of the head and hand, it exhibits a distinct similarity to the somatotopic representation on the cerebral cortex (according to Penfield and Rasmussen; **Fig. 1.5**).

In contrast to this, body acupuncture has no direct, neurologically defined reflex relationship between a point or pathway and certain organs or body regions, with the exception of the *shu* and *mu* points.

The points used in both body acupuncture and ear acupuncture can be demonstrated through their diminished skin resistance. As emphasized above, we must bear in mind that ear acupoints can only be identified when irritated as a result of disturbed function or injury of the corresponding organ, whereas body acupoints can be located at any time.

In body acupuncture, certain needle sensations, such as the *de qi* sensation or propagated sensation along the channel (PSC), may often be induced and can be interpreted as a sign that acupuncture treatment will be successful. Ear acupuncture does not show such reactions.

With both procedures, more active points or zones can be identified on the body side affected by symptoms than on the opposite side. This stems from the twofold crossing of reflex paths between auricle, brain, and target organ or body area, respectively.

In ear acupuncture, compared with body acupuncture, it is relatively easy to obtain a diagnostic orientation and to use it therapeutically. Orientation results from directly identifying the irritated reflex zones based on changes to the skin (such as scaling, reddening, or other inflammatory symptoms) as well as sensitivity to pressure and diminished skin resistance. This requires more involved diagnostic procedures in body acupuncture.

Needling, electrostimulation, and laser may be used in both procedures as a method of stimulation. Cupping and moxibustion are, however, reserved for body acupuncture in view of the differentiation and density of the ear points, which makes targeted application on the ear impossible.

A general statement regarding the effectiveness of the two methods is not possible in view of indication-dependent priorities. For example, the domain of ear acupuncture, and therefore its special effectiveness, lies mainly in the area of acutely painful disorders, which, in terms of Chinese medicine, is the area of *yang* diseases. Here, body acupuncture may be effective too, but this seems to be more effective primarily in the area of chronic or chronically reoccurring diseases. In many cases, a combination of both procedures is sensible.

There are no differences with respect to the duration of treatment, which may take about 20 to 45 minutes per session, and the treatment intervals or frequencies of treatment sessions, which depend on the patient's constitution and the type of disease.

Ear acupuncture, compared with body acupuncture, can be learned within a relatively short time. The theoretical basis can be acquired within a few weeks, and intensive practical training lasting only several months is necessary to achieve

Somatotopic acupuncture

Referring to information
(concentration)

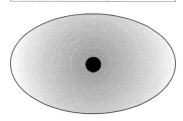

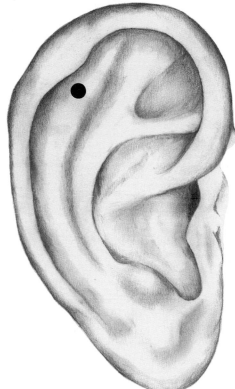

Referring to informative-binary system:
Yes/no (either/or) principle

Points can be identified only while irritated

On

Off

Body acupuncture

Referring to energy
(field of tension)

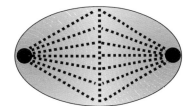

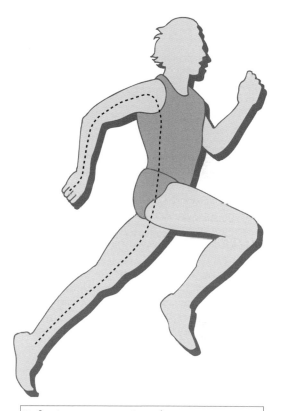

Referring to energetic-endosomatic system:
Energy flow principle

Points can be verified at any time

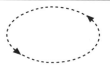

Fig. 1.4 Binary system vs. energetic system.

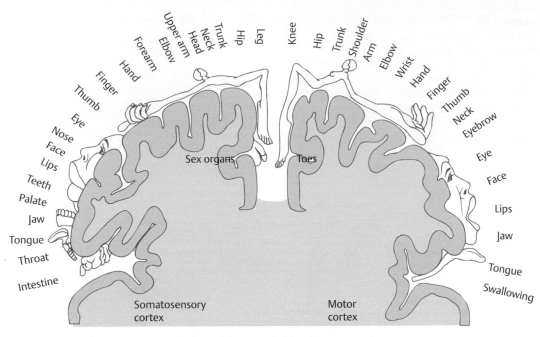

Fig. 1.5 Zones of representation (adapted from Penfield and Rasmussen).

meaningful treatment results. On the other hand, several years of practical experience with body acupuncture are usually required to attain mastery of this technique.

Ear acupuncture has distinct advantages regarding its practical application. Unlike body acupuncture, it does not require the patient to undress either completely or partially for treatment. Furthermore, those body areas that cannot be treated locally with body acupuncture because of wounds, bandages, swellings, or extreme pain can be treated through the auricular reflexes via remotely located ear points.

In contrast, body acupuncture has the advantage of generally working without technical accessories. The experienced therapist finds the points solely through exact localization and palpation. To find points on the auricle, however, at least pressure probes, styli, or the acupuncture needle itself are required. Probing with the acupuncture needle—the *very point technique* of Gleditsch (Grüsser et al 2005)—is usually reserved for the experienced therapist. Simple electrical search instruments for finding points and determining the diminished skin resistance are further useful to safely locate each of the irritated ear points because

of their delicacy, dense arrangement, and state of irritation.

For both acupuncture systems, the *mechanism of action* is via activation of the body's own homeostasis and, ideally, will lead to healing rather than just quick pain relief. It is assumed that the body's natural healing mechanisms themselves are reactivated through the targeted positioning of a stimulus, thus restoring the original symptom-free interaction of body functions.

Adverse effects in terms of a treatment-induced interference with health are not known with either ear acupuncture or body acupuncture. The only exception is a rather comfortable numbness or tiredness immediately after treatment. However, these effects regularly disappear within a few hours and should be taken as a positive sign, namely, as a treatment-induced expression of the body's ability to regulate itself.

1.5 Laterality

Laterality in the medical sense refers to the laterodominant specialization of the human brain. It can be recognized in certain body functions that are also laterodominant, such as left- or right-handedness as an expression of integrative and coordinative performances of the brain. Interesting insights into this topic have been provided by American scientists, such as Deutsch and Ornstein, who verified empirical observations through systematic scientific investigations. According to them, the left hemisphere of the brain is more responsible for the rational, verbal, and mathematical capacities of a right-handed person, whereas the right hemisphere represents more the nonverbal (visual or intuitive) creative capacities of a person. Truly left-handed individuals—constituting approximately 2 to 5% of the population—show an inverted dominance of the cerebral hemispheres, although the results obtained in this respect are not uniform.

The laterodominant specialization of the human brain is related to individual speech development (Ornstein), and hence obviously also to different cultural environments. This explains the widespread right-handedness in Western civilizations, where rational thinking is expected and promoted almost exclusively, compared with less developed civilizations and populations from Asian region, where imaginative, intuitive thinking is prevalent and where, even today, pictographs are used for writing.

The almost opposite specializations of the two cerebral hemispheres are obviously associated with endogenous self-regulating mechanisms that aim for some adjustment or harmonization of both areas in order to ensure a more balanced expression of life. Exogenous influences on laterality, such as re-education of left-handedness and the suppression or neglect of talents, may interfere with the body's innate regulating processes that aim for adjustment and may lead to pathological reactions within the organism. How interferences with laterality manifest themselves on the auricle in the form of different positions of irritation at the corresponding zones of representation has not yet been investigated scientifically; this question needs to be further studied in order to be settled.

Thus, laterality is of minor importance to ear reflexology. Based on the knowledge put forward, one might assume that the ear sending stronger informative signals is always assigned to the more inactive—and in Western culture usually more intuitive—hemisphere of the brain. Again, this must be understood as an expression of endogenous regulating mechanisms aiming for an adjustment of rational and intuitive capacities in the sense of ambidexterity.

In ear acupuncture, therefore, we often find that the reactivity of zones of representation is distinctly contralateral (with respect to the dominant hemisphere) for many different symptom complexes that can be characterized as psychosomatic in the widest sense. In contrast, all traumatically or nonpsychically characterized diseases of the body are projected onto the homolateral auricle (with respect to the location of the disease) and hence should be treated primarily from this side. Nevertheless, there are also additional irritated zones on the nondominant auricle, and these can be included in the treatment.

In all cases of uncertain laterality that cannot be established unconsciously and intuitively as right- or left-handedness by means by the hand-clapping test, treatment may be carried out on both auricles without any problems.

For orientation purposes during daily practice, both auricles are usually examined independently of laterality for the presence of reacting points, and needling is started on the more informative side.

Within the scope of its distinct specialization, which employs magnetic fields, frequency modulation, and color filters, the French auriculotherapy of Nogier places particular emphasis on the phenomenon of laterality and on the way it may be influenced by a "laterality control point." This emphasis should, however, be met with reservations. Furthermore, it should be considered that the patient may possibly be manipulated when the holistic appreciation of his or her emotional/mental personality is neglected in favor of high-tech diagnostics for which the objective scientific basis is still pending.

1.6 Indications and Contraindications

Indications. It is well known that not all symptoms can be treated equally well or successfully with a single therapeutic procedure. Like body acupuncture, ear acupuncture has its limitations with respect to treatment options. In order to employ the procedure successfully, understanding these limitations is all the more important, the more differentiated and restricted the spectrum of a procedure.

We may assume that, based on a functioning microsystem in the widest therapeutic sense, ear acupuncture has a supportive or alleviating effect in almost all physical ailments or diseases, and that it can also be used in combination with other methods. On this basis alone, however, the therapist would not do justice to the strong points of ear acupuncture. On the one hand, these relate mainly to the so-called *yang* diseases as described in Chinese medicine. On the other hand, they relate to the so-called acute diseases in the approach of Western medicine, such as acutely painful symptoms of the motor system (e.g., lumbago–sciatica syndrome, myalgia) as well as acutely traumatic states, neuralgia, or cephalalgia.

Furthermore, certain forms of addiction, such as nicotine addiction and craving for food, seem to represent a popular topic for treatment. However, I would like to stress that ear acupuncture has its limitations as an effective but solely supportive method of treatment.

Contraindications. It is absolutely necessary to distinguish between relative and absolute contraindications.

Relative Contraindications
- Pain of unknown origin.
- Painful malignant diseases.

During Pregnancy
- Ovary point (23).
- Uterus point (58).
- Genital areas.

Absolute Contraindications
- Life-threatening diseases.
- Extraordinary sensitivity to local pressure, or inflammation of reflex zones or points.
- Inflammation or injury of the entire auricle.

1.7 Side Effects and Complications

Side effects. The only uncomfortable side effect known in ear acupuncture is so-called primary aggravation, which is rare and not of a serious nature. It represents a kind of progression of the patient's original symptoms and usually subsides within a few hours. On the one hand, this primary aggravation indicates that the therapeutic approach was correct; on the other hand, it demonstrates that the stimulus chosen by the therapist was too strong.

Complications. The rare but mostly avoidable complications that may occur in connection with ear acupuncture must be taken seriously.

> **! Caution**
> - Vasovagal attack (increased risk when treating in the area of the concha and antihelix).
> - Local infection.

Uncritical and careless needling of the most densely vagally innervated region around the auditory canal carries the risk of a vasovagal attack that may lead to potentially fatal situations if the patient has an underlying primary disease. This must be prevented by adequate positioning of the patient and by diagnosing serious primary heart diseases.

A further complication associated with serious consequences is the risk of local infection, which occurs particularly after unclean and traumatic needling. Certain stimulation techniques for which continued monitoring by the physician is not possible (e.g., the use of permanent needles or pellet plasters) and traumatic subcutaneous puncture techniques (e.g., insertion of a "wet" needle between the skin and the cartilage layer) may lead to local infections, including the rare but ultimately harmful perichondritis.

As there are no compelling indications for these high-risk needle techniques, the therapist is under obligation to provide a particularly comprehensive explanation for their use.

1.8 Nomenclature

Despite the relatively short period of the development of and systematic approach to ear acupuncture, different and partially conflicting nomenclatures have been adopted. In the 1960s, Nogier started to provide each point with a name, but then he turned to his own numbering system in the 1980s, after König and Wancura had introduced the Chinese numbering of ear points to Europe through their publications in the early 1970s (Lange 1985). The Chinese, too, had originally used names for the points, as is evident from ancient Chinese ear panels and their symbolic illustrations (see **Fig. 1.6**). Today, some of these points or zones still have a number as well as a name; e.g., the name of point 55 is the *shen men* point (Divine Gate point).

The numerical nomenclature of Nogier did not survive, and in practice, two systems stood their ground: the predominantly numerical nomenclature of the Chinese school and the name-oriented nomenclature of Western auriculotherapy, which can largely be traced back to Nogier. The points often have very promising pseudoscientific names (e.g., interferon point) or names analogous to medications, and this gives the impression that there are no therapeutic limits to ear acupuncture. The effectiveness of these points, as proved in practice, does not correspond to their naming and should be understood merely as a clue pointing in the proper direction.

A nomenclature for auriculotherapy agreed upon in Seoul in 1987 by the World Health Organization (WHO) describes—primarily in the Chinese style—approximately 43 ear points or zones following the so-called WHO Code. The WHO Conference on Nomenclature of Ear Points in Lyon in 1970, at which Nogier was especially acknowledged, did not yield definitive results. This step toward internationalization is certainly welcome and promotes the worldwide exchange of research data. However, it is of little importance for practical work as this code is much too complicated.

A promising attempt at finding a nomenclature came from the University of California, Los Angeles (UCLA), United States of America. The leading author was Oleson (1990), who subdivided the auricle into small zones (**Table 1.1**). According to their anatomical positions, these zones are assigned to an alphanumerical code, in which the letters reflect the initials of the Latin-derived anatomical names (**Fig. 1.7**). The position and size of each of these zones—which spread like a net over the auricle—are difficult to define with respect to their size, and hence were chosen arbitrarily. As with the reflex zones, they require a more precise anatomical description and definition.

We do not yet have the experience to decide whether this subdivision will prove successful and can be applied to the three-dimensional structure of the auricle. Nevertheless, the UCLA nomenclature seems to be much more practical and meaningful in terms of its logic and reproducibility than the WHO Code, especially with respect to the international exchange of experience. It is hoped, therefore, that this idea will be discussed and worked on further at one of the next meetings of the WHO Task Force for Standardization of Acupuncture Nomenclature. For the benefit of internationalization, the present book includes a list of English terms or codes, as well as an overview of the UCLA subdivision into zones. We highly recommend that colleagues who are interested in the international exchange of experience familiarize themselves with the English terms listed and/or the WHO or UCLA code of ear acupuncture.

In practice, the coexistence of the more descriptive Western nomenclature and the mainly numerical nomenclature of the Chinese school has so far proved successful. This kind of practice-oriented nomenclature should be familiar to everyone practicing ear acupuncture. In some cases, certain alphanumerical modifications of the nomenclature have developed out of practical need. For example, Lange (1985) carried out a sensible modification for the occiput point (29) and points 29a, 29b, and 29c, which are located on the postantitragal line and were in part described by Chinese, and in part by Western, ear acupuncturists. Here, a distinct process of integration can be seen in Western ear acupuncture.

Table 1.1 Comparison of the current internationally used nomenclatures, and division into zones

Body area	Auricular area	World Health Organization code	University of California, Los Angeles, zone
Ear center	Helix	MA-H1	H1
Chinese rectum	Helix	MA-H2	H2
Chinese urethra	Helix	MA-H3	H3
External genitals	Helix	MA-H4	H3
Anus	Helix	MA-H5	H2
Ear apex	Helix	MA-H6	H7
Chinese heel	Antihelix	MA-AH1	A17
Chinese ankle	Antihelix	MA-AH2	A17
Chinese knee	Antihelix	MA-AH3	A18
Chinese hip	Antihelix	MA-AH4	A19
Buttocks	Antihelix	MA-AH5	A6
Sciatic nerve	Antihelix	MA-AH6	A7
Chinese sympathetic nerve	Antihelix	MA-AH7	A9
Chinese cervical vertebrae	Antihelix	MA-AH8	A1, A2
Chinese thoracic vertebrae	Antihelix	MA-AH9	A3, A4
Neck	Antihelix	MA-AH10	A10, A11
Chest	Antihelix	MA-AH11	A12
Fingers	Scapha	MA-SF1	SF1
Wrist	Scapha	MA-SF2	SF2
Elbow	Scapha	MA-SF3	SF3
Shoulder	Scapha	MA-SF4	SF5
Chinese clavicle	Scapha	MA-SF5	SF6
Divine Gate	Triangular fossa	MA-TF1	TF1
Eye	Lobule	MA-L1	L5
Chinese external nose	Tragus	MA-T1	T3
Apex of tragus	Tragus	MA-T2	T1
Chinese larynx/pharynx	Tragus	MA-T3	ST2
Subcortex	Antitragus	MA-AT1	WT4
Lung	Inferior concha	MA-IC1	C15
Trachea	Inferior concha	MA-IC2	C17
Endocrine zone	Inferior concha	MA-IC3	WT5
Triple burner	Inferior concha	MA-IC4	C18
Mouth	Inferior concha	MA-IC5	C1
Esophagus	Inferior concha	MA-IC6	C2
Cardiac orifice	Inferior concha	MA-IC7	C3
Duodenum	Superior concha	MA-SC1	C5
Small intestine	Superior concha	MA-SC2	C6
Appendix	Superior concha	MA-SC3	C6
Large intestine	Superior concha	MA-SC4	C7
Liver	Superior concha	MA-SC5	C13
Pancreas/gallbladder	Superior concha	MA-SC6	C12
Chinese ureter	Superior concha	MA-SC7	C9
Bladder	Superior concha	MA-SC8	C9

Source: World Health Organization nomenclature, Seoul, 1987, adapted from Oleson (1990).

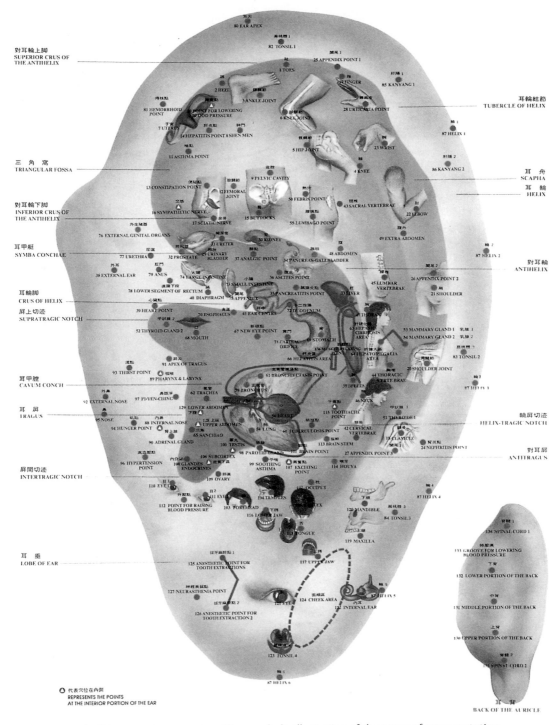

Fig. 1.6 Early Chinese ear topography with a symbolic illustration of the zones of representation.

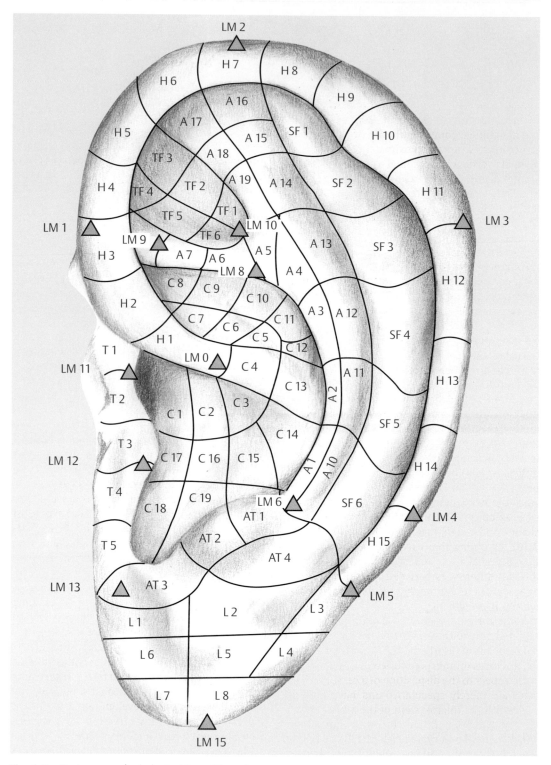

Fig. 1.7 Ear topography (adapted from Oleson).

2   Anatomy of the Outer Ear (Auricle)

2.1   Anatomical Nomenclature

General remarks. The auricle is an oval elastic structure of subtemporal position between the mandibular joint and the mastoid. This oval structure measures approximately 60 to 65 mm along its vertical longitudinal axis, while its horizontal diameter is approximately 30 to 35 mm. The basic structure is formed of elastic cartilage and is covered by perichondrium. The lobule of the auricle (earlobe) consists of soft, highly fatty connective tissue.

The anatomical structure (relief) of the auricle is complicated despite its constant features, making it necessary to look in detail at the anatomical makeup of the auricle. Only by doing so can we gain enough experience to find and reliably describe the reflex zones and points in relation to the anatomical structure.

Furthermore, it would be pointless to try to learn ear acupuncture solely from the book and its two-dimensional illustrations. Rather, it is important to put the theoretical foundations to practical use as soon as possible and to do this under the guidance of an experienced practitioner, using either an ear model or an auricle in vivo. It cannot be emphasized enough how difficult it is to be properly oriented so that important zones and points can be reliably located, since the unchanging basic structure of the auricle exhibits a surprisingly diverse variety of shapes and reliefs (see color plates, **Figs. 2.3–2.10**). Assuming that each person possesses an unmistakable ear relief of their own, with additional differences between the left and right ears, we can undoubtedly talk about an *individual ear physiognomy*.

Some authors assign special importance to ear physiognomy with respect to a person's individual disposition (Markgraf 1982). Such far-reaching attempts to interpret auricular physiognomy with respect to the disposition of a person's character are merely speculative and have nothing to do with the microsystem of the auricle. It is a fact, however, that the auricle has an unusual origin in terms of embryology and that its distinctly individual relief undergoes only minor changes after birth.

Lateral surface of auricle. This surface at the front of the ear shows a constant structure, the anatomy of which is described as follows (**Fig. 2.1**).

A kind of brim, the **helix**, borders the ear. The structure begins at the root of the helix, or **crus of the helix**. This is located in the middle of the deepest plain of the auricle, the concha, and subdivides the concha into an upper part, the **superior concha**, and a lower part, the **inferior concha**; the latter represents the region around the **acoustic meatus**.

The section following the crus of the helix is called the ascending helix; this culminates at the highest point of the convex ear margin in the **apex of the helix**. The dorsal part of the helix, also called the descending helix, finally turns, in a soft transition via the helical tail, into the **lobule**. In the upper part of the descending helix, there is often a visible and palpable protrusion, the **darwinian tubercle**. This modification, which can be found as the tip of the ear in animals, is a developmental rudiment in humans. Nevertheless, it is important as a point of reference and a reflex zone.

A cartilaginous protrusion, the antihelix, runs parallel to the helix; as a quasi-vertical axis and counterpart to the helix, it contributes considerably to the characteristic image of the ear's relief. In its cranial part, the antihelix forks into two roots, the **inferior antihelical crus** and the **superior antihelical crus**. Both roots together surround a concave depression, the **triangular fossa**, which is cranially bordered by the ascending helix. The plain between antihelix and helix is called the **scapha**; this turns caudally into the lobule.

Toward the face, above the acoustic meatus and running vertically between the ascending helix and the attachment of the lobule, we find a cartilaginous protrusion, the **tragus**. This may be unicuspid or bicuspid and has its counterpart in a cartilaginous conical protrusion, the **antitragus**, from which it is separated by the **intertragic notch**. Reaching over the acoustic meatus, the tragus represents the developmental rudiment of a valve that originally served to close the entrance to the external auditory canal.

The antitragus is demarcated from the end of the antihelix by the small **postantitragal fossa**, which represents an important area for ear

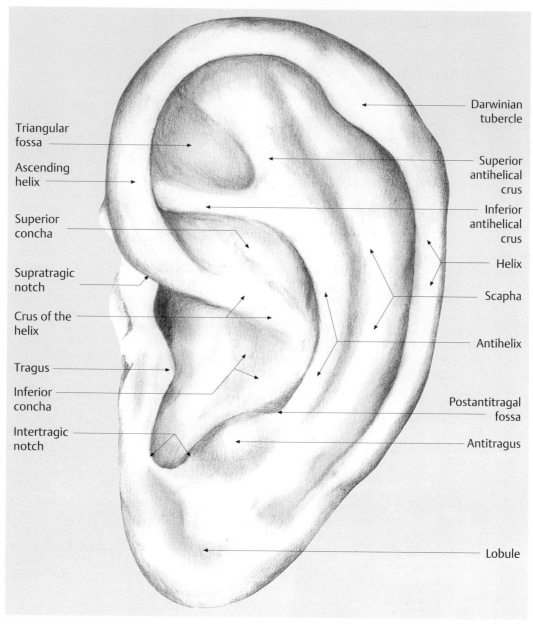

Fig. 2.1 Lateral surface of the auricle—overview of anatomy.

acupuncture. The tragus is cranially demarcated from the helix by a small groove, the **supratragic notch**.

Medial surface of auricle. Because of the regions attached to the cranial bone, the visually and palpably accessible portion at the back of the ear is much smaller. The negative relief of the medial

surface (**Fig. 2.2**) shows the same structures as the lateral surface, with the exception of:

- Those portions of the superior and inferior conchae that are close to the acoustic meatus.
- The ascending helix at the attachment of the ear to the facial skin.
- The tragal portion of the intertragic notch.

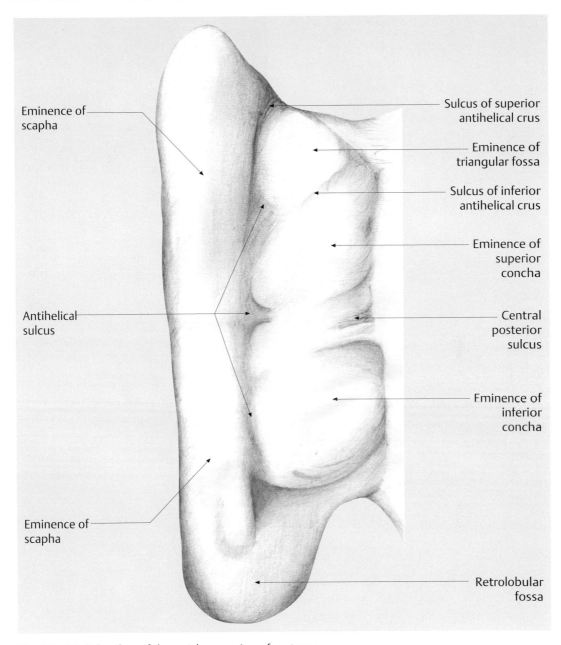

Eminence of scapha

Sulcus of superior antihelical crus

Eminence of triangular fossa

Sulcus of inferior antihelical crus

Eminence of superior concha

Antihelical sulcus

Central posterior sulcus

Eminence of inferior concha

Eminence of scapha

Retrolobular fossa

Fig. 2.2 Medial surface of the auricle—overview of anatomy.

The depressions of the lateral surface present themselves as eminences, the projections as grooves. The scapha corresponds to a protrusion on the medial surface of the ear, the **eminence of the scapha**. This turns into a small concave depression in the lobule portion, the **retrolobular fossa**, which again corresponds to the slight protrusion of the lobule at the front. Parallel to the eminence of scapha runs a groove corresponding to the antihelix at the front, the **antihelical sulcus**. The antihelical bifurcation on the lateral surface has its mirror image on the medial surface in the form of a groove-like apical continuation of the antihelical sulcus, the **sulcus**

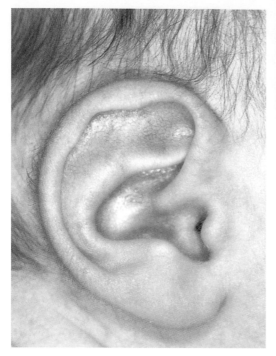

Fig. 2.3 Ear of an infant.

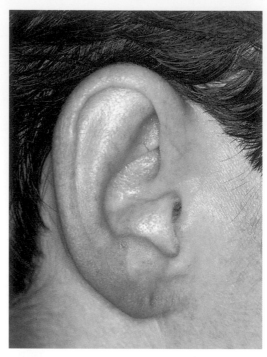

Fig. 2.4 Prominent superior antihelical crus.

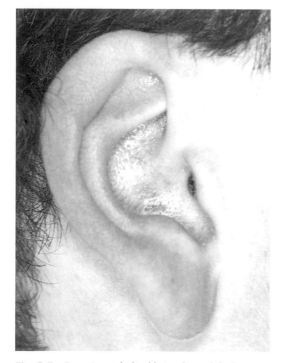

Fig. 2.5 Prominent helical brim, large lobule.

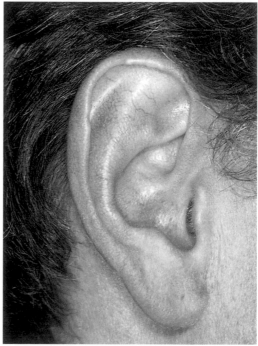

Fig. 2.6 Narrow helical brim, partially attached lobule.

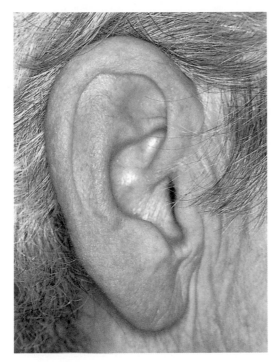

Fig. 2.7 Fleshy auricle, contour interruption of inferior antihelical crus.

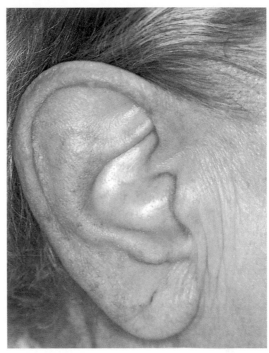

Fig. 2.8 Rudimentary antitragus, crus of helix missing.

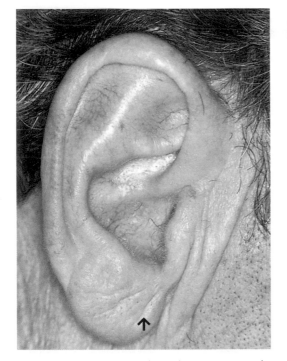

Fig. 2.9 "Stress groove," (arrow) antitragus poorly developed, postantitragal fossa hardly visible.

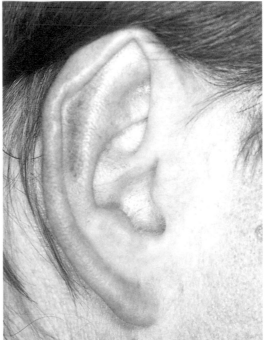

Fig. 2.10 Completely attached lobule; helical brim with two kinks, continuing until it almost reaches the lobular transition to the facial skin.

Table 2.1 Corresponding areas on the outer ear

Medial surface of auricle	Lateral surface of auricle
Eminence of scapha	Scapha
Antihelical sulcus	Antihelix
Sulcus of superior crus	Superior antihelical crus
Eminence of triangular fossa	Triangular fossa
Sulcus of inferior crus	Inferior antihelical crus
Eminence of superior concha	Superior concha
Central posterior sulcus	Crus of helix
Eminence of inferior concha	Inferior concha
Retrolobular fossa	Auricular lobule

of the superior crus. The inferior antihelical crus presents itself on the medial surface as the **sulcus of the inferior crus**, which demarcates the **eminence of the triangular fossa** caudally. Further down follow portions of the superior concha in the form of a slight protrusion, the **eminence of the superior concha**. Separated by a groove-like depression corresponding to the crus of the helix on the lateral surface, called the **central posterior sulcus**, the **eminence of the inferior concha** continues caudally, again in the form of a slight protrusion (**Table 2.1**).

The anatomical structure of the medial surface of the auricle can be easily traced by guiding the thumb along the back of the ear and the index finger along the lateral surface of the auricle like a pair of tongs. This comparison by palpation illustrates the relationship between the contours at the back and the familiar relief in front of the ear.

2.2 Embryology and Innervation

General remarks. The development and shaping of the external ear—the auricle, which serves as an ear trumpet—begin during the 6th week of embryogenesis. The first branchial cleft remains open, while all other clefts are closing. The final shape of the auricle is gradually formed from the dorsal section of the first branchial cleft as well as from six mesenchymal condensations, three of these appearing at each external auditory canal. The fusion of these knobs is a complicated process; as a result, the auricular structure often shows variations, and auricular anomalies are also common.

Regions of innervation. According to the publications by Nogier P, (1976) expanded by the "*loci auriculo medicinae*" which are mainly based on work of Bourdiol in the 1970s, there are three regions of innervation on the lateral surface of the auricle. The nerve supply of the auricle derives from:

- The cervical plexus.
- A part of the third branch of the trigeminal nerve.
- The vagus nerve.

The large auricular branch of the superficial cervical plexus supplies sensory fibers to the lobule and to part of the brim of the helix up to the darwinian tubercle. The superior concha and inferior concha, along with the deepest part of the crus of the helix, are innervated by the auricular branch of the vagus nerve, with a particularly dense supply of nerve fibers around the acoustic meatus. The remaining portion of the external ear, i.e., the ascending helix, part of the crus of the helix, tragus and antitragus, triangular fossa, and scapha, lies in the sensory region that is innervated by the auriculotemporal branch of the mandibular nerve (third branch of the trigeminal nerve).

The medial surface of the auricle is primarily innervated by motor fibers from the large auricular branch of the superficial cervical plexus.

These fields of innervation cannot be clearly demarcated from one another but merge together in intermediate zones of more or less mixed nerve supplies. According to Durinjan, three more major nerves and their branches are thought to be involved in innervation of the auricle. The first German-language publication of Umlauf's work, in the *Deutsche Zeitschrift für Akupunktur* (DZA, *German Journal of Acupuncture*; Umlauf 1988), states that five nerves innervate the auricle:

- One branch of the cervical plexus.
- The trigeminal nerve.
- The intermediate nerve, which is part of the facial nerve.
- The glossopharyngeal nerve.
- The auricular branch of the vagus nerve.

The areas innervated by the nerves involved show extensive overlapping, with the result that none of the areas is solely supplied by one nerve.

Peuker's neuroanatomical study, published in the DZA (Peuker 2003), shows that the auricle is innervated by four nerves of branchiogenic as well as somatogenic origin. According to this study, the auricular nerve (branch of the vagus nerve), the great auricular nerve (branch of the cervical plexus), and the auriculotemporal nerve (branch of the trigeminal nerve) are involved laterally and largely overlap, but at no point do all three of them overlap. Medially, in addition to the auricular branch of the vagus nerve and the great auricular nerve, the lesser occipital nerve is involved, covering almost 50% of the area. According to Peuker, the vagus nerve supplies not only the concha, but also almost the entire antihelix.

This study brings into question the auricular innervation models that have so far been held valid. Future research into the neuroanatomical and neurophysiological fundamentals of ear acupuncture may help to clarify this. The unusual representation of the vagus nerve in the auricle is common to all innervation models, as is its consideration in everyday practice (see Chapter 1.7, Side Effects and Complications). Due to the pronounced presence of the vagus nerve in these areas, they are considered risk zones as there is an increased danger of inducing a vagovasal collapse through needle stimulation.

Representations. The parts of organs and tissues originating from the three embryonic germ layers—endoderm, mesoderm, and ectoderm—are mainly represented according to the areas of innervation (**Fig. 2.11**):

- Representations of the **endoderm**-derived intestinal organs are located in the plain of the concha, which is innervated by the vagus nerve.

- Representations of **mesoderm**-derived body components, such as the skeleton, muscles, connective tissue, and also ureter and uterus, are located in the part of the auricle that is innervated by the trigeminal nerve.
- The **ectoderm**-derived structures, such as the brain, nervous system, skin, and epithelia of the sensory organs, are assigned to the area of lobule and helical rim up to the darwinian tubercle that is primarily innervated by the superficial cervical plexus.

2.3 Overview of Zones of Representation

General remarks. We owe the description of the topography of the auricle to Nogier, who deduced it from combined views of embryogenesis and innervation of the auricle, as well as from germ layer assignments and from the reflex relationships he had researched. The result is the familiar image of the inverted embryo (**Fig. 2.12**), which serves as an aid for orientation on the auricle. The embryolike somatotopic representation with its disproportions depending on receptor density and innervation reminds us of the Penfield and Rasmussen's homunculus (see **Fig. 1.5**), which illustrates the representation of the body's organs and their parts in the cerebral cortex.

This image facilitates orientation on the auricle. The two axes are roughly provided by the anatomical structures: the antihelix (vertical axis) represents the projection of the spinal column, while the crus of the helix (horizontal axis) represents the level of the diaphragm. With the aid of these two axes, a swift and reliable location of representation zones is made possible, and hence also the location of reactive points. The head with the sensory organs is represented caudally, the extremities by contrast cranially.

Assignments. The representation zone of the spinal column is projected onto the antihelix. Starting with the projection of the atlas of the cervical spine just above the postantitragal fossa, the zone is divided cranially into the thoracic and lumbar parts of the spine and ends with the sacral region at the end of the inferior antihelical crus. According to the Chinese school, however, the cranial region ends at the bifurcation of the two antihelical crura.

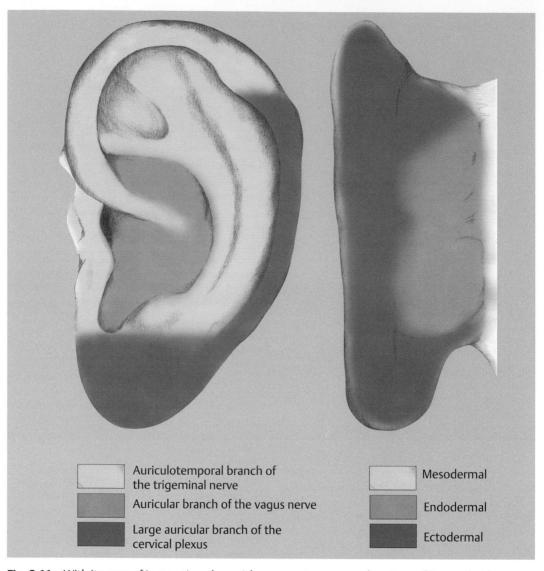

Auriculotemporal branch of the trigeminal nerve	Mesodermal
Auricular branch of the vagus nerve	Endodermal
Large auricular branch of the cervical plexus	Ectodermal

Fig. 2.11 With its areas of innervation, the auricle represents organs and portions of tissues that have originated from the three embryonal germ layers.

The representation zones of the ligaments, muscles, and joints of the upper extremity are projected onto the region of the scapha, between the antihelix and the helix. The hand and wrist are represented at the level of the darwinian tubercle, and individual fingers and the thumb are represented close to the apex of the helix. The lower arm, elbow joint, upper arm, and shoulder follow caudally.

The bent leg is projected onto the superior antihelical crus and into the triangular fossa, where we also find the reflex zone of the foot with its ankle joint, forefoot, and toes. The reflex zones of the toes border onto the ascending helix.

Located in the inferior concha are the projection points of the thoracic organs, such as the lungs, trachea, esophagus, and heart (although in this context the heart is not to be viewed as an organ).

The reflex zones of the abdominal organs are located in the superior concha. Those of the intestinal organs are represented close to the

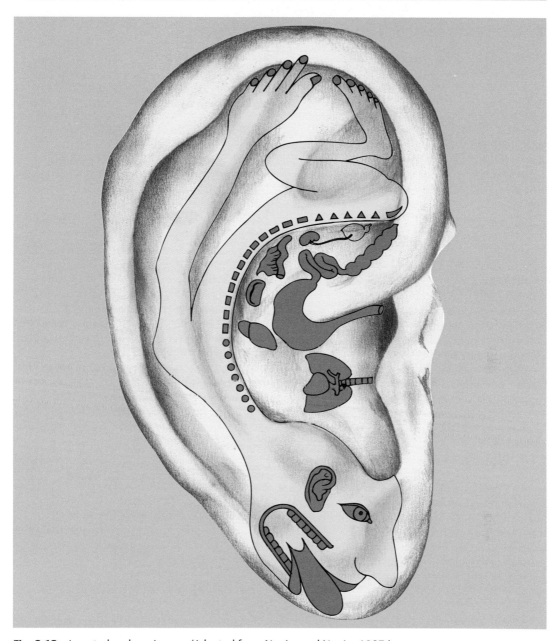

Fig. 2.12 Inverted embryo image. (Adapted from Nogier and Nogier 1987.)

crus of the helix at the floor of the concha. The remaining organs of the abdomen, such as the liver, pancreas, gallbladder, urinary bladder, and kidneys, are projected at the level of the superior concha close to the antihelix, in a caudal to cranial direction in the sequence listed here.

The inner side of the intertragic notch contains several points with gland-specific effects. According to Chinese nomenclature, this reflex area is also described as the endocrine zone (22).

3　Systematic Localization of Points on the Auricle

Based on the anatomical structures and reference points described in the previous chapter, the reliable points and zones of representation are now presented in detail. They are described with regard to their location and range of indications in a didactically meaningful order.

The overview on the opposite page (**Fig. 3.1**) will help with the topographical assignment of points.

3.1　Lateral Surface of Auricle (Front of Ear)

3.1.1　Supratragic Notch

External Ear Point ___ 20 (Fig. 3.2)
Location. In a depression of the upper ventral part of the tragus, toward the face, just before the ascending helix.

Toward the face, approximately 3 to 4 mm further up the ascending helix, we find the frustration point and, in the direction of the concha, on the dorsal part of the tragus, we find the interferon point (**Fig. 3.2**).
Indication. External otitis, beginning perichondritis, othematoma.

Heart Point ___ 21 (Fig. 3.2)
Location. Slightly below the external ear point (20), a short distance from the transition of the tragus crest toward the face.
Indication. Functional heart problems, paroxysmal tachycardia associated with psychovegetative syndrome (see also Heart Zone [100], p. 55).

Interferon Point (Fig. 3.2)
Location. At the center of the supratragic notch.
Indication. Predisposition to chronic infection, chronic infection. Supportive in malignant diseases, allergies.

Frustration Point (Fig. 3.2)
Location. Approximately 0.5 cm from the intertragic notch toward the face, along the skinfold between the helix and the face.

Indication. Psychological stress, susceptibility to addictive forms of behavior.

3.1.2　Tragus

Apex of Tragus Point ___ 12 (Fig. 3.3)
Location. On the upper dorsal part of the tragal tip.
Indication.
Acts to relieve pain, especially in feverish inflammatory diseases, according to Chinese indications, also effective in strabismus.

ACTH Point
(Adrenal Gland Point) ___ 13 (Fig. 3.3)
Location. Midway between the tragal tip (the caudal tip in patients with a double-tipped tragus) and the lowest point of the intertragic notch, on its crest.
Indication. Especially effective in inflammatory and degenerative diseases of the locomotor system (e.g., rheumatoid diseases of the joints, arthrosis), including acute episodes. Allergic bronchial asthma, pollinosis, allergic skin diseases, chronic fatigue.

External Nose Point ___ 14 (Fig. 3.3)
Location. In the middle of the tragus, at the transition toward the facial skin.
Indication. According to Chinese experience, effective in inflammations of the external nose (e.g., furunculosis, acne vulgaris) (questionable effectiveness).

Larynx/Pharynx Point (Chinese) ___ 15 (Fig. 3.3)
Location. On the upper part on the inside of the tragus, roughly opposite the apex of tragus point (12).
Indication. Pharyngitis, laryngitis (aphonia), tonsillitis, aphthous stomatitis.

! *Caution*

Danger of patient collapsing (vicinity of the external acoustic meatus).

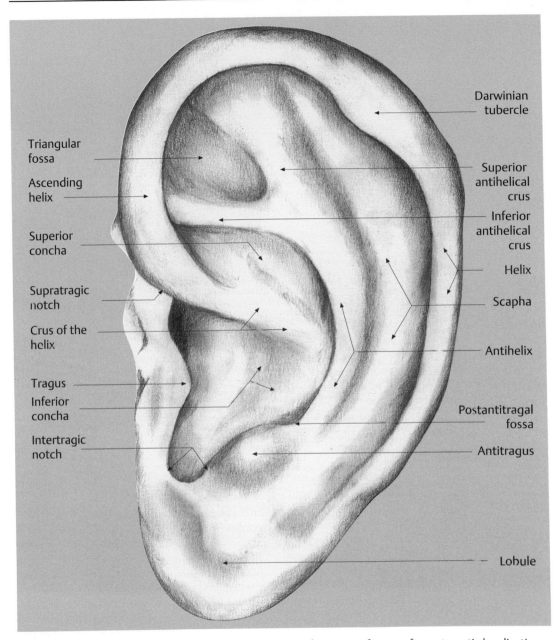

Triangular fossa

Ascending helix

Superior concha

Supratragic notch

Crus of the helix

Tragus

Inferior concha

Intertragic notch

Darwinian tubercle

Superior antihelical crus

Inferior antihelical crus

Helix

Scapha

Antihelix

Postantitragal fossa

Antitragus

Lobule

Fig. 3.1 Lateral surface of auricle—anatomy with topographic page references for systematic localization of points.

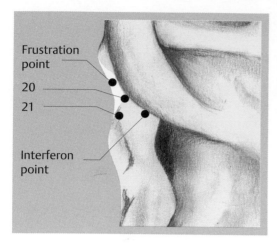

Fig. 3.2 Supratragic notch.

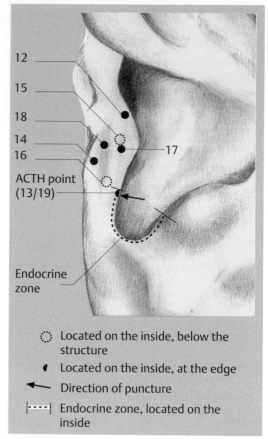

⟨◌⟩ Located on the inside, below the structure

◀ Located on the inside, at the edge

← Direction of puncture

|----| Endocrine zone, located on the inside

Fig. 3.3 Tragus.

Inner Nose Point ___ 16 (Fig. 3.3)

Location. On the underside of the tragus, i.e., in the roof of the acoustic meatus, from the outside: at the level of the centerpoint between the tragal tip and the ATCH point. Direction of needle insertion: from the acoustic meatus.

Indication. Allergic rhinitis, sinusitis, epistaxis, pollinosis.

Thirst Point ___ 17 (Fig. 3.3)

Location. Below the tip of the tragus in the direction of the transitional fold toward the facial skin.

Indication. Dryness of the mouth (questionable effectiveness).

Hunger Point ___ 18 (Fig. 3.3)

Location. In the lower part of the tragus in the direction of the transitional fold toward the facial skin.

Indication. Anorexia, bulimia following indigestion or disturbed metabolism (e.g., diabetes mellitus, pancreatic disease) (questionable effectiveness).

> ┌─ *Practical Tip* ─────────────
> This point is rarely found to be irritated in obesity and is rarely used.

Antihypertension Point ___ 19 (Fig. 3.3)

Location. In the lower third of the caudally slanting part of the tragus, further toward the concha.

This is no longer listed in the more recent Chinese literature; it is probably identical to the adrenal gland point (13; same localization).

According to the French School (Nogier 1969), this is the location of the adrenal gland point, named the "ACTH point" by Nogier's followers.

Indication. Increased blood pressure.

Assuming that acupuncture has a regulating and harmonizing effect in terms of the activation of endogenous physiological control mechanisms, this point may also be indicated in predisposition to hypotensive dysregulation (questionable effectiveness).

3.1.3 Intertragic Notch

ACTH Point (Adrenal Gland Point) __ 13 (Fig. 3.4)
(See p. 24.)

Endocrine Zone __ 22
Location. This zone (initially described by the Chinese School) lies on the inside of the crest along the concave intertragic notch. It begins with the ACTH point (see p. 24) and ends with the ovary point (23).

Nogier distinguished three points in this zone:
- The *parathyroid gland point* on the floor of the inferior concha at the transition to the actual triple burner zone of the Chinese School.
- The *pituitary gland point* slightly dorsal to the parathyroid gland point.
- The thyroid gland point, or TSH point.

Indication. Apart from the TSH point, experience shows that the above subdivisions cannot be seen as having this specificity. Therefore, the indications listed include only general disturbances of endocrine function, such as the ones also described by the Chinese School: disorders resulting from endocrine disturbances (e.g., menopause, dysmenorrhea); chronic inflammation of the skin, lungs, joints; and thyroid gland dysfunction.

TSH Point (Thyroid Gland Point) (Fig. 3.4)
Location. The point defined by Nogier as the thyroid-specific portion of the endocrine zone occupies the more ventrocranial part of the endocrine zone.
Indication. Adjuvant therapy in thyroid-specific disorders, such as thyroiditis, hypothyroidism, and hyperthyroidism.

Ovary Point (Gonadotropin Point) __ 23
Location. This zone occupies the center of the crest of the intertragic notch that ends toward the antitragus partially on the inside of the antitragus, and partially slightly to the outside toward the lobule.
Indication. Dysmenorrhea, menorrhagia and metrorrhagia, menopausal complaints, menstrual migraine, infertility and sexual neurosis in men and women, impotence, frigidity.

Eye Points __ 24 a and 24 b (Fig. 3.4)
Location. Point 24 a: In the skinfold of the intertragic notch, at the transition toward the face (approximately midway between the ACTH and TSH points).

Point 24 b: In the skinfold/transition of the notch toward the lobule, midway between the TSH and ovary points.
Indication. Adjuvant in myopia, astigmatism, optic atrophy, and macular degeneration.

3.1.4 Antitragus

Points 26, 27, 28, and 32 have proved ineffective and are therefore not discussed here.

Thalamus Point __ 26 a (Fig. 3.5)
Location. On the inside of the antitragus, in the middle of the baseline at its transition to the concha. Virtually opposite the sun point (35) on the outside of the antitragus (basally).
Indication. Adjuvant in severe, acute, and chronic states of pain (e.g., in the locomotor system, head, malignant diseases, phantom limb pain).

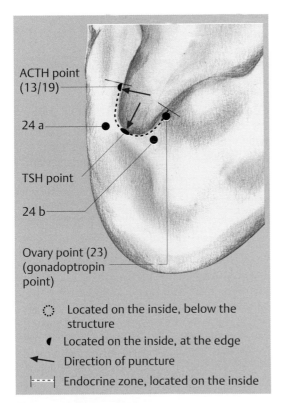

ACTH point
(13/19)

24 a

TSH point

24 b

Ovary point (23)
(gonadoptropin
point)

◌ Located on the inside, below the structure

◖ Located on the inside, at the edge

← Direction of puncture

├---┤ Endocrine zone, located on the inside

Fig. 3.4 Intertragic notch.

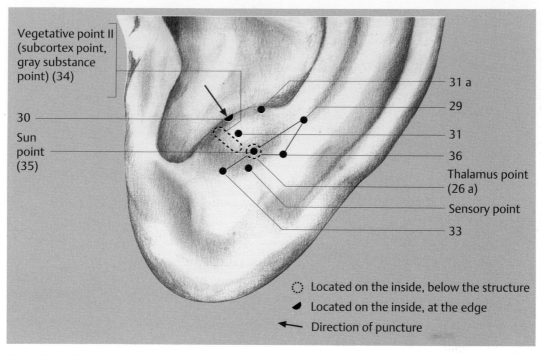

Vegetative point II
(subcortex point,
gray substance
point) (34)

30

Sun
point
(35)

31 a

29

31

36

Thalamus point
(26 a)

Sensory point

33

◌ Located on the inside, below the structure

◖ Located on the inside, at the edge

← Direction of puncture

Fig. 3.5 Antitragus.

It also has a sedative effect.

Also adjuvant in residual symptoms after apoplexia, such as partial hemiparesis and dyslalia.

Parotid Gland Point ____ 30 (Fig. 3.5)
Location. At the tip of the antitragus.
Indication. Parotitis—also as a prophylactic in combination with the *shen men* point (55)—susceptibility to infections resulting from immunodeficiency (if necessary, in combination with the interferon point), and for symptomatic alleviation of pruritus.

Asthma Point (Dyspnea Point) ____ 31 (Fig. 3.5)
Location. Below the tip of the antitragus on the outside of the antitragus, approximately halfway between the tip and the base of the outside of the antitragus.
Indication. Adjuvant in bronchial asthma, dyspnea, and thoracic oppression associated with functional complaints. If applicable, also adjuvant while quitting smoking.

Cough-Relieving Point ____ 31 a (Fig. 3.5)
Location. Between the parotid gland point (30) and postantitragal notch, slightly below the connecting line between them, next to the brainstem point.
Indication. Acute and chronic dry cough of any origin.

The point has an antitussive (alleviating) rather than a cough-relieving effect.

Forehead Point ____ 33 (Frontal Skull Point, according to Nogier) (Fig. 3.5)
Location. In the ventral portion of the antitragal baseline (the "sensory line" according to Nogier), below the ovary point (23). Also located on this sensory line are sun point (35) and occiput point (29).
Indication. Frontal headache, sinusitis. Adjuvant in insomnia, vertigo.

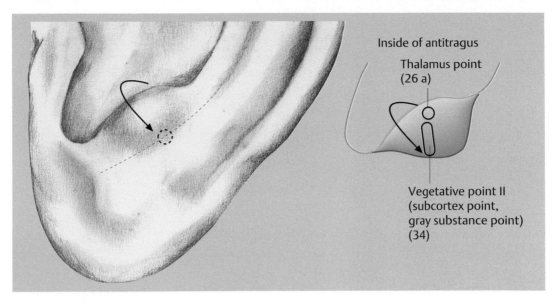

Fig. 3.6 Inside of antitragus.

Vegetative Point II (Subcortex Point, Gray Substance Point) ___ 34 (Fig. 3.6)
Location. On the inside of the antitragus, in the triangle of the ovary point (23), thalamus point (26 a), and antitragal tip (parotis point).
Indication. Acute and chronic inflammations associated with pain. Depressive mood, psychovegetative syndrome.
    Adjuvant in convulsive disorders.

► Harmonizing and sedative effect in situations of psychological stress. In the literature, vegetative point II and the subcortex or gray substance point are sometimes listed as different points located next to each other. However, experience shows that they occupy the same area. ◄

Sun Point ___ 35 (Fig. 3.5)
Location. On the outside of the antitragus, in the center of its baseline, right opposite the thalamus point (26 a).

► The sun point is the central point of the sensory line (29, 35, 33). ◄

Indication. Acute and chronic cephalalgia, particularly migraine; insomnia, vertigo.

Sensory Point (Fig. 3.5)
Location. Below the sun point (35) and the forehead point (33), forming the lower angle of an almost isosceles-shaped triangle with these points.
Indication. Adjuvant in neuralgiform complaints, such as cervico-occipital neuralgia, trigeminal neuralgia, glossalgia.

Roof Point (Crown of Head Point) ___ 36 (Fig. 3.5)
Location. Ventral and caudal to the occiput point (29). This point represents the lower tip of another isosceles triangle, which it forms with points 29 and 35.
Indication. Cephalalgia, drowsiness, cervico-occipital neuralgia, intercostal neuralgia. If necessary, use in combination with the sensory point.

3.1.5 Postantitragal Fossa

Brainstem point ___ 25 (Fig. 3.7)
Location. On the edge of the postantitragal fossa, between the antitragus and antihelix.
Indication. Cephalalgia, meningeal irritation, concomitant symptoms of neurological and psychological disorders (e.g., multiple sclerosis, cyclothymia).

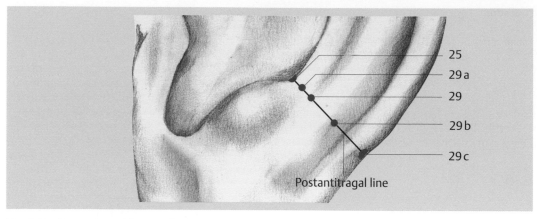

25
29 a
29
29 b
29 c

Postantitragal line

Fig. 3.7 Postantitragal fossa with postantitragal line.

Occiput Point (Pad Point) ___ 29 (Fig. 3.7)

Location. On or near (approximately 2 mm away from) the postantitragal line. This is an imaginary line that runs to the dorsal edge of the helix, which it crosses at a right angle (**Fig. 3.7**) below the postantitragal fossa halfway between the notch and the intersection with the ending of the scapha; see also Jerome Point (29 b).

Indication. Pain of all kinds, especially neuralgia and cephalalgia. Because of its sedative component, it is also used in bronchial asthma, inflammatory diseases, psychovegetative exhaustion, tendency to collapse, and vertigo; also in diseases of the nervous system and convalescent therapy.

Representing the dorsal end point of the sensory line (29, 35, 33), this important point has a wide range of indications.

Kinetosis Point (Nausea Point) ___ 29 a (Fig. 3.7)

Location. Located on the postantitragal line halfway between brainstem point 25 at the postantitragal fossa and occiput point 29.

Indication. Inner ear dizziness (the point is usually part of von Steinburg's line of vertigo), therapy and prophylaxis of motion sickness or kinetosis (e.g., while travelling by sea or air); if necessary, use in combination with the relaxation point (Jerome point, 29 b) to treat fear of flying.

Jerome Point (Relaxation Point) ___ 29 b (Fig. 3.7)

Location. Located on the postantitragal line defined by the postantitragal fossa, brainstem point (25), and occiput point (29), at the intersection with the scapha at the transition to the lobule.

Indication. Relaxation of the striated muscles, reflex muscle tension caused by emotions or pain, e.g., in connection with diseases of the locomotor system (e.g., spinal syndrome, lumbago–sciatica syndrome). Harmonization and sedation in conditions of emotional stress, disturbed sleep, or difficulty falling asleep, Possible use by alternating every 1 or 2 days with the opposite point on the medial surface of the ear, which is supposed to be effective in problems relating to sleeping through the night.

> **Practical Tip**
> The corresponding point on the medial surface of the ear is indicated for difficulty with sleeping through the night (dysphylaxia).

Craving Point ___ 29 c (Fig. 3.7)

Location. Directly on the intersection of the postantitragal line at an approximate right angle to the dorsal helix–lobule rim.

> **Practical Tip**
> The needle is inserted from dorsal toward the rim of the lobule, which is splinted between the thumb and index finger.

Indication. Adjuvant in treatment for addiction (e.g., nicotine addiction, obesity). We owe to Lange (1985) the meaningful alphanumerical naming of the points with the guiding number 29, all of which are located on the imaginary line from the postantitragal fossa. His approach documents the importance of these connected points as components of an imaginary line (see Chapter 4.4 vertigo line) as well as the importance of individual acupuncture treatment for the head region.

3.1.6 Lobule

The lobule is subdivided into nine fields for the sake of easier orientation (**Fig. 3.8**, **Fig. 3.9**). The following approach has proved successful in practice:

1. An imaginary horizontal line is drawn from PT1, located on the lobule, approximately 0.5 cm ventrocaudally to the lowest concavity (intertragic notch), and on to the dorsal rim of the lobule. This corresponds with the upper delineation of the lobule.

2. Keeping this upper boundary in mind, the center of the lobule can be located. This is the "eye point" (caution: piercing). One of the nine fields of the lobule is positioned around this eye point.

3. This level can also be subdivided to give additional fields ventrally and dorsally. The three fields are of approximately the same size.

Starting again from the central field (the eye point), the "tonsils field" can be found on a vertical line caudally and the "mouth field" cranially.

4. On the level of the tonsils field, there are additional fields ventrally and dorsally containing corresponding points. The same applies to the level of the mouth field. The size of the fields is chosen in relation to the size of the individual lobule, and the fields should be roughly equal.

5. The fields are numbered from I to IX, starting with the facial field I (below the intertragic notch), and moving dorsally and downward.

These fields serve as a basic orientation to facilitate the localization of their respective points. In practice, it has not proved successful to delineate these fields with the aid of pseudo-geometrical lines derived from variable anatomical structures.

PT1 (Formerly Antiaggression Point) (Fig. 3.8)
Location. On the lobule, approximately 0.5 cm ventrocaudally to the lowest concavity of the intertragic notch, in the upper nasal quarter of field I.
Indication. As a psychotropic point (PT) in psychological disorders, psychological strain, e.g., irritability, aggressive and suppressed aggressive behavior, addictive disorders.
Adjuvant in chronic disorders (e.g., chronic polyarthritis), malignant diseases—relating to the aspect of "Why me?"

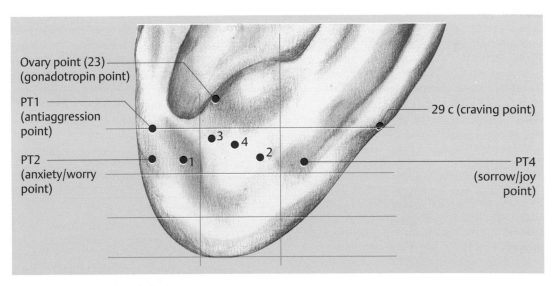

Fig. 3.8 Points on the lobule.

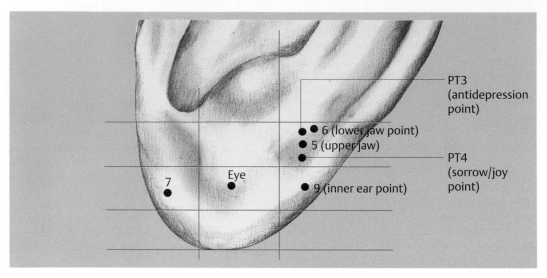

PT3
(antidepression
point)

● ● 6 (lower jaw point)
● 5 (upper jaw)
●
PT4
(sorrow/joy
7   Eye   point)
● ●
● 9 (inner ear point)

Fig. 3.9   Points on the lobule.

Note. In cases of possibly violent aggressive behavior, the corresponding area at the back of the ear should be investigated and, if irritated, included in the therapy.

In milder forms of aggressiveness, no sensitivity will be found here.

PT2 (Formerly Anxiety/Worry Point) (Fig. 3.8)
Location. The point is located approximately 0.5 cm below PT 1 in the lower nasal quarter of field I.
Indication. Anxiety under concrete life-threatening circumstances, but also undefined anxiety, lack of drive (e.g., in depression). Fears about something, worry over someone.

Note. In right-handed people, mainly the right ear should be treated for anxiety, and the left ear for worry. In left-handed people, this should be the other way around.

PT4 (Formerly Sorrow/Joy Point) (Fig. 3.8)
Location. In the lower dorsocaudal quarter of field III, approximately at the same level as PT2.
Indication. Depressive mood, including lack of drive, diminished interest in life or disrupted enjoyment of life, sorrow.

Note. According to Nogier, lack of drive, diminished interest in life, or disrupted enjoyment of life is supposed to be treated in right-handed people primarily via the right ear, while sorrow is supposed to be treated via the left ear as an adjuvant. In left-handed people, this should be done the other way around.

Tooth Point ___1 (Fig. 3.8)
Location. In field I of the lobule.
Indication. Analgesia during tooth extractions, toothache.

> **Practical Tip**
>
> Needling of this point alone has little effect, but it has proved rather successful in combination with the following points: upper jaw point (5), lower jaw point (6), and the other tooth point (7), as well as the occiput point (29) and *shen men* point (55). Furthermore, here in the cartilage-free area of the lobule, any inundation of these areas with local anesthetic carries only a low risk of infection and is allegedly more effective than puncture alone.

According to Russian studies (Portnov 1979), needling of these points in combination with electrostimulation is equally as effective as using local anesthesia, but it seems to be more costly and time-consuming.

Upper Palate Point ___2 (Fig. 3.8)
Location. In the lower dorsal quarter of field II (on a vertical line above the eye field).
Indication. Aphthous stomatitis, trigeminal neuralgia, periodontosis.

Lower Palate Point ___3 (Fig. 3.8)
Location. In the upper ventral quarter of Field II.
Indication. Trigeminal neuralgia, periodontosis, aphthous stomatitis, pharyngitis.

Tongue Point—4 (Fig. 3.8)
Location. In the center of field II, lying together with the upper palate point (2) and the lower palate point (3) roughly on a diagonal line running through field II from the upper ventral to the lower dorsal corner.
Indication. Glossalgia (caution: contraindicated in cases of pernicious anemia), disturbed sense of taste, glossitis, stomatitis.

Upper Jaw Point (Chinese) ___5 (Fig. 3.9)
Location. Approximately in the center of field III.
Indication. Arthralgia of the jaw joint (temporomandibular joint syndrome), toothache, also during tooth extraction, periodontosis, trigeminal neuralgia.

Upper Jaw Point (According to Nogier) (Fig. 3.10)
Location. Located on the scapha (**Fig. 3.10**) between the Jerome point and PT3 (antidepression).

Indication. Pain in the jaw joint (temporomandibular neuralgia).

Lower Jaw Point (Chinese) ___6 (Fig. 3.9)
Location. Slightly above and dorsal to the upper jaw point 5, at the upper horizontal border of field III.
Indication. Toothache, also during tooth extraction, trigeminal neuralgia, parotitis.

Lower Jaw Point (According to Nogier) (Fig. 3.10)
Location. See Upper Jaw Point above.
Indication. Pain and inflammation in the area of the mandibular joint.

PT3 (Formerly Antidepression Point) (Fig. 3.9 and Fig. 3.10)
Location. Ventral and caudal to the Jerome point (29 b) at the ending of the scapha, at the intersection with the imaginary horizontal line between PT1 and the craving point (29 c) or lower cranial quarter of field III.
Indication. Depressive mood, reactive depression, disturbed sleep.

Tooth Point ___7 (Fig. 3.9)
Location. On the lobule, in the center of field IV of the lobule.
Indication. Toothache. Has an alleviating effect in cases of tooth extraction.

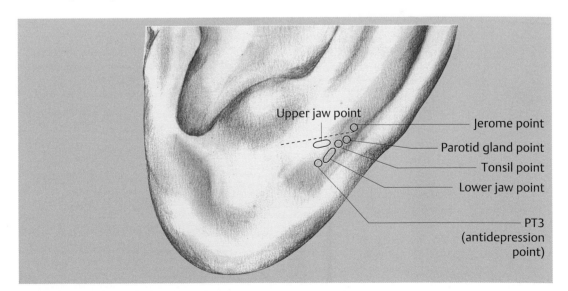

Fig. 3.10 Zones of representation according to Nogier.

Eye Point ____8 (Fig. 3.9)

Location. In the center of the subdivided lobule (see above), in the center of field V.

▶ The eye point is often sacrificed to jewelry (piercing). However, this is not detrimental to the health of the eye or to the power of vision. ◀

Indication. Adjuvant in external diseases of the eye (e.g., conjunctivitis); supportive in cephalalgia and neuralgia, particularly when localized around the eye socket and behind the eyeball. Abducens nerve palsy.

Inner Ear Point ____9 (Fig. 3.9)

Location. In the center of field VI.
Indication. Adjuvant in vertigo, tinnitus, impaired hearing.

> ─ **Practical Tip** ─
> If necessary, use in combination with the sensory line.

Master Omega Point (Fig. 3.11)

Location. In the upper dorsal quarter of field VII, above the analgesia point. The vertical line drawn in the figure, which connects the omega points, is considered a memory aid for the omega points and is not suitable for locating these points.
Indication. Psychological/mental harmonization in severe chronic illnesses (e.g., pain syndromes, malignant neoplasm). Helps to accept the suffering.

Analgesia Point (Fig. 3.11)

Location. In the lower ventral quarter of field VII, at the caudal rim of the lobule. In cases of facially adnate lobules, the point is located in the skinfold toward the face.
Indication. Severe pain syndromes of all kinds, particularly in the head region, preferably in combination with the thalamus point (26 a).

Tonsil Point (Chinese) ____10 (Fig. 3.11)

Location. In the center of field VIII (on a vertical line below the eye field) on the lobule.
Indication. Acute and chronic diseases of the tonsils, pharyngitis.

> ─ **Practical Tip** ─
> If necessary, use in combination with the mouth zone (84).

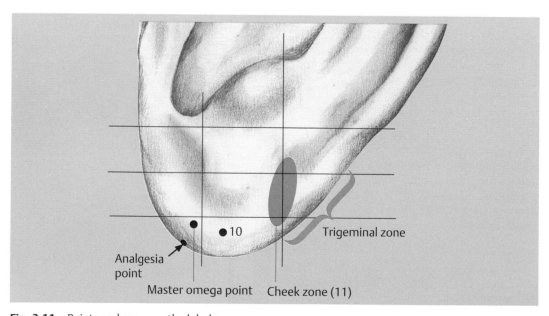

Fig. 3.11 Points and zones on the lobule.

Tonsil Point (According to Nogier) (Fig. 3.10)

Location. Located between the Jerome point (29 b) and PT3 (formerly the antidepression point) at the ending of the scapha.

Indication. The same as for the Chinese tonsil point above.

Cheek Zone ——11 (Fig. 3.11)

Location. The narrow oval zone covers the border between fields V and VI and also expands to a small extent into fields II and III as well as fields V and VIII.

Indication. Trigeminal neuralgia, facial paresis, myofascial facial pain.

> ┌─ *Practical Tip* ─
> If necessary, use in combination with the upper jaw point (5) and lower jaw point (6).

Trigeminal Zone (According to Nogier) (Fig. 3.11)

Location. On the dorsal rim of the lobule, expanding over the dorsal borders of fields VI and IX.

Indication. Trigeminal neuralgia, myofascial facial pain.

The needle is inserted from the dorsal direction toward the rim (similar to the craving point).

> ┌─ *Practical Tip* ─
> This zone is needled by using the sieving method, i.e., several needles being inserted in close proximity. Bleeding in the form of a microbloodletting may be allowed until it stops spontaneously close to the time of needle removal.

3.1.7 Antihelix

Chinese acupuncture as well as Western auriculotherapy views the antihelix as the projection area of the spinal column and uses it accordingly for diagnosis and treatment. The Chinese school describes pointlike areas analogous to the individual sections of the spinal column, whereas French/Western ear acupuncture views the entire antihelix as a reactive reflex area.

On the ridge of the antihelix, the bony structures of the spinal column—the individual vertebrae—are projected as a continuous chain. According to Nogier's mnemonic aid, the projections take place from the bottom to the top: Following the cervical spine in the caudal region of the antihelix and the thoracic spine in the middle region of the antihelix, we find the lumbar spine and the sacral region extending onto the inferior antihelical crus up to the brim of the helix.

The chain of points for the vertebrae (**Fig. 3.12**) begins with the atlas point (C1), which is located cranially just above the postantitragal fossa. Subsequent points for the cervical spine join in regular sequence up to the C7 to T1 transition. This is located approximately at the level where a dorsally elongated line from the helical crus crosses the middle portion of the antihelix.

Then follows the chain of points for the thoracic spine, with T1 to T12 in the adjacent middle portion of the antihelix up to the beginning of the inferior antihelical crus. It ends there with the thoracolumbar T12 to L1 transition approximately at the level where a vertical line from the tip of the triangular fossa crosses the inferior antihelical crus.

Next follows the region of the lumbar spine with the projections of L1 to L5 on the inferior antihelical crus. The transition (L5 to S1) to the lumbosacral region is located approximately in the middle of the inferior antihelical crus. Finally, still on the inferior antihelical crus, the sacrum and coccyx are projected toward the brim of the helix.

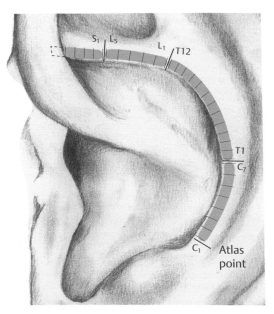

Fig. 3.12 Projection area of the spine.

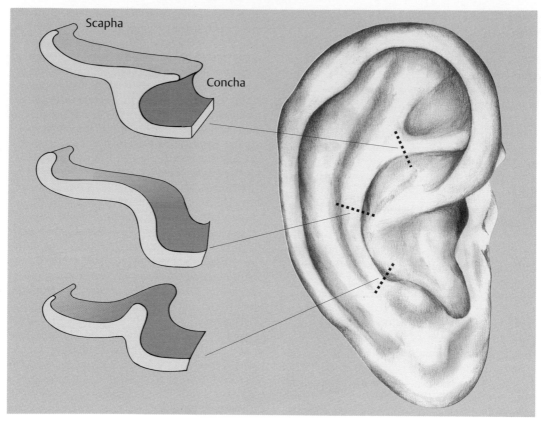

Fig. 3.13 Changes in the antihelical relief.

The threefold change in the antihelical relief (**Fig. 3.13**) provides some guidance for demarcating the distinct sections of the projection of the spinal column.

In the area of the cervical spine, the antihelix exhibits a sharper, yet still rounded, contour. At the C7 to T1 transition, it is transformed into a soft-curved relief that dominates the entire projected region of the thoracic spine. At the T12 to L1 transition, however, this shape transforms into a sharp-edged ridge that ultimately ends below the brim of the helix.

Antihelix—Zones of Representation According to Chinese Specifications

Based on the aforementioned subdivision, Chinese ear acupuncture describes so-called maximum points within the individual sections for the spinal column, which are named after the individual spinal segments and, again, are numbered. However, these maximum points, to which

special organs or regions of organs are assigned, are only vaguely described with respect to their location within the sections of the spinal column projections.

Furthermore, according to the Chinese school, the projection of the spinal column covers a shorter distance, namely, from the postantitragal fossa up to the antihelical bifurcation into crura. As a result, the individual sections of the spinal column are shifted: similar to the Western concept, the cervical spine is projected onto the antihelix with the C7 to T1 transition at the level of the crus of helix, whereas Nogier's thoracic stretch from T6 to T12 (close to the triangular fossa) is occupied, according to the Chinese concept, by projections of the lumbar spine and the sacral and coccygeal vertebrae.

Cervical Spine Zone ____37 (Fig. 3.14)
Location. In agreement with the Western school of ear acupuncture, this is in the caudal area of the antihelix.

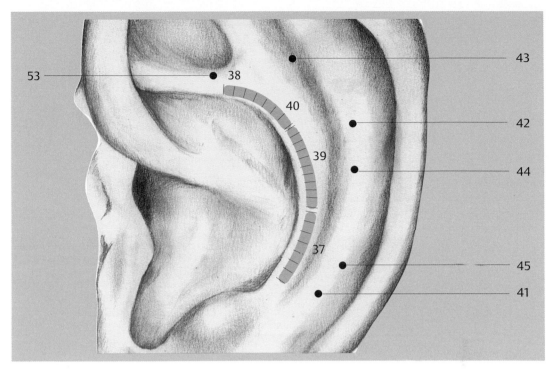

Fig. 3.14 Zones of representation and localization according to Chinese specifications.

Indication. Cervical syndrome, cervical spine whiplash injury.

Sacral Spine Zone (Coccyx Zone) ___ 38 (Fig. 3.14)
Location. Close to the antihelical bifurcation into the two crura.
Indication. Lumbago, intercostal neuralgia.

Thoracic Spine Zone ___ 39 (Fig. 3.14)
Location. This zone occupies approximately the area designated T1 to T6 in the Western concept.
Indication. Intercostal neuralgia.

Lumbar Spine Zone ___ 40 (Fig.3.14)
Location. Adjacent to the thoracic spine zone (39), passing without demarcation into the sacral spine zone (38).
Indication. Lumbago.

Located a little further dorsally, slightly below the antihelical ridge in the direction of the scapha and matching the segments, we find the organ-related master points mentioned previously. They are described as follows:

Neck Point ___ 41 (Fig. 3.14)
Location. At the level of the point for C1, near the scapha.
Indication. Cervical syndrome.

Thorax Point ___ 42 (Fig. 3.14)
Location. Approximately at the level of the cranial end of the thoracic spine zone (39).
Indication. Thoracic oppression, intercostal neuralgia, herpes zoster, mastitis, sternocostal syndrome.

Abdomen Point ___ 43 (Fig. 3.14)
Location. Above of the upper portion of the lumbar spine zone (40).
Indication. Abdominal complaints.

Mammary Gland Point ___ 44 (Fig. 3.14)
Location. Approximately at the level of the crus of helix, but slightly dorsal to the antihelical ridge, in the direction of the scapha.
Indication. Pain in the breast as a result of root irritation in the corresponding segment. Mastodynia, insufficient lactation, mastitis.

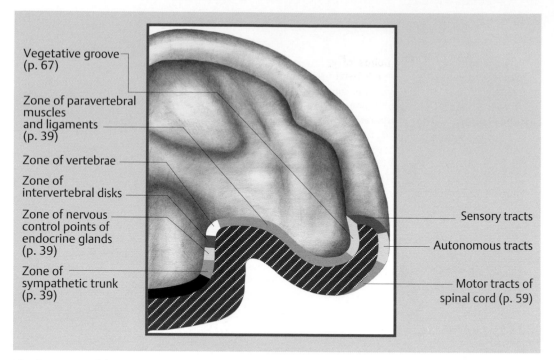

Vegetative groove (p. 67)

Zone of paravertebral muscles and ligaments (p. 39)

Zone of vertebrae

Zone of intervertebral disks

Zone of nervous control points of endocrine glands (p. 39)

Zone of sympathetic trunk (p. 39)

Sensory tracts

Autonomous tracts

Motor tracts of spinal cord (p. 59)

Fig. 3.15   French/Western zones of representation, horizontally outlined.

Thyroid Gland Point ___ 45 (Fig. 3.14)

Location. Approximately at the level of the first third of the cervical spine projection onto the antihelix, near the scapha.

Indication. According to Chinese experience, dysfunction of the thyroid gland. According to Western experience, it is more effective as a segmental collective point in root irritation in the area of cervical segments C2, C3, and C4.

Buttocks Point ___ 53 (Fig. 3.14)

Location. Slightly dorsal to the sciatica zone (52) on the inferior antihelical crus, almost belonging to the sciatica zone.

Indication. As for the sciatica zone (52); see page 46 and **Fig. 3.20**.

Antihelix—Zones of Representation According to French/Western Specifications

In contrast to the isolated antihelical master points of Chinese ear acupuncture, which have fixed indications, the French school arrived in the 1970s at a segment-oriented interpretation of the antihelical areas for both diagnostics and therapy (**Fig. 3.15**). This interpretation arose from the finding that the neuromuscular functional components of the spinal column are projected not only onto the antihelix, but also, in a horizontal arrangement, onto the remaining auricle.

According to this **horizontal subdivision,** narrow parallel zones of projections are located in the region of the antihelix and remaining auricle; these run longitudinally while taking into account that the antihelical relief changes vertically.

It is conspicuous that the zones for control points and those for the chain of ganglia are described in great detail, whereas the remaining zones are not specified in a similar way. For didactic reasons, we will first present an overview of the individual zones on the entire auricle and then discuss them again in greater detail together with the corresponding anatomical structures.

The following zones of representation are found in the region of the antihelical wall:

- **Zone of representation of vertebrae:** On the ridge of the antihelix.

- **Zone of intervertebral disks:** In the antihelical wall (toward the concha), slightly below the ridge.
- **Zone of nervous control points of endocrine glands** (see also p. 40 and **Fig. 3.16**): Just below the zone of intervertebral disks, in the antihelical wall dropping toward the concha.
- **Zone of sympathetic trunk/paravertebral chain of sympathetic ganglia** (see p. 41): Still in the antihelical wall, just before its transition to the plain of the concha (the projection area of the inner organs).
- **Zone of paravertebral muscles and ligaments** (see scapha, p. 41): Begins slightly below the antihelical ridge (toward the brim of the helix) and expands dorsally as a plain area into the scapha almost below the brim of the helix and up to the superior and inferior crus (see the shaded area in **Fig. 3.15**).
- **"Vegetative groove"** (zone of origin of sympathetic nuclei, according to Lange [1985]; see scapha, p. 49): Adjacent to the zone of paravertebral muscles and ligaments, immediately below the brim of the helix (see the dotted line in **Fig. 3.22**).
- **Zone of spinal cord** (see helix/helical brim, p. 49): Its **motor tracts** are projected on the medial surface of the helix and its **sensory tracts** on the lateral surface of the helical brim. Between these are the **autonomous tracts** (which are insignificant). On the vertical level, the zone begins at the level of the postantitragal fossa and ends approximately at the level of the projection of the carpus.

In analogy to the vertical segmentation of the spinal column into its individual segments and to its approximate assignment of vertebrae, the position of the projection zones of the individual intervertebral disks can be roughly determined. Furthermore, the control points for the endocrine glands and those for the ganglia of the sympathetic trunk can also be located.

Antihelix—Zone of Nervous Control Points of Endocrine Glands

Parathyroid Gland Point (Fig. 3.16)
Location. Approximately at the level of C5 to C6.
Indication. Adjuvant in secondary hyperparathyroidism in connection with malabsorption, pregnancy, chronic renal insufficiency; in hypoparathyroid tetany, and parathyroid gland lesions following strumectomy.

Thyroid Gland Point (Fig. 3.16)
Location. Just before the C7 to T1 transition, at the level of C6 to C7.
Indication. Adjuvant in dysfunction of thyroid gland, especially in cases of residual complaints not eliminated by proper thyroid medication.

> ── *Practical Tip* ──
> Can be combined with endocrine zone (22) or the TSH point.

Thymus Gland Point (Fig. 3.16)
Location. At the level of T1 to T2.
Indication. Disturbed immune system (e.g., allergic diathesis, pollinosis), and also chronic predisposition to infections.

> ── *Practical Tip* ──
> Depending on the indication, in combination with the following points: interferon point (see **Fig. 3.2**), allergy point (78), ACTH point (adrenal gland point, 13) (see **Fig. 3.3**), shen men point (55).

Mammary Gland Point (Fig. 3.16)
Location. Approximately at the level of T5.
Indication. Disturbed lactation, premenstrual mastodynia.

▶ Although the breast is not considered to be an endocrine gland, it is assigned to this reflex area. ◀

Endocrine Pancreas Point (Fig. 3.16)
Location. Cranial and close to the mammary gland point, at the level of T6.
Indication. Adjuvant in type 2 diabetes mellitus, paroxysmal hypoglycemia.

Adrenal Gland Point (Fig. 3.16)
Location. Just before the antihelical change in relief, i.e., before the T12 to L1 transition at the level of T11 to T12.
Indication. Chronic fatigue, tiredness, hypotension, paroxysmal hypoglycemia. See also the adrenal gland ACTH point (13) (see **Fig. 3.3**).

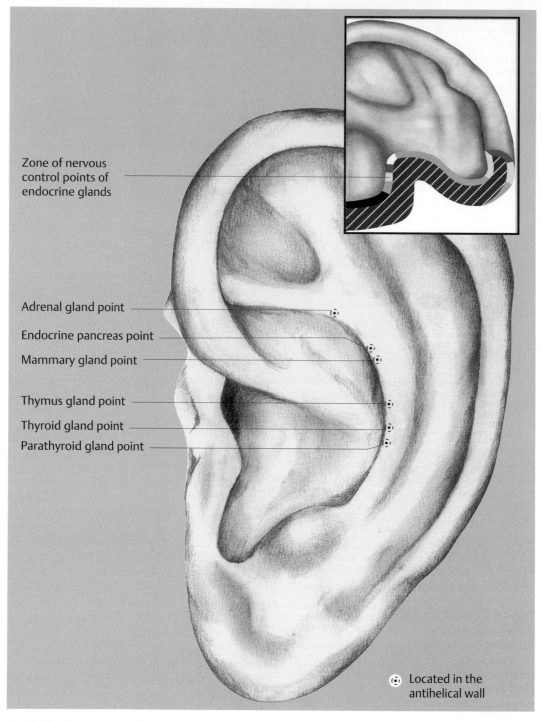

Zone of nervous control points of endocrine glands

Adrenal gland point

Endocrine pancreas point

Mammary gland point

Thymus gland point

Thyroid gland point

Parathyroid gland point

Located in the antihelical wall

Fig. 3.16 Nervous control points of endocrine glands.

Cardiac Plexus Point (According to Nogier) (Wonder Point) (Fig. 3.17)

Location. At the level of the C3 projection, in line with the inferior concha at the transition to the antihelical wall.
Indication. See page 56 (**Fig. 3.17**, **Fig. 3.26**).

Bronchopulmonary Plexus Point (According to Nogier) (Fig. 3.17)

Location. At the upper rim of the inferior concha at the level of the end of the helix, between the projections of the heart (100) and cardia (86).

Zone of Sympathetic Trunk/ Paravertebral Chain of Sympathetic Ganglia

The zone of paravertebral sympathetic chain of sympathetic ganglia runs alongside the zone of nervous control points of the endocrine glands, close to the concha and parallel to the antihelix, just before its transition to the concha. Here, the projections of the three cervical ganglia are important for ear acupuncture (**Fig. 3.17**, **Fig. 3.18**).

Superior Cervical Ganglion Point (Fig. 3.17)

Location. Just before the transition of the antihelical wall to the concha, approximately at the level of the atlas point (C1).
Indication. Has a regulating effect on the cervical sympathetic trunk, lacrimation, blood flow, and sweating of the face.

Middle Cervical Ganglion Point (Fig. 3.17)

Location. Slightly cranial to the superior vertebral ganglion at the level of the projection of C5 to C6.
Indication. Disturbed regulation of blood pressure, disturbed blood supply to the facial area.

Inferior Cervical Ganglion Point (Cervicothoracic Ganglion Point, Stellate Ganglion Point) (Fig. 3.17)

Location. In the zone of sympathetic trunk, approximately at the level of the projection zone of C7 to T1.
Indication. Has a regulating influence on the thoracic portion of the sympathetic trunk; migraine, unilateral cephalalgia, cervico-occipital neuralgia, cervicobrachialgia, hyperemesis gravidarum, Sudeck's atrophy.

Thyroid Plexus Point (Fig. 3.17)

Location. In the zone of sympathetic trunk, at the level of the projection zone of T2.
Indication. Adjuvant in thyroid gland dysfunction (questionable effectiveness).

Thymic Plexus Point (Fig. 3.17)

Location. In the zone of the sympathetic trunk, approximately at the level of the projection of T2 to T3.
Indication. Predisposition to infection, allergies.

Supposedly, it harmonizes the sympathetic control of the arterial supply to the thymus (questionable effectiveness).

Adrenal Plexus Point (Fig. 3.17)

Location. In the zone of sympathetic trunk, at the level of the projection of T12.
Indication. The undefinable nerve and ganglion plexus of the paravertebral chain of sympathetic ganglia is represented within the zone of sympathetic trunk, between the individually listed plexus points in the projection area of T1 to L2/L3. Irritated points appear along this stretch (e.g., in vasospastic diseases or neuralgia), and may be included in the therapeutic approach (questionable effectiveness).

3.1.8 Scapha

As stated before, the area of the scapha is the **zone of paravertebral muscles and ligaments** (**Fig. 3.19**).

According to experience with Chinese ear acupuncture, the *joint points*, or *master points*, of the locomotor system are found in this region. For better orientation, we remind the reader again of the stylized concept of Nogier's inverted embryo and the disproportional projection onto the auricle. The resulting representation of the extremities in the cranial part of the auricle is remarkably wide-ranging. Thus, the upper extremity with the shoulder, arm, and hand is projected onto the scapha, with the hand represented at the apical part of the scapha and the shoulder at the level of the helical crus in the middle portion of the scapha. By contrast, the lower extremity occupies mainly the region of the superior antihelical crus, triangular fossa, and inferior antihelical crus, as well as the origin of both crura.

The joint points in the zone of paravertebral muscles and ligaments assigned to the locomotor system have been largely established by the

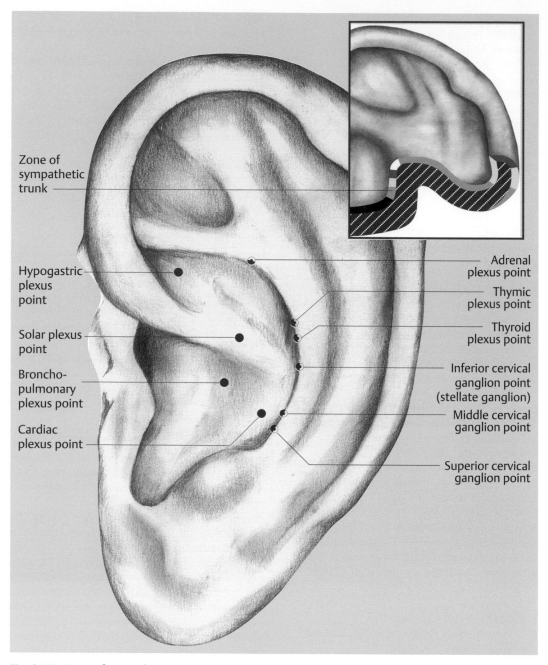

Zone of sympathetic trunk

Hypogastric plexus point

Solar plexus point

Broncho-pulmonary plexus point

Cardiac plexus point

Adrenal plexus point

Thymic plexus point

Thyroid plexus point

Inferior cervical ganglion point (stellate ganglion)

Middle cervical ganglion point

Superior cervical ganglion point

Fig. 3.17 Zone of sympathetic trunk/paravertebral chain of sympathetic ganglia and plexus points.

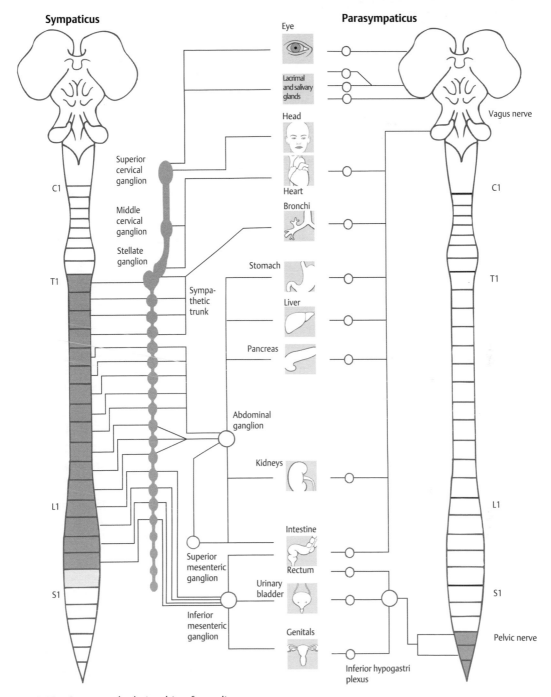

Sympaticus

Parasympaticus

C1

T1

L1

S1

Superior
cervical
ganglion

Middle
cervical
ganglion

Stellate
ganglion

Sympa-
thetic
trunk

Abdominal
ganglion

Superior
mesenteric
ganglion

Inferior
mesenteric
ganglion

Eye

Lacrimal
and salivary
glands

Head

Heart

Bronchi

Stomach

Liver

Pancreas

Kidneys

Intestine

Rectum

Urinary
bladder

Genitals

Vagus nerve

C1

T1

L1

S1

Pelvic nerve

Inferior hypogastri
plexus

Fig. 3.18 Segmental relationship of ganglia.

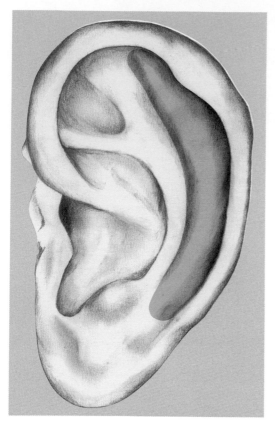

Fig. 3.19 Zone of paravertebral muscles and ligaments.

as a functional unit of the body as a whole, including its neuromuscular and tendinous parts; it stands to reason that potential diseases make themselves known not only in a circumscribed fashion via localized reflex zones. The neighboring and participating structures of the microsystem react with it as well and, depending on the severity of the disease, irritation will be more or less dominant. Accordingly, treating the maximally irritated point—either the Chinese one or the French description, sometimes even both—will guarantee the best therapeutic success possible. The quarrel over different localizations of points or different zones of representation for certain tissue parts in individual organs is futile; only the therapeutic outcome is important.

The segmental diagnostic and therapeutic approach of the French school fits in well with these considerations because it covers reflex zones, not only according to their accurate localization, but also with respect to their status of irritation, so that areas defined inadequately or not at all may be recognized as being affected and may be treated. This approach is therefore very successful, in particular, when the locomotor system is disturbed.

Points and Reflex Zones of the Locomotor System on the Scapha, Antihelical Crura, and Triangular Fossa

To obtain a better idea of the locomotor system, it is treated here as a general structure under the heading *scapha* (**Fig. 3.20**). With this in mind, the projections of the anatomical structures in question are once again listed. The osphyalgia point (54) and the clavicle point (63) are not discussed here: the osphyalgia point is no longer listed in the most recent Chinese ear topographies, and the clavicle point is of no therapeutic importance.

Toe Zone ____ 46 (Fig.3.20)
Location. The big toe is located in the upper ventral corner of the superior antihelical crus. All the other toes, including the little toe, are located along the upper ventral border of the triangular fossa. The localization of the toe zone according to the French school is identical, although perhaps shifted slightly in a caudal direction.

Chinese school but, in part, also by the French/Western school of ear acupuncture. As a result, the localizations given for individual joints may differ. However, this is hardly important in practice because, for maximal efficiency of the therapy, the point indicated in a given case may be found through the patient's history, the clinical findings, and the area of maximal irritation. The latter applies above all to purely local traumas and degenerative diseases of the locomotor system.

In general, however, it is recommended to use primarily the segment-oriented diagnostics and therapy of the French school—synonyms are segment therapy, ear geometry, and vegetative groove according to Lange (1985)—and to search only secondarily for locally irritated points of the affected zones of joints and bones. Each body part, and hence also each joint, must be viewed

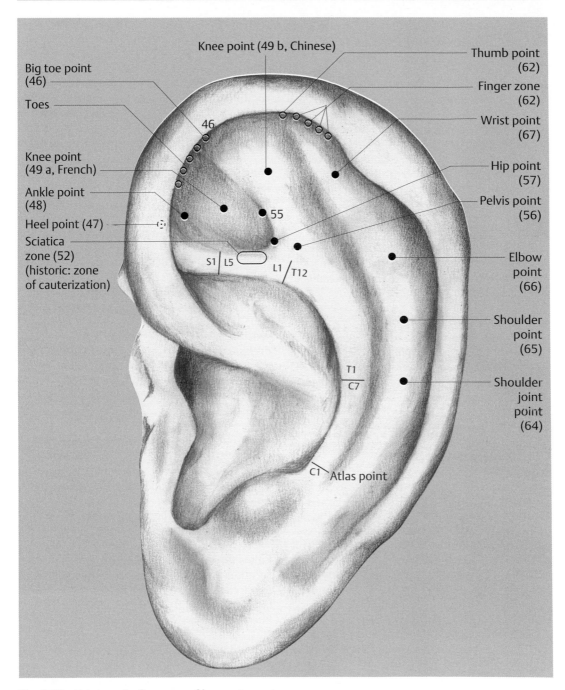

Knee point (49 b, Chinese)

Thumb point (62)

Big toe point (46)

Finger zone (62)

Toes

Wrist point (67)

46

Knee point (49 a, French)

Hip point (57)

Ankle point (48)

Pelvis point (56)

Heel point (47)

55

Sciatica zone (52) (historic: zone of cauterization)

S1 | L5

L1 / T12

Elbow point (66)

Shoulder point (65)

T1 / C7

Shoulder joint point (64)

C1 Atlas point

Fig. 3.20 Points and reflex zones of locomotor system.

▶ Apart from the point for the big toe, the reflex zones for individual toes cannot be demarcated from one another as individual points. ◀

Indication. Pain in the toe region (e.g., in hallux valgus), hammer toe, podagra.

Knee Point ___ 49 a and 49 b (Fig. 3.20)

Location. Point 49 a: According to the French school, this point is located exactly in the center of the triangular fossa where it is deepest.
Point 49 b: According to the Chinese school, the reflex zone for the knee joint is found in the middle of the superior antihelical crus, in terms of its length and width.
Indication. For points 49 a and 49 b: Pain in the knee joint resulting from trauma, inflammation, degenerative changes (arthrosis); adjuvant in physiotherapeutic mobilization.

Practical Tip

The French knee point (49 a) is favoured as effective for symptoms originating from the system of capsules, ligaments, and muscles, while the Chinese knee point (49 b) is mainly effective in degenerative joint troubles referable primarily to bones and cartilage.

Calcaneus Point (Heel Point) ___ 47 (Fig. 3.20)

This point is no longer described in recent Chinese ear topographies.
Location. According to the French school, this lies in the lower ventral corner of the triangular fossa, beneath the brim of the helix, approximately at the level of the ankle joint projection.
Indication. Pain in the area of the heel bone as a result, for example, of periostitis or a heel spur.

Hip Joint Point ___ 50 (Fig. 3.20)

According to recent Chinese ear topographies, this point corresponds to the hip point (57) (see below).

Sciatica Zone ___ 52 (Fig. 3.20)

Location. Approximately at the level of the lumbar spine projection, in the flat part of the transition from the inferior antihelical crus to the triangular fossa.

Indication. Lumbago, lumbago–sciatica syndrome, residual symptoms after intervertebral disk surgery.

Buttocks Point ___ 53 (see Fig. 3.14)

Location. Slightly dorsal to the sciatica zone on the inferior antihelical crus, almost belonging to the sciatica zone.
Indication. See Sciatica Zone, page 46 (52).

Shen Men Point ("Divine Gate Point") ___ 55 (Fig. 3.20)

Location. In the concavity of the triangular fossa; locate the point by starting from the antihelical bifurcation of the crura, the "tip of the fossa," at the lower margin of the superior antihelical crus, slightly cranially and toward the concavity.
Indication. The *shen men* point is one of the most important analgesic points on the auricle.

Because of its antiphlogistic and analgesic/sedative effect, it is particularly indicated for all diseases of the locomotor system as well as in the therapy of addiction (see the National Acupuncture Detoxification Association concept).

Adjuvant in allergic pruritus, bronchial asthma, insomnia.

Hip Point ___ 57 (Hip Joint Point, was 50) (Fig. 3.20)

Location. Both points are located at the areas of bifurcation of the antihelical crura, ventral to the tip of the fossa.
Indication. Pain in the region of hip or hip joint (e.g., in coxarthrosis).

Pelvis Point ___ 56 (Fig. 3.20)

Location. At the bifurcation of the two antihelical crura, close to the hip point (57).
Indication. Pain in the region of the pelvis and hip.

▶ This point is no longer listed in the most recent Chinese ear topographies, but its localization is the same as that of the French hip/pelvis point. ◀

Finger Zone ___ 62 (Fig. 3.20)

Location. On the scapha under the helical brim, close to the intersection of the upper edge of the superior antihelical crus and the helical brim.

The thumb is represented on the upper dorsal corner of the superior antihelical crus, close to or under the helical brim.
Indication. Pain in the region of fingers and thumb, as a result of trauma and inflammation.

Shoulder Joint Point ___ 64 (Fig. 3.20)
Location. On the scapha at the level of the intersection of an imaginary almost horizontal line ("diaphragm line") through the zero point (see Notch, Root of the Helix see **Fig. 3.1**) of the lower edge of the crus of helix.
Indication. Stiffness in the shoulder, distortion of the shoulder joint, humeroscapular periarthritis.

Shoulder Point ___ 65 (Fig. 3.20)
Location. On the scapha, within the area for the zone of paravertebral muscles and ligaments at the level of the supratragic notch.
Indication. As above for the shoulder joint point (64).

Elbow Point ___ 66 (Fig. 3.20)
Location. On the scapha, at the level of the intersection of an imaginary horizontal line through the bifurcation of the two antihelical crura.

! *Caution*

Do not be guided by the direction that the inferior antihelical crus runs in, as in vivo it may run obliquely.

Indication. Epicondylitis, distortion, bursitis.

Upper Arm Point (Not Illustrated)
This projection area does not have a number and is derived from the French topography.
Location. Between the shoulder point (65) and elbow point (66) (**Fig. 3.20**).
Indication. Adjuvant in pain in shoulder or elbow joint, cervicobrachial syndrome, upper arm complaints.

Wrist Point ___ 67 (Fig. 3.20)
Location. On the scapha, obliquely above the bifurcation of the antihelical crura.
Indication. Distortions and contusions of the wrist, tendinitis.

Additional Points on the Scapha, Triangular Fossa, and Antihelical Crura

In the region of scapha, triangular fossa, and antihelical crura there are additional zones and points that are not assigned to the locomotor system (**Fig. 3.21**).

Lower Arm Point (Not Illustrated)
Like the upper arm point, this projection area is derived from the French topography.
Location. In the region between the wrist point (67) and elbow point (66) (see **Fig. 3.20**).
Indication. Brachial syndrome, tendovaginitis. Adjuvant in cervicobrachial syndrome, epicondylitis.

Vegetative Point I ___ 51 (Autonomic Point, Sympathetic Point) (Fig. 3.21)
Location. On the inferior antihelical crus at the intersection with the protruding helical brim of the ascending helix, usually slightly covered by the helical brim.
Indication. Autonomic disorders, harmonizes the autonomic nervous system.
Adjuvant in various kinds of colic and abdominal pain (caution: ascertain the cause).

Uterus Point ___ 58 (Fig. 3.21)
Location. In the upper ventral corner of the triangular fossa, hidden under the helical brim.
Indication. Adjuvant in dysmenorrhea, metrorrhagia, tocolysis, impotence, psychosomatic symptoms in the region of the locomotor system.

Blood Pressure Control Point ___ 59 (Fig. 3.21)
Location. At the intersection of the superior antihelical crus and the edge of the helical brim, slightly toward the fossa.
Indication. Adjuvant in arterial hypertension.

Practical Tip

If necessary, use in combination with the antihypertension point (19) or ACTH point (13), or with the thalamus point (26 a).

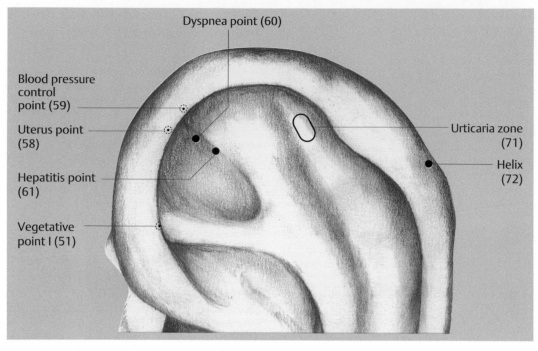

Fig. 3.21 Points on the scapha, triangular fossa, and antihelical crura.

Dyspnea Point ___ 60 (Fig. 3.21)
Location. In the triangular fossa, at almost the same level as the uterus point (58) and below the blood pressure control point (59).
Indication. Adjuvant in bronchial asthma, in chronic obstructive bronchitis.

> ─ **Practical Tip** ─
> If necessary, use in combination with the asthma point (31), ACTH point (13), endocrine zone (22), vegetative point I (51), and broncho-pulmonary plexus point (in the inferior concha).

This area is rarely found to be irritated and is therefore little used (questionable effectiveness).

Hepatitis Point ___ 61 (Fig. 3.21)
Location. In the triangular fossa, at roughly the same level as the urticaria zone (71) and below the dyspnea point (60) but dorsal to the latter and closer to the edge of the superior antihelical crus.
Indication. Adjuvant in hepatitis, cholecystitis (questionable effectiveness).

> ─ **Practical Tip** ─
> If necessary, use in combination with the liver zone (97) in the inferior concha.

Urticaria Zone ___ 71 (Fig. 3.21)
Location. In the region of the cranial scapha, between the darwinian tubercle and the intersection of the dorsal edge of the superior antihelical crus and the brim of the helix.
Indication. Urticaria (caution: contraindicated in Quincke's edema), insect bites, pruritus.

> ─ **Practical Tip** ─
> If necessary, use in combination with parotid gland point (30) (see **Fig. 3.5**) and parotid gland point (according to Nogier).

Appendix Points I ___ 68, II ___ 69, III ___ 70 (Not Illustrated)
Location. In Chinese ear topographies, these three additional points are listed on the scapha.
Indication. Chronic and acute appendicitis, according to Chinese ear acupuncture. (No reported experience.)

**Tonsil Points I ___ 73, II ___ 74,
III ___ 75, Liver Points I ___ 76, II ___ 77
(Not Illustrated)**
Location. Aligned on the brim of the helix.
Indication. Diseases of the tonsils or the liver, respectively, according to Chinese ear acupuncture. (Rarely used in the West.)

▶ The appendix points, tonsil points, and liver point I/II are not viewed by the Western or French school in the sense of fixed localizations but rather as secondary points or pseudolocalizations. They may also be summarized as lymphatically active points. Hence, in the context of segment therapy, one or even several of these pseudolocalizations should sometimes be included, if indicated by the state of irritation (questionable effectiveness). ◀

**"Vegetative Groove" (Zone of Origin
of Sympathetic Nuclei, Zone of
Intermediolateral Nuclei, According to
Lange)**
Location. This narrow band runs along the dorsal edge of the scapha just beneath the brim of the helix, parallel to the zone of paravertebral muscles and ligaments. Both zones merge without distinct demarcations approximately at the level of the brim of the helix. The groove beneath the helical brim, originally described by Nogier and Bourdiol as the zones of neurovegetative spinal cord centers, starts at the level of the postantitragal fossa and extends toward the darwinian tubercle. The neurovegetative groove according to Lange continues toward the intersection of inferior antihelical crus and ascending helix beneath the brim of the helix.
Indication. Segment-related symptoms, such as conditions associated with pain, neuralgia; initial orientation for building up the line of treatment with respect to ear geometry according to Nogier (segment therapy).

**Zone of Paravertebral Muscles and
Ligaments (Fig. 3.22)**
Location. This two-dimensional zone of representation expands from the downward slope of the antihelix into the scapha, covering the scapha completely in the cranial and caudal directions, and also covering parts of the superior and inferior antihelical crura up to the edge of the

triangular fossa. The region represents mostly segment-oriented reflex zones of the paravertebral neuromuscular units and the corresponding ligament portions. It includes the Chinese joint points, or master points, of the locomotor system and is also an important component for building up a treatment line as defined by Nogier's ear geometry.
Indication. Diseases of the locomotor system, segment-related conditions associated with pain, such as neuralgia, functional abdominal or thoracic complaints.

3.1.9   Helix and Helical Brim

Helix Points ___ 72 (Fig. 3.23)
Location. The area of the helix includes six points that have no individual names. These are located at regular intervals along the brim of the helix, starting at the darwinian tubercle and continuing to the deepest point on the lower edge of the lobule.
Indication. According to the Chinese school, these points were originally described for orientation only. However, according to König and Wancura's book on Chinese ear acupuncture (1998), they are indicated in the suppression of inflammation, fever, infection of the upper respiratory tract, and other conditions.

The indications listed for the appendix points and tonsil points on the scapha (see p. 48) apply to these points as well.

**Tip of Ear Point (Allergy Point) ___ 78
(Fig. 3.23)**
Location. This point can be easily located by folding the auricle in such a way that the dorsal helical brim runs parallel to the tragus, and then flattening the resulting "cylinder" at the upper end. The fine fold formed at the tip of the ear marks the area in question with reasonable accuracy.
Indication. Adjuvant in disorders of the immune system, such as allergies (e.g., pollinosis), bronchial asthma, urticaria, predisposition to infection, and immunodeficiency. The sedative component of this point certainly plays a role in the treatment of hypertension, while the analgesic and antifebrile effect prevails in febrile illnesses.

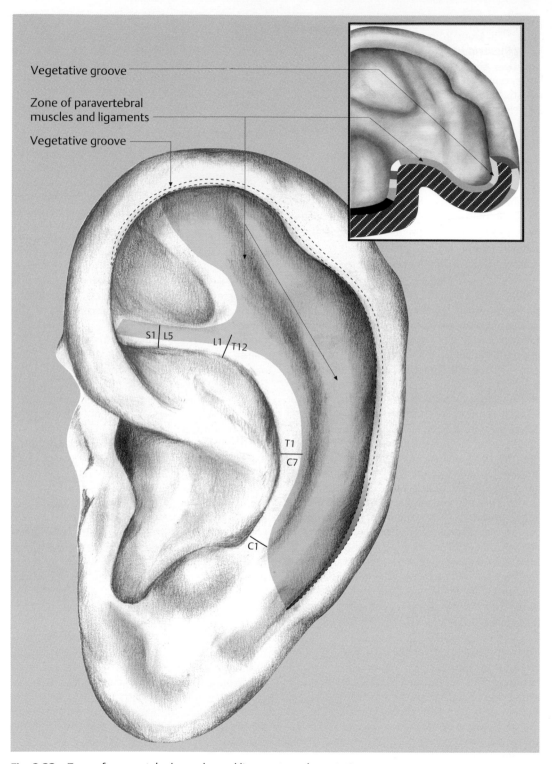

Fig. 3.22 Zone of paravertebral muscles and ligaments and vegetative groove.

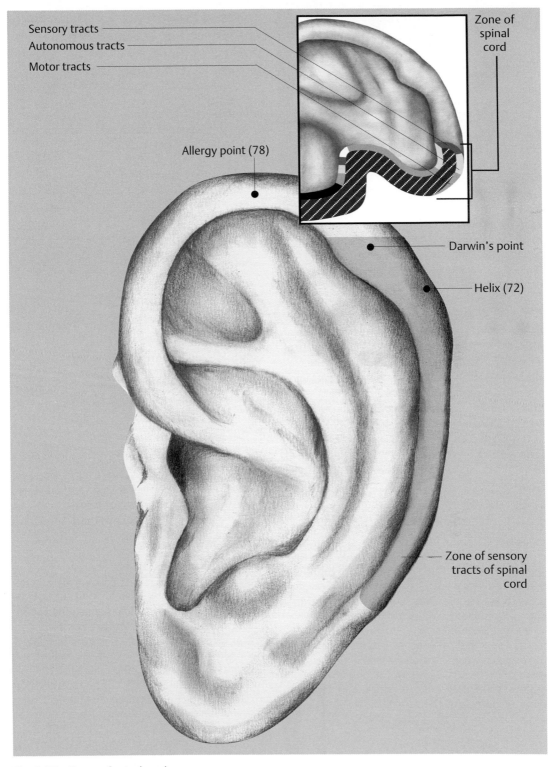

Sensory tracts

Autonomous tracts

Motor tracts

Zone of spinal cord

Allergy point (78)

Darwin's point

Helix (72)

Zone of sensory tracts of spinal cord

Fig. 3.23 Zones of spinal cord.

▶ If bleeding occurs upon withdrawal of the needle, it makes sense to let the bleeding continue as a microbloodletting, thus enhancing the effect. According to observations made in recent years in the course of allergy treatment, puncturing this point from the inside of the helical brim is supposed to be more effective. ◀

Darwin's Point (Fig. 3.23)

Location. On the darwinian tubercle, if present, which is usually well visible and palpable.
Indication. Adjuvant in arthritic joint problems of the extremities (questionable effectiveness).

Zone of Spinal Cord (Fig. 3.23)

Location. Spanning horizontally from the edge of the helical brim to the dorsolateral part of the helix and vertically from the darwinian tubercle to the postantitragal fossa.

▶ This zone represents the somatosensory fibers of the spinal cord corresponding to the individual sections of the spinal column along the vertical segmentation. Accordingly, the projections of the cervical nerves are found at the level of the projections of C1 to C7 on the lateral surface of the helix, while those of the corresponding motor tracts are found on the medial surface of the helix. ◀

Indication. Segment-related painful syndromes (e.g., postherpetic neuralgia, intercostal neuralgia).

3.1.10 Ascending Helix

French/Western auriculotherapy and Chinese ear acupuncture differ significantly in their specifications for this region of representation. Since 1978, this area has been further categorized by the French school and has led to the discovery of additional reflex zones.

Mutual examination of the research results has not resulted in a reconciliation of the varying points of view, let alone in concurring assessments. Since insufficient information is available regarding the preferable specifications, localizations of points on the ascending helix are presented here in terms of both schools.

Zones of Representation According to Chinese Ear Acupuncture

External Genitals Point ___ 79 (Fig. 3.24)

Location. On the ascending helix, slightly above the intersection of the inferior antihelical crus and the ascending helix.
Indication. Inflammation of the genitals, impotence (questionable effectiveness, as yet no personal experience).

Urethra Point ___ 80 (Fig. 3.24)

Location. Slightly below the intersection of the inferior antihelical crus (if it runs horizontally) and the ascending helix.
Indication. Ischuria, urethritis, nocturnal enuresis (questionable effectiveness, as yet no personal experience).

Zones of Representation According to French/Western Ear Acupuncture (Auriculotherapy)

Genital Region Point (Bosch Point According to Nogier) (Fig. 3.24)

Location. Slightly above the supratragic notch on the ascending helix, but at its lower edge, at the level of the weather point.
Indication. Sexual neurosis, impotence, dyspareunia, migraine.

▶ Nogier's naming of this point refers to the painting The *Garden of Earthly* Delights by Hieronymus Bosch, which may be admired in the Prado in Madrid. A detail of this painting shows a little devil piercing exactly this area with a lancet. ◀

Weather Point (Fig. 3.24)

Location. Roughly in the middle on the ascending helix. To be found exactly in in the middle of an imaginary vertical line connecting the intersection point (on the rim of the ascending helical brim) which is formed by another imaginary, almost horizontal, line (caution: does not always run horizontal to the inferior crus). This line runs through the pelvis/hip representation crossing the rim of the ascending helical brim (see intersection point above). From there the imaginary vertical line leads to the middle of the supratragic notch and the point is to be found at approximately half way along the line.

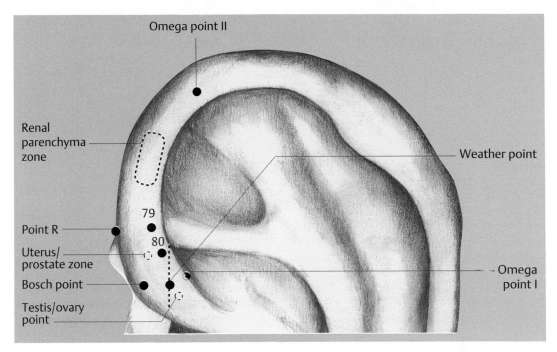

Fig. 3.24 Points/zones on the ascending helix.

Indication. Vegetative point: Complaints triggered by hypersensitivity to changes in atmospheric conditions; disorders such as migraine, cephalalgia, insomnia, recurring posttraumatic pain.

Testis/Ovary Point (According to Nogier) (Fig. 3.24)

Location. Inside the cranial wall of the ascending helix, immediately at its emergence from the superior concha.

Indication. Infertility, oligomenorrhea.

Prostate/Uterus Point (According to Nogier) (Fig. 3.24)

Location. At the level of the urethra point (80) but on the inside of the ascending helix or helical brim, above the testis/ovary point.

Indication. Menstrual disorders, prostatitis, impotence.

Renal Parenchyma Zone (According to Nogier) (Fig. 3.24)

Location. On the inside of the ascending helix between the upper and lower demarcations of the triangular fossa.

Indication. Adjuvant in diseases of the renal parenchyma (e.g., glomerulonephritis,

renal insufficiency at the stage of compensated retention).

Omega Point I (Fig. 3.24)

Location. Inside the upper edge of the ascending helix, approximately at the level of the weather point, sometimes rather on the inside of the ascending helix.

Indication. This point belongs to the group of vegetative, or autonomic, points. Disorders of the autonomic nervous system resulting from metabolic diseases and environmental factors (e.g., amalgam fillings).

Omega Point II (Fig. 3.24)

Location. On the brim of the ascending helix, ventral to the allergy point (78) (see **Fig. 3.23**), slightly above the intersection of the lower edge of the superior antihelical crus and the rim of the helix.

Indication. The omega point II belongs to the group of psychotropic points. It acts in a harmonizing and balancing way in personality disorders associated with disturbed relationships to the surrounding environment. This includes false emotional behavior directed toward other people, as well as objects (e.g., ruthlessness toward other people and destructive tendencies toward objects). The range of indications includes continuous aggression resulting from disturbed relationships and from other causes.

Point R (According to Bourdiol; Bourdiol Point, Psychotherapeutic Point) (Fig. 3.24)
Location. Right at the ventral edge of the ascending helix, at the transition to the facial skin, at the level of the intersection of the inferior antihelical crus and ascending helix.
Indication. As this belongs to the group of the so-called psychotropic points, it is used in psychosomatic syndromes, such as bronchial asthma, ulcerative colitis, Crohn's disease, chronic recurrent gastrointestinal ulcer, neurodermatitis, psoriasis. This area seems to act by harmonizing the interaction of the two cerebral hemispheres once a disturbed interaction of the hemispheres has developed, for example as a result of emotional traumas, severe chronic diseases, or persistent conflict situations.

▶ The name "psychotherapeutic point" comes from this point's ability to uncover emotions. Bourdiol (1982) observed this during his research on ear geometry and pointed out that there should be a well-founded bond of trust between physician and patient in order to cushion possible emotional reactions or the resolution of emotional blocks during confidential conversations. ◀

Frustration Point (Fig. 3.2)
Location. Approximately 3 to 4 mm from the external ear point (20) (see **Fig. 3.2**) toward the face on the rim of the ascending helix.
Indication. Belongs to the group of so-called psychotropic points. Psychological strain, tendencies toward addictive behavior.

3.1.11 Crus of Helix

Diaphragm Point ___ 82 Point Zero (According to Nogier) (Also Called Singultus Point, Start Point of Solar Plexus Zone) (Fig. 3.25)
Location. Located in a palpable small notch in the ascending helix just before the transition to the helical crus. The notch can be best located with the help of a stirrup-shaped exploring probe or a spherical dental filler. If there is no notch, it can be located approximately at the intersection

between a perpendicular drawn from the thoracolumbar transition (antihelix—inferior crus) and the helical crus.
Indication. According to the Chinese school: menstrual disorders, hemorrhagic diseases (hemostatic effect), singultus (hiccups). According to the French/Western school: abdominal pain (spasmolytic effect), hiccups. Fear of examinations, stage fright, functional stomach disorders.

According to the Western view, adjuvant in autonomic imbalance resulting from severe chronic or wasting diseases.

▶ This zone is seen as the physiological and geometric center of the auricle and is the starting point of Nogier's lines of treatment (see also ear geometry, segment therapy). ◀

Furthermore, according to French/Western specifications, the general sensitivity of the auricle—i.e., any lack of reflexes (insensitivity) or any exaggerated reflexes (hypersensitivity)—is supposed to be easily influenced here. Accordingly, point zero (82) should be pricked with a silver needle in cases of hypersensitivity (a calming effect), but with a golden needle in cases of hyposensitivity (a stimulating effect). After a short waiting period, the auricle should be searched again for irritated points (questionable effectiveness).

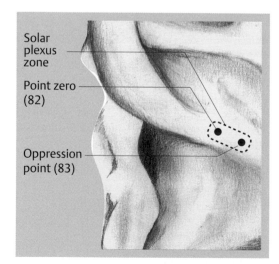

Fig. 3.25 Solar plexus zone and its points.

Oppression Point ___83 (Also Called Solar Plexus End Point of Solar Plexus Zone, Bifurcation Point) (Fig. 3.25)

Location. On the crus of the helix, usually on top of a small nodule, just before the transition to the plain of the concha.

Indication. Enuresis, according to the Chinese view. Otherwise, irritable stomach, examination anxiety, stage fright, functional stomach complaints.

3.1.12 Inferior Concha

Based on the concept of the upside-down embryo, it can be deduced that parts of the digestive tract (such as the mouth and esophagus), parts of the respiratory tract (including the plexus points), as well as the autonomic reflex portions of the heart will be projected on the inferior concha (the reflex zone of the heart, according to Nogier).

Mouth Zone ___84 (Throat Zone) (Fig. 3.26)

Location. In the corner of the acoustic meatus and the ascending helix, but on the plain of the concha.

Indication. Adjuvant in addictions (e.g., nicotine addiction), stomatitis (e.g., aphthous stomatitis), paresis of the facial nerve.

Larynx Zone (Not Illustrated)

Location. At the lower dorsal margin of the acoustic meatus.

Indication. Aphonia, laryngitis, dysphagia.

Trachea Zone ___103 (Fig. 3.26)

Location. This zone lies dorsal to the larynx zone and mouth zone (84); it is located between the center of the inferior concha and the dorsal edge of the acoustic meatus.

Indication. Adjuvant in tracheobronchitis, asthmoid diseases of the respiratory system.

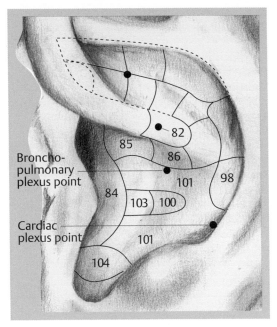

Fig. 3.26   Inferior concha: zones and plexus points of the internal organs.

Esophagus Zone ___85 (Fig. 3.26)

Location. This zone extends as a narrow band, starting from the mouth zone (84) along the lower edge of the helical crus and ending at the beginning of the lower third of the helical crus at the transition to the cardiac orifice zone (86).

Indication. Hyperemesis, reflux esophagitis, dysphagia. (Caution: ascertain the cause.)

Cardiac Orifice Zone (Cardia Zone) ___86 (Fig. 3.26)

Location. Adjacent to the esophagus zone (85) at the lower edge of the dorsal third of the crus of the helix.

Indication. Cardiospasm, functional epigastric discomfort, nausea, bloating.

Heart Zone ___100 (Vegetative Zone) (Fig. 3.26)

Location. In the center of the inferior concha at its deepest point.

Indication. Autonomic lability, insomnia, depressive mood, vegetatively induced arrhythmia of the heart (e.g., tachycardia), paroxysmal palpitations, angina pectoris; the point does not relate

3 Systematic Localization of Points on the Auricle

to the heart as an organ: heart (see medial surface of the auricle, p. 64).

Cardiac Plexus Point (According to Nogier) (Wonder Point) (Fig. 3.26)

Location. At the level of the C3 projection, on the plain of the inferior concha at its transition to the antihelical wall.

Indication. Hypersensitivity of the autonomic nervous system associated with symptoms such as a tendency to collapse in response to fright and anxiety. Hyperhidrosis. For further indications, see Heart Zone, page 55 (100).

> — **Practical Tip** —
> The heart zone (100) and cardiac plexus point have very similar ranges of indications and should be included in the treatment according to their state of irritation.

Lung Zone ___ 101 (Fig. 3.26)

Location. The specifications for this area have been corrected in view of earlier Chinese ear topographies (König and Wancura 1998). The main part of this area is located below the heart zone (100), reaching toward the caudal transition of the inferior concha to the antihelix; its dorsal demarcation is the spleen zone (98). The spleen zone (98) is represented mainly on the left auricle.

Indication. Adjuvant in bronchial asthma, chronic obstructive lung disease, any kind of addiction, bronchitis, and emphysema. According to the Chinese school, also adjuvant in skin diseases, used as the main zone for anesthesia by ear acupuncture.

Bronchopulmonary Plexus Point (According to Nogier) (Fig. 3.26)

Location. At the upper margin of the inferior concha at the level of the crus of helix, between the heart zone (100) and cardiac orifice zone (86).

Indication. Adjuvant in bronchospastic conditions (e.g., asthmoid bronchitis), bronchial asthma, hyperventilation syndrome, chronic obstructive pulmonary disease.

Triple Burner Zone ___ 104 (Fig. 3.26)

Location. A relatively wide area caudal to the acoustic meatus, in the inferior concha between the lower part of the tragus and the antitragus.

Indication. In accordance with the meaning of the triple burner zone in Chinese medicine, indicated in chronic obstipation, predisposition to edema.

The definition of this area derives from the attempt of the Chinese school to apply traditional Chinese concepts of body acupuncture to the auricular microsystem and, in this way, deduce therapeutic approaches (see König and Wancura, 1998).

So far, the author has been unable to obtain corresponding reproducible results from practical experience (questionable effectiveness).

Spleen Zone ___ 98 (Fig. 3.26)

Location. According to the Chinese specification, on the dorsal edge of the inferior concha at the level of the C1 to T5/T6 projection, but only on the left auricle.

Indication. Meteorism (tympanites), urinary incontinence, dyspepsia (questionable effectiveness).

3.1.13 Superior Concha

Stomach Zone ___ 87 (Fig. 3.27)

Location. A relatively extensive area with a wide central part, surrounding the transition of the helical crus to the concha like a collar. The zone borders on the cardiac orifice zone (86) with a small part in the inferior concha, while the larger part lies in the superior concha.

Indication. Acute and chronic recurring gastritis, lack of appetite, eating disorders, nausea, obesity.

> — **Practical Tip** —
> If applicable, adjuvant in headache and excessive strain syndromes.

Duodenum Zone ___ 88 (Fig. 3.27)

Location. This area borders the stomach zone (87) cranioventrally, running as a narrow zone in a ventral direction.

Indication. Adjuvant in duodenitis, duodenal ulcers, chronic cholecystitis.

Small Intestine Zone (Jejunum/Ileum Zone) ___ 89 (Fig. 3.27)

Location. A continuation of the projection of the digestive tract in a ventral direction, adjacent to

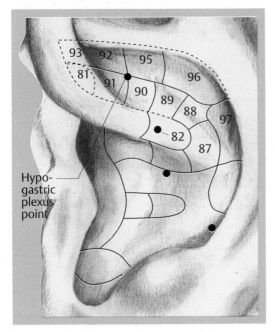

Fig. 3.27 Superior concha: zones and plexus points of the internal organs.

the duodenum zone (88), bordering caudally on the middle third of the crus of the helix.
Indication. Adjuvant in fermentative dyspepsia, diarrhea, Crohn's disease.

Large Intestine Zone (Appendix Zone IV) —— 90
Sigmoid—Rectum —— 91 (Fig. 3.27)
Location. An elongated area adjacent to the small intestine zone (89) that runs parallel to the helical crus on the floor of the superior concha and reaches beneath the ascending helix at the intersection of inferior antihelical crus and ascending helix, the hemorrhoid zone (81).
Indication. Chronic obstipation, colitis, hemorrhoids (hemorrhoid zone), diarrhea.
Adjuvant in ulcerous colitis.

▶ The appendix zone IV (90), which is separately listed by the Chinese school, is proportionately assigned by Western ear acupuncture to the adjacent areas of the small intestine zone (89) and large intestine zone (91). ◀

It should be remembered that, with any symptoms from the digestive organs, the corresponding gut sections should be predominantly explored for points of maximal irritation.

Urinary Bladder Zone —— 92 (Fig. 3.27)
Location. In the superior concha above the large intestine zone (91) and bordering on the inferior antihelical crus.
Indication. Urinary incontinence, cystitis, nocturnal enuresis, irritated bladder, lumbago (see segment therapy, p. 67).

Prostate Zone —— 93 (According to the Chinese School) (Fig. 3.27)
Location. Ventral to the urinary bladder zone (92), in the angle between the ascending helix and inferior antihelical crus, on the floor of the superior concha.
Indication. Prostatitis, ischuria, urinary incontinence (questionable effectiveness).

Kidney Zone —— 95 (Fig. 3.27)
Location. This zone lies dorsal to the urinary bladder zone (92) and parallel to the inferior antihelical crus on the floor of the superior concha at its upper margin.
Indication. Adjuvant in functional diseases of the urogenital tract, including adrenal glands. Lumbago, dysmenorrhea, migraine. According to Chinese medicine, also indicated in tinnitus, ear diseases, hair loss, fractures.

▶ The Chinese school localizes the urethra point (94) right on the border between the urinary bladder zone (92) and kidney zone (95), However, this point should be viewed as part of the kidney zone and is of little practical importance. ◀

In certain conditions (e.g., urolithiasis), the entire kidney zone exhibits maximal irritation of the above-mentioned points (see Hypogastric Plexus Point).

Hypogastric Plexus Point (Fig. 3.28)
Location. In the ventral part of the superior concha, at the border between the urinary bladder zone (92), kidney zone (95), and large intestine zone (90, 91).
Indication. Ureteral colic, renal colic, colosigmoidal diverticulitis, colonic colic.

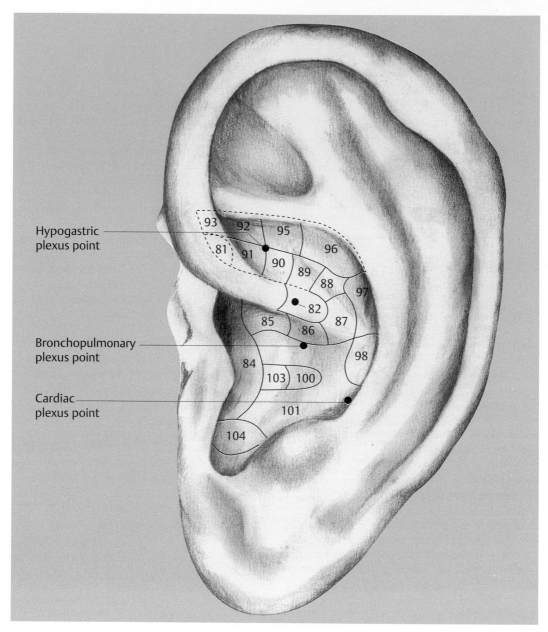

Hypogastric
plexus point

Bronchopulmonary
plexus point

Cardiac
plexus point

Fig. 3.28 Concha: complete overview of zones of the internal organs and plexus points.

▶ The localization corresponds to the projection zone of the inferior mesenteric ganglion according to Bourdiol (1980); this supplies an identical area (such as the descending colon and the organs of the small pelvis) and consists of sympathetic and parasympathetic fibers. ◀

Pancreas/Gallbladder Zone ____96 (Fig. 3.27)
Location. This relatively extensive reflex zone lies in the upper region of the superior concha, parallel to the antihelix, just before its transition to the inferior antihelical crus, opposite the duodenum zone (88) and the small intestine

zone (89). The zone is demarcated ventrally by the kidney zone (95) and dorsally by the liver zone (97).

Here, too, interpretations from the Chinese and French/Western ear acupuncture differ. According to the Chinese concept, the gallbladder is represented only on the right auricle and the pancreas only on the left auricle, both under the same number (96).

By contrast, French/Western auriculotherapy localizes only parts (such as the body and tail) of the pancreas in the left superior concha, while the head of the pancreas and the gallbladder are assigned to the right superior concha (Bourdiol 1980), in agreement with the position of the organs in the body relative to sagittal cross-sections.

Indication. Digestive disorders, chronic recurrent pancreatitis, cholecystitis, cholelithiasis.

Liver Zone ⎯⎯ 97 (Fig. 3.27)

Location. Toward the antihelix, dorsal to the stomach zone (87) in the transition from the superior concha to the inferior concha.

The area varies in size depending on the organ's position in the body; hence, it is larger on the right auricle than on the left auricle, where it makes room for the neighboring pancreas/gallbladder zone (96) and spleen zone (98) (inferior concha).

Indication. Adjuvant in hematological diseases (e.g., anemia), hepatopathy, addictions (e.g., abuse of alcohol or medication), intercostal neuralgia.

According to Chinese medicine, also indicated in eye diseases (questionable effectiveness).

"Hemorrhoid" Zone ⎯⎯ 81 (Fig. 3.27)

Location. Beneath the helical brim, on the floor of the superior concha in continuation with the large intestine zone (91).

Indication. Hemorrhoidal complaints, anusitis, anal fissure, obstipation.

▶ The original localization of the rectum zone (81) according to the Chinese specification is on the ascending helix; because of a lack of correlation, it was abandoned in favor of the zone described above. ◀

3.2 Medial Surface of Auricle (Back of Ear)

Although the lateral surface of the auricle is more important with regard to diagnosis and therapy, and the reflex zones of the lateral surface apply to the majority of diseases (provided they are deemed treatable by ear acupuncture), the projection fields of the medial surface (see **Fig. 2.2**) should be included in the therapeutic approach.

Orientation on the medial surface is more complicated for the physician, and treatment less comfortable for the patient. However, the use of a combination of reflex points on the lateral and medial surfaces often results in decisive therapeutic breakthroughs (e.g., in joint disease). Corresponding to the positions on the lateral surface of the auricle, the projection zones are found immediately opposite on the medial surface. In view of the broad-based attachment of the auricle to the cranium, the negative reliefs of some of the anatomical structures are missing on the medial auricular surface. These include the intertragic notch, the tragus, the supratragic notch, and parts of the helical crus, as well as the ventral portions of the triangular fossa and inferior antihelical crus. For this reason, the corresponding reflex zones are not found on the medial surface of the auricle.

While the sensory parts of individual reflex zones are projected on the lateral surface of the auricle, the motor parts are primarily represented in the corresponding reference zones of the medial surface. Consequently, the master points on the medial surface of the auricle can intensify the therapeutic stimuli already applied to the corresponding positions on the lateral surface. It is therefore obvious to include them in therapy, especially in diseases of the locomotor system and the joints.

3.2.1 Overview

General remarks. Usually found immediately opposite their corresponding sensory projections on the lateral surface of the auricle, the motor projections take the form of slightly smaller areas on the medial surface. For example, the motor fibers of the **spinal cord** are projected on the dorsal rim of the helical brim, while the sensory parts are represented on the lateral part of the helical brim.

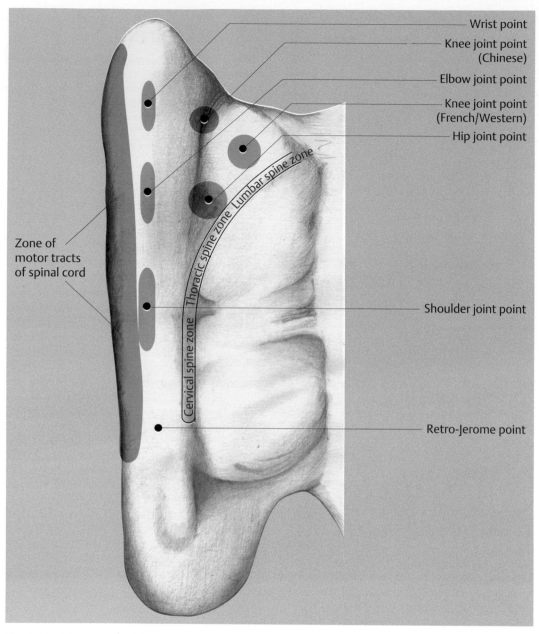

Fig. 3.29 Motor parts of the locomotor system on the medial surface of the auricle.

The motor parts of the **upper extremities** are projected on the eminence of the scapha. The lower demarcation can be found approximately on a linear elongation of the central posterior sulcus, while the upper demarcation is at the intersection of the eminence of the scapha and the cranial end of the sulcus of the superior antihelical crus. As is the case on the lateral surface of the auricle, the zones of the fingers and hand are located in the cranial region, while those of shoulder and shoulder joint are in the caudal region of this projection zone.

The motor parts of the **lower extremities** are projected on the eminence of triangular fossa next to the cranial region of the eminence of the scapha and partly also on the sulci of the inferior and superior antihelical crura. Differentiation in this zone of representation corresponds to the representation zone on the lateral surface of the auricle. For example, the sensory part of the French/Western knee joint point (49 a) is found on the lateral auricular surface in the center of the triangular fossa, while its motor component is in the center of the eminence of the triangular fossa on the medial surface (**Fig. 3.29**).

Practical Tip

Apply a pinch grip: using the index finger and thumb—with their tips directly opposing one another— tentatively pinch the auricle, so that points can be located on the medial surface by using the lateral surface as a guide to orientation.

The **inner organs** are projected on the lateral surface of the auricle with their zones of representation in the superior and inferior conchae, on the medial surface on the eminence of the superior and inferior conchae, respectively, and also on the central posterior sulcus—provided the corresponding zones exist on the medial surface in view of the broad-based attachment of the auricle, or at least are present in a reduced form (see **Fig. 3.30**).

3.2.2 Systematics of Reflex Zones

Chinese School

The zones of representation described below are derived from the Chinese school. The letter "m" stands for "medial."

Here, the same considerations apply as discussed earlier; i.e., multiple areas identified for one body area have been registered as master points without being true reference points. Consequently, they qualify in practice only as supportive or enhancing points that are not routinely detectable, even if clinical symptoms are present.

In the most recent Chinese literature, the topography of these areas is described in relatively vague or fragmentary terms. Presumably, the results are too unconvincing to allow precise specifications.

Kidney Point ___ 95 m (Fig. 3.30)
Location. At the lower edge of the eminence of the inferior concha, at the transition to the lobule.
Indication. Insomnia, vertigo, cephalalgia, dysmenorrhea (questionable effectiveness).

Liver Point ___ 97 m (Fig. 3.30)
Location. On the eminence of inferior concha close to the antihelical sulcus, opposite the liver zone (97) proper of the lateral surface of the auricle.
Indication. Lumbago, thoracic oppression, joint problems (questionable effectiveness).

Spleen Point ___ 98 m (Fig. 3.30)
Location. At the same level as the liver point (97 m), at the upper edge of the eminence of the inferior concha, close to the central posterior sulcus.
Indication. Fermentative dyspepsia, abdominal complaints referable to meteorism. Adjuvant in diarrhea (questionable effectiveness).

Lung Point ___ 101 m (Fig. 3.30)
Location. At the upper edge of the eminence of the inferior concha, at the same level as the liver point (97 m) and the spleen point (98 m), close to the attachment of the auricle and below the central posterior sulcus.
Indication. Skin diseases as understood in Chinese medicine, bronchial asthma (questionable effectiveness).

Heart Point (organ) ___ 100 m (Fig. 3.30)
Location. At the upper edge of the eminence of the triangular fossa, almost in the antihelical sulcus of the superior antihelical crus.
Indication. Adjuvant in sleeping disorders, cephalalgia, glossitis as understood in Chinese medicine (questionable effectiveness).

Antihypertension Groove ___ 105 m (Fig. 3.30)
Location. This groove-type area is located at the beginning of the inferior groove of the crus.
Indication. Adjuvant in hypertension.

Practical Tip

This hypertension-lowering groove is most effectively needled as microbloodletting.

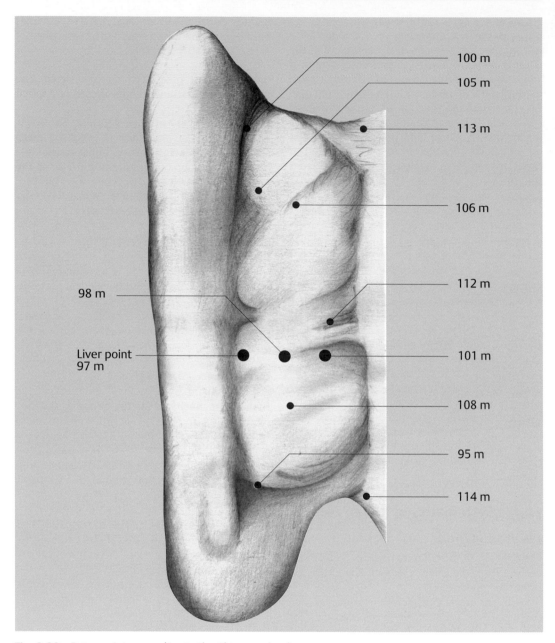

100 m
105 m
113 m
106 m
112 m
98 m
Liver point
97 m
101 m
108 m
95 m
114 m

Fig. 3.30 Retro points according to the Chinese school.

Upper Back of Ear Point ___ 106 m (Fig. 3.30)

Location. On top of a small cartilaginous tubercle at the upper edge of the eminence of the superior concha.

Indication. Pain in the back, lumbago, skin diseases as understood in Chinese medicine (questionable effectiveness).

Lower Back of Ear Point ___ 108 m (Fig. 3.30)

Location. In the center of the eminence of the inferior concha.

Indication. Pain in the back (e.g., thoracic vertebrae syndrome), pain in the shoulder.

Vagus Nerve Branch Point (Also Called Retro-Point Zero) __ 112 m (Fig. 3.30)

Location. In the central posterior sulcus, at the level of the helical crus on the lateral surface of the auricle.

Indication. Cephalalgia, swelling of the nasal mucosa in rhinitis (little effectiveness in my experience; see also Retro-Point Zero).

Adjuvant in bronchial asthma.

Upper Ear Attachment Point __ 113 m (Fig. 3.30)

Location. At the transition between the sulcus of the superior antihelical crus and the attachment of the auricle.

Indication. Cephalalgia, abdominal pain. (Caution: ascertain the cause.)

Adjuvant in bronchial asthma, paresis (see also Lower Ear Attachment Point 114 m) (questionable effectiveness).

Lower Ear Attachment Point __ 114 m (Fig. 3.30)

Location. Close to the caudal curvature of the sulcus of the inferior concha, at the transition between the lobule and the attachment of the auricle.

Indication. Cephalalgia, abdominal pain.

Adjuvant in bronchial asthma, paresis (see also Upper Ear Attachment Point 113 m) (questionable effectiveness).

French/Western School

The French/Western ear acupuncture (auriculotherapy) described by Nogier and Bourdiol (1980) is committed to a more precise topography. As is the case with the lateral surface of the auricle, orientation is provided by the representation zone of the spinal column, (see **Fig. 3.29, Fig. 3.30**) which is projected in the antihelical sulcus. The zone that stretches from here to the attachment of the ear and includes the eminences of the inferior and superior conchae accommodates the sensorimotor representation fields of the inner organs. Located on the eminence of the scapha, between the antihelical sulcus and the rim of the helical brim, and on the eminence of the triangular fossa and in the sulcus of the superior antihelical crus, respectively, are the motor projection fields of the upper and lower extremities, namely, the joint points of the hand, elbow, and shoulder, and the joint points of the knee and hip, All joint points are found opposite the corresponding projections on the lateral surface of the auricle. Again, the pinch grip (thumb and index finger) is applied for orientation.

Furthermore, the somatomotor part of the spinal cord with its motor tracts is projected on the dorsal rim of the helix at the transition to the eminence of the scapha, demarcated cranially by the darwinian tubercle and caudally by the intersection of postantitragal fossa and the rim of helix (according to Kropej 1977; see ear plate).

Synthesis Point (According to Nogier) (Not Illustrated)

Location. At the attachment of the ear, in a small groove formed below the central posterior sulcus; it is visible when pressing the lower half of the auricle slightly toward the face.

Indication. For strengthening the constitution (e.g., in cases of cerebral palsy, toxic exposures, predisposition to infections) (questionable effectiveness).

Retro-Thalamus Point (Fig. 3.31)

Location. Opposite the thalamus point (26 a) of the lateral surface of the auricle.

Indication. Adjuvant in severe pain syndromes (e.g., malignant diseases, severe neuralgia, joint problems).

Retro-Antiaggression Point (Fig. 3.31)

Location. Directly opposite the corresponding point of the lateral surface of the auricle (see pinch grip, p. 61).

Indication. Adjuvant in conditions of psychological strain, in conditions with suppressed aggression.

Retro-Jerome Point (Fig. 3.31)

Location. Directly opposite the Jerome point (29 b) of the lateral surface of the auricle, i.e., on the back of the postantitragal fossa (see pinch grip, p. 61).

Indication. Adjuvant in insomnia, especially in difficulty with sleeping through (dysphylaxia).

Retro-Point Zero (Fig. 3.31)

Location. In the central posterior sulcus opposite point zero (82) (see **Fig. 3.25**) of the lateral

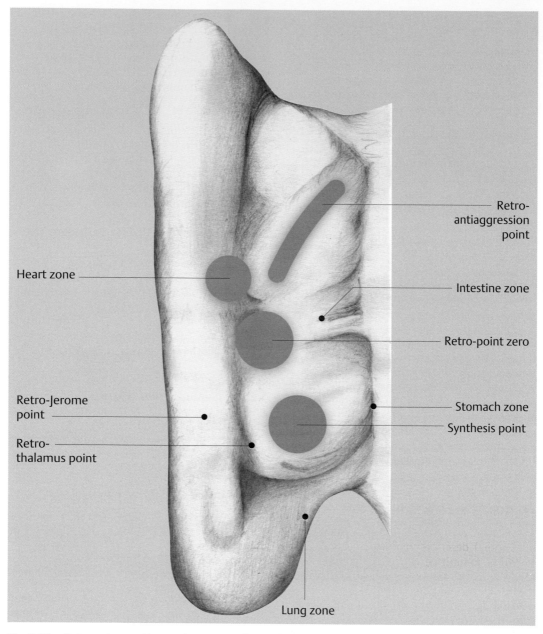

Heart zone

Retro-Jerome point

Retro-thalamus point

Retro-antiaggression point

Intestine zone

Retro-point zero

Stomach zone

Synthesis point

Lung zone

Fig. 3.31 Retro points and internal organs on the medial surface according to the French/Western school.

surface of the auricle. On account of its location, this point probably corresponds to the vagus nerve branch point 112 m (see **Fig. 3.30**) (see pinch grip, p. 61).

Indication. Spasmolytic effect in abdominal spasmodic conditions; effective in combination with point zero of the lateral surface of the auricle (e.g., acute gastroenteritis, functional abdominal complaints).

4 Special Points and Treatment Areas

The following is a summary of points and areas that are frequently combined in daily practice. For orientation, they are assigned particular directions of action and will be explained in detail beyond this classification.

4.1 Analgesic Points

These points first and foremost include those areas that are distinguished by their varying analgesic effect.

Shen Men Point —— 55 (Fig. 4.1)

This is located at the upper edge of the triangular fossa. It is effective as a general pain point with additional antiphlogistic effect. It is used, in particular, when diseases of the locomotor system have become inflammatory or are derived from trauma. Because of its analgesic action, this point is also effective in the treatment of addictions (see Treatment of Addictions, Chapter 9.11).

> **— Practical Tip ——**
> In Chinese ear acupuncture, this point is the only general pain point and is used in almost all pain syndromes. Hence, it makes sense to include this point, depending on its state of irritation, in the therapy of special disorders such as migraine.

Thalamus Point —— 26 a (Fig. 4.1)

This point is located on the inside of the antitragus at its base. It represents the corresponding brain part and its function as the central portal of entry and filter of all afferent pain signals. It is only important in serious conditions involving generalized pain. Thus, its range of applications applies mainly to severe chronic pain syndromes, pain associated with malignant diseases, phantom limb pain, and other severe pain conditions (e.g., an acute migraine attack or acute sciatica).

▶ Irritation of this point is usually only detectable in severe pain conditions related to the disorders referred to above. ◀

Occiput Point —— 29 (Fig. 4.1)

This is located in the postantitragal fossa. It belongs to a special group of points (29 a, 29 b, and 29 c) as well as to the sensory line. Apart from its analgesic effect, it has a calming and sedative effect, and it harmonizes the mind.

> **— Practical Tip ——**
> A special feature is its particular effectiveness in headaches of various origins, including tension headaches, as well as neuralgiform pain syndromes in the region of the face and head.

Forehead Point —— 33 (Fig. 4.1)

This is located at the ventral end of the sensory line (29, 35, 33) (see **Fig. 4.3**). It is effective for headaches affecting the forehead (e.g., sinusitis, concussion, neuralgia). It acts as an adjuvant in sleep disorders and nonsystemic vertigo.

Vegetative Point II —— 34 (Subcortex Point, Gray Substance Point) (Fig. 4.1)

This is located on the inside of the antitragus ventral to the thalamus point. This zone carries a special status among the analgesic points. It is also very effective in conditions involving chronic pain, including rheumatoid arthritis and chronic neuralgia, as well as in systemic vertigo, tinnitus, and hyperemesis gravidarum. It acts as an adjuvant in diabetic polyneuropathy.

Sun Point —— 35 (Fig. 4.1)

The sun point is located on the outside of the antitragus in its base, as the central point of the sensory line. This point is extraordinarily effective, particularly for parietal headaches and migraines; it is the point of first choice when treating any one of this assortment of symptoms.

> **— Practical Tip ——**
> Because of its pronounced effectiveness, the sun point (35) is the starting point in the treatment of acute migraine attacks, particularly in combination with the occiput point (29) and thalamus point (26 a).

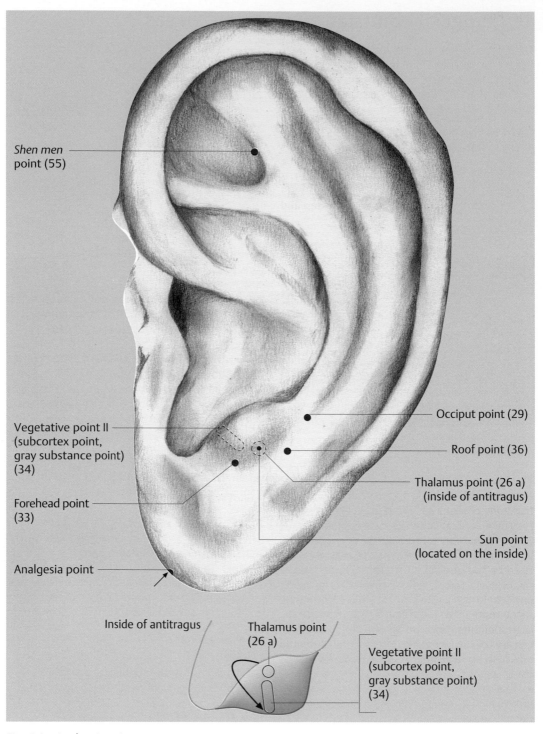

Fig. 4.1 Analgesic points.

Roof Point ——36 (Fig. 4.1)

Located below the occiput point (29), this point has a relatively narrow range of indications; its analgesic effect relates to the parietal area of the skull. For this reason, it is only important as an auxiliary point in certain types of cephalgia.

Retro-Thalamus Point (see Fig. 3.1)

This is located opposite the thalamus point (26 a) (identify it using a pinch grip) of the lateral surface of the auricle. This point is used for the same spectrum of indications as the thalamus point. It can be applied effectively when alternated with the thalamus point in malignant diseases and when short or daily treatment intervals are required.

Analgesia Point (Fig. 4.1)

This point is located at the ventral edge of the lobule at the level of the "ventral quadrant" of the ear, slightly ventral and caudal to the master omega point. The analgesia point, which is derived from Nogier's approach, is effective in indications listed for the thalamus point (26 a). In severe pain conditions, it is usually combined with the thalamus point (26 a) and also with the retro-thalamus point (see **Fig. 3.31**).

4.2 Vegetative Groove
(According to Lange)

The vegetative groove is located at the edge of the scapha beneath the helical brim. This projection zone of the origin of sympathetic nuclei (or intermediolateral nuclei, 31) was recognized by Lange as an indicator zone for the segmental demarcation of diseases or pain syndromes as defined by Nogier's ear geometry, and was labeled the vegetative groove. Our own practical experience confirms that the most sensitive points are found more often in this zone rather than in the corresponding region of the helix. Especially in diseases of the locomotor system, this allows the novice to produce impressive therapeutic results using segment therapy (formerly ear geometry) in this area. Nogier and Bourdiol defined this groove as the zone of neurovegetative centers of the spinal cord, without realizing that these can be regarded as diagnostic guide points (due to their higher sensitivity) and as vegetative control points indicative of the diseased segment (because they are more effective than the points

on the helix, the representation zone of the spinal cord). Based on each disturbed or irritated point in this zone, a modified segment therapy can be developed. This is achieved by drawing an imaginary line that connects the irritated point with point zero (diaphragm point, 82, according to the Chinese school) (**Fig. 4.2**). This line serves as a segmental line of treatment, along which, in analogy to Nogier's ear geometry, several additional irritated points are often found up to the helical brim and therefore may be included in the therapy. The following take-home message applies to the vegetative groove:

▶ Embarking on diagnosis and therapy for a locomotor system disease is simple and effective when using the segmental approach. ◀

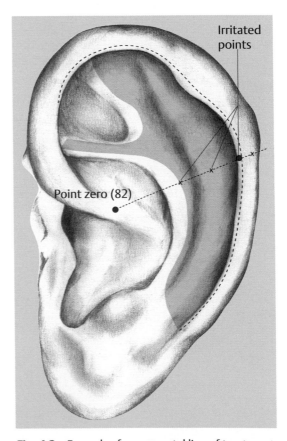

Fig. 4.2 Example of a segmental line of treatment between the vegetative groove/point zero and reactive points (small crosses) in the zone of paravertebral muscles and ligaments of the spinal cord.

4.3 Sensory Line

The sensory line described by Nogier is located at the base of the antitragus at the transition to the lobule. Its course is defined by the following three points: occiput point (29), sun point (35), and forehead point (33) (**Fig. 4.3**).

Nogier's original specifications relate to a short, elongated zone around the sun point (35) that runs parallel to the base of the antitragus. He described this as being effective especially for tinnitus.

Apart from this, treatment through the sensory line is also effective in cephalalgia. This line of treatment is especially important in cases of cephalalgia triggered by extraordinary irritation of the sensory nerve center, hence its name, through either the eyes, the ears, or the nose (e.g., migraines triggered by odor or noise).

Furthermore, the sensory line is used in combination with segment therapy (formerly ear geometry) in headaches originating from the vertebrae. Here, it enables a simple and reliable therapeutic approach when embarking on individualized headache therapy.

4.4 Vertigo Line

The identification of the so-called vertigo line (**Fig. 4.3**) can be traced back to a publication, in 1981, from the 12th World Congress of Ear, Nose, and Throat (ENT) Specialists in Budapest. The paper was presented by the Drs Pildner von Steinburg, ENT specialists from Munich, under the title "Central vestibular dysfunction—its treatment by acupuncture as a selective reflex therapy." The vertigo line contains grouped points on the auricle that can normalize the dysfunction of vestibular neurons through reflexes. The points can be found on two lines that lie roughly perpendicular to each other. One line runs almost horizontally on the inside of the antitragus, just below its upper rim (the dotted line in **Fig. 4.3**). The other line intersects the first line at the level of the postantitragal fossa. It is identical to the postantitragal line until it intersects with the scapha (Jerome point, 29 b). The postantitragal line then continues in direction of the dorsal helix and crosses it at a right angle.

On both of these imaginary lines, three or four irritated points can be detected in certain

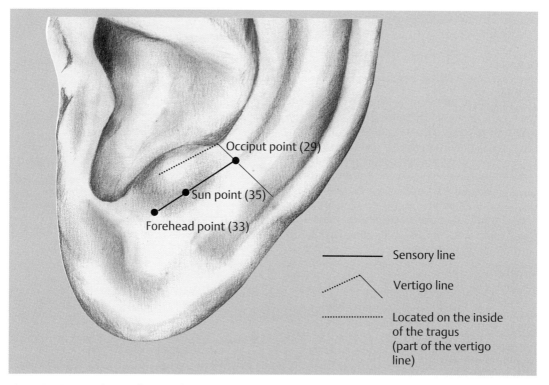

Occiput point (29)

Sun point (35)

Forehead point (33)

——— Sensory line

········ Vertigo line

·············· Located on the inside of the tragus (part of the vertigo line)

Fig. 4.3 Sensory line and vertigo line.

diseases, particularly in vestibular vertigo (i.e., systemic and directional forms of vertigo), but often also with concomitant symptoms (such as cervical syndrome, conditions resulting from craniocerebral trauma, and those arising after an acute, sudden loss of hearing). Needle stimulation at these irritated points quickly causes the vestibular dysfunction to subside.

It is certainly no coincidence that the vertigo line can be demonstrated within the areas of the inner antitragal surface and the postantitragal line, both of which are densely covered with reflex zones. The irritated areas are often identical with defined points, such as the brainstem point (25), kinetosis point (29 a), occiput point (29), or Jerome point (29 b).

In all other types of vertigo, treatment via the vertigo line is not effective. For example, with conditions that belong to the spectrum of non-systematic vertigo, the sensory line or other individually applicable areas of ear somatotopy should be considered.

4.5 Vegetative Points

These points on the auricle are reflex zones that are effective in harmonizing the autonomic nervous system (**Fig. 4.4**). They should be monitored for their state of irritation, especially when the clinical picture includes, as is often the case, concomitant, individually pronounced vegetative–dystonic symptoms, irrespective of their primary or secondary nature. The vegetative points are also detectable in autonomic disorders that cannot be assigned to any specific syndrome, and they are therefore therapeutically useful. Vegetative point I (51), vegetative point II (subcortex), and the heart zone (100) are particularly effective in harmonizing the autonomic nervous system. They are named accordingly and show certain differences with regard to their specific effects.

Vegetative Point I___51 (Fig. 4.4)
This is located on the inferior antihelical crus at the intersection with the brim of the ascending helix. It is effective as an adjuvant point, mainly in dysfunctions of the intestine and cardiovascular system, as well as in pulmonary dysfunctions. In addition, it is often used in dysmenorrhea, fertility disorders in both sexes, and addictive disorders.

Vegetative Point II/Subcortex—34 (See Gray Substance Point) (Fig. 4.4)
Located on the inside of the antitragus, this point has similar indications for use. In addition, however, this point is of special importance in the treatment of acute and chronic pain, as well as chronic diseases in general, tinnitus, and conditions following stroke.

Note. Both reflex zones—vegetative Points I and II—are major accompanying points in the treatment of addictions.

Heart Zone ___100 (Fig. 4.4)
This is located in the center of the inferior concha. According to the assignments of ear somatotopy, this point is not regarded as a representation zone of the heart as an organ per se, but instead represents its autonomic sensory function. Therefore, this point is indicated in the treatment of autonomic lability in patients with sleeping disorders and for intermittent states of inadequate agitation, symptoms such as inadequate fright and anxiety-induced tachyrhythmias, collapse dispositions, hyperhidrosis, and paroxysmal tachycardia, as well as related organ dysfunctions.

At this juncture, the following points should again be listed: occiput point (29) and Jerome point (29 b). Although their function in the field of autonomic disorders is only adjuvant, they do have a accompanying harmonizing effect on the vegetative system due to their principal specific action.

Occiput Point ___29 (Fig. 4.4)
This point is located in the postantitragal fossa. Due to its accompanying vegetative effect, it is included in the treatment approach for numerous (not just pain-dominated) diseases, including vertigo and circulatory instability (also listed with Analgesic Points, see Chapter 4.1).

Jerome Point ___29 b (Fig. 4.4)
This point is located at the intersection of the postantitragal line and scapha. Its main range of indications includes sleeping disorders, as well as feelings of tension (as it has a muscle-relaxing effect). It often turns out to be irritated in very different conditions. It is not a vegetative point, but with its accompanying harmonizing effect on the

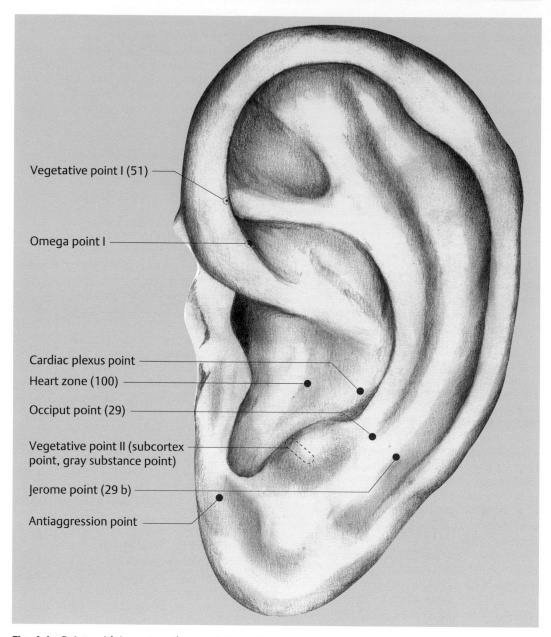

Fig. 4.4 Points with impact on the vegetative system.

Vegetative point I (51)

Omega point I

Cardiac plexus point

Heart zone (100)

Occiput point (29)

Vegetative point II (subcortex point, gray substance point)

Jerome point (29 b)

Antiaggression point

vegetative system, it often provides a supporting, vegetatively harmonizing impulse in painful clinical conditions (e.g., lumbago–sciatica syndrome, intercostal neuralgia, cervico-occipital neuralgia), as well as in globus hystericus, hiccups, and hyperhidrosis.

Cardiac Plexus Point (According to Nogier) (Wonder Point) (Fig. 4.4)

The cardiac plexus point is located in the inferior concha close to the wall of the antihelix, at the level of the C3 projection. This vegetative point is used for the same indications as the heart zone

(100) and can be combined with this point (see p. 55).

Omega Point I (Fig. 4.4)

Located inside the upper edge of the ascending helix, close to the weather point, this is not a distinct vegetative point. However, it may be detected in vegetative disorders of the autonomic nervous system resulting from metabolic diseases and environmental factors.

Weather Point (Fig. 3.24)

Located on the ascending helix, this is definitely a specific vegetative point in cases of hypersensitivity to changes in atmospheric conditions. It is used in all disorders triggered by this individual sensitivity (e.g., postsurgical pain, phantom pain, insomnia, cephalalgia, and particularly migraine).

4.6 Psychotropic Points

In connection with this subject, it is important to also refer to the section "Laterality" (see p. 8). When using the psychotropic points, lateral dominance of the cerebral hemispheres and its representation in auricular somatotopy is supposed to play an important role (Fig. 4.5). Furthermore, it should be recalled that treatment of these points supports the attempt of the two (dominant and nondominant) hemispheres to achieve harmonization in life, i.e., a kind of inner satisfaction (caution: not self-satisfaction).

In all mental disorders that compromise these attempts, the psychotropic zones of the auricle are found to be irritated and therefore provide a therapeutic opportunity to intervene in a stabilizing or harmonizing way. Depending on their psychosomatic effects, they may also positively affect organ function.

General monitoring of all psychotropic points for their state of irritation is reliable in mental or psychotropic disorders and allows for the proper choice of therapeutic points. Hence, the final selection usually corresponds to the patient's psychogenesis and medical history. This approach avoids the difficult considerations and laborious research necessary for selecting the proper reflex zones. Thus, it seems consistent and reasonable to speak in relatively neutral terms of "psychotropic zones," which, in appropriate circumstances,

may include several psychotropic (PT) points. These points are numbered consecutively and, irrespective of their suggestive original names (the verification of which may be problematic), may be included in the therapeutic concept.

- The psychotropic zone on the **ventral** part of the lobule, below the intertragic notch, includes the following psychotropic points:
  - PT1 = (formerly antiaggression point).
  - PT2 = (formerly anxiety/worry point).
- In the psychotropic zone on the **dorsal** part of the lobule, at approximately the same levels as PT1 and PT2, the following psychotropic points can be found:
  - PT3 = (formerly antidepression point).
  - PT4 = (formerly sorrow/joy point).

PT1 (Fig. 4.5)

From among a multitude of ear points, only PT1 is detectable in almost all patients with mental and psychosomatic disorders. It is located slightly inferior to the intertragic notch.

Presumably, even the healthy-looking people of our civilized world suffer from a disturbance of this kind as a result of our lifestyle. Unfortunately, the initial, even simplistic, name of the point does not do justice to its wide range of indications.

Certainly, the indications derived from the symptom of "aggression" predominate, but the point is also extremely helpful as an adjuvant in less spectacular symptoms or diseases (e.g., functional heart problems, cephalalgia, concentration and sleeping disorders, as well as dysfunction of temperature perception).

PT2 (Fig. 4.5)

PT2 is located below the antiaggression point (PT1, in field I of the lobule). This point is mainly indicated for the resolution of justifiable anxiety attacks. In right-handed individuals, this zone is on the right ear. In case of a vague, undefined form of anxiety ("angst"), a zone named the "worry point" is present at the same location on the left ear (field I of the lobule, below the antiaggression point). In left-handed individuals, these correlations are suggested to be reversed. From personal experience, however, this is a dubious differentiation.

When the symptoms are less prominent, this zone may not be reactive at all.

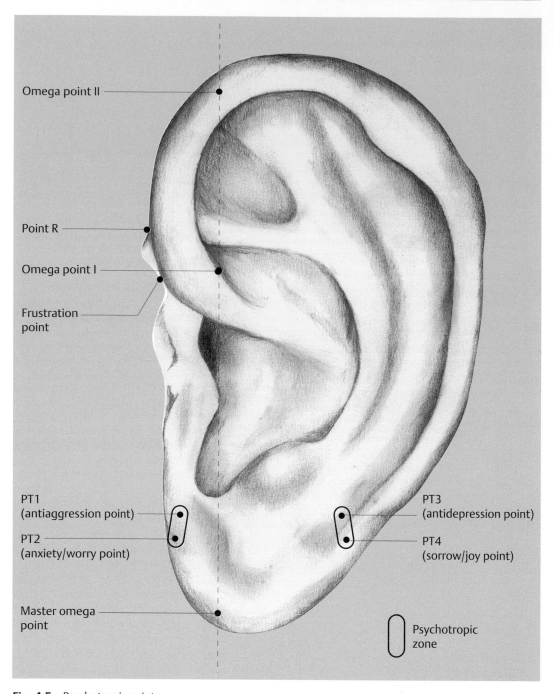

Fig. 4.5 Psychotropic points.

▶ Therefore, this zone should only be included in therapy when all other irritated reflex zones have been exhausted. ◀

PT3 (Fig. 4.5)

PT3 is located almost at the same level as the antiaggression point, but in the area of the intersection of the scaphal ending and the lobule, below the Jerome point (29 b). It is irritated in depressive states and depressions resulting from stressful living conditions (e.g., following tragic events). This point may be useful as an adjuvant in so-called endogenous depression, possibly in combination with other psychotropic points.

Note. Treatment should preferably always be carried out in collaboration with a competent psychiatric colleague.

PT4 (Fig. 4.5)

PT4 is located at the same level as PT2 but on the dorsal part of the lobule, slightly more dorsally than and below the antidepression point—a psychotropic reflex area. This area carries the alternative name of the "sorrow/joy" point, depending on the individual's handedness: in right-handed individuals, the point is supposedly assigned to the emotional state of joy, and in left-handed individuals to that of sorrow.

This differentiation is dubious and from personal experience inexplicable. It also needlessly complicates the selection of this point.

Omega Point II (Q II) (Fig. 4.5)

Located on the brim of the ascending helix, this lies ventral to the allergy point (78) (see **Fig. 3.23**).

This point belongs to the group of psychotropic points and has a harmonizing and balancing effect in personality disorders with disturbed relationships to the surrounding environment. This includes psychological misconduct with regard to people as well as property (e.g., recklessness toward people, destructive tendencies toward property). Prolonged aggression based on this or other origins is part of the indications.

Master Omega Point (Fig. 4.5)

This is located in the upper dorsal quarter of field VII, above the analgesia point, and is definitely one of the psychotropic points. It can be detected in personalities who are burdened by severe diseases (e.g., malignoma, pain syndromes, chronic polyarthritis, multiple sclerosis, etc.), are unable to cope, and cannot accept their suffering. The use of this point supports psychological and mental harmonization and acceptance of the suffering (see **Fig. 3.11**).

Point R (According to Bourdiol) (Psychotherapeutic Auxiliary Point) (Fig. 4.5)

Located at the ventral edge of the ascending helix, in the facial skinfold at the level of the intersection of the inferior and superior antihelical crura. This psychotropic point has a very particular characteristic. The name *psychotherapeutic auxiliary point* is based on the psychologically revealing nature of this point, which Bourdiol discovered during his research on ear geometry. He points out that the use of this point requires a sound bond of trust between physician and patient in order to process possible psychological reactions, resolving psychological blockages during a confiding conversation.

Its range of indications includes its adjuvant use in psychosomatic syndromes, such as bronchial asthma, ulcerative colitis, Crohn's disease, chronic recurrent gastrointestinal ulcer, neurodermatitis, and psoriasis.

Needling of this point supposedly harmonizes the interaction between the two cerebral hemispheres when this has been disturbed (e.g., due to psychological trauma, severe chronic diseases, or prolonged situations of conflict).

Practice

5   Introduction

The success of any therapeutic approach largely depends on the proper selection of indications, and this principle—commonplace in medical practice—should be borne in mind for any therapeutic procedure. It is especially important to follow this principle in ear acupuncture; the reflex zones of the auricle allow one to apply therapeutic stimuli to any organ or body part without achieving the maximal effect that is possible when proceeding strictly as indicated by the diagnosis. It is exactly this possibility of always achieving a certain therapeutic effect that may tempt someone into treating a complete range of diseases with ear acupuncture, more or less according to the "principle of a watering can." The fact that the reflex relationships of the auricular microsystem, while certainly surprisingly complex, are not uniformly formed for all illnesses or syndromes is often disregarded, but this fact should always be kept in mind during therapy.

Hence, the most important step in achieving a therapeutic result is an accurate diagnosis or an identification of the appropriate syndrome.

If these basic considerations or criteria are ignored, the outcome of the therapy will be moderate, or even so poor that the therapist will find little encouragement and will most likely soon give up the procedure.

▶ **The diagnosis is arrived at according to the following aspects:**

- Does the syndrome belong to the sphere of indications defined for ear acupuncture?
  - As the therapeutic method of first choice?
  - Only in combination with other therapies, e.g., body acupuncture?
  - Only as a complementary therapy?
- Is the syndrome acute or chronic?
  - The main areas of indications for ear acupuncture are acute and acutely recurring diseases.
- Does the patient's constitution and/or sensitivity permit successful treatments?
  - If necessary, pretreat with medication and/or body acupuncture.
  - If necessary, wait until a better time can be chosen.

- Clarification and consideration of obstacles to therapy:
  - In acute inflammation, e.g., due to piercing in an area important to somatotopy.
  - Presence of scars (interference field according to Huneke).
  - Status following otoplasty.
  - Blockages. ◀

5.1   Patient History

Some of the aforementioned criteria can only be reliably established by a thorough analysis of the patient's history. As in any field of medicine, one of the most important building blocks in diagnostic and therapeutic approaches is the physician's diagnostic skill in relation to a specific procedure. This applies also to acupuncture and ear acupuncture, even when there is already a diagnosis in terms of Western medicine or when the patient is presenting with such a diagnosis.

It is recommended that the practitioner review the Western diagnosis, including the patient's history, according to the descriptive system of Chinese medicine and also to interpret it as a proper complex of symptoms, or syndrome. In this way, it is easier—especially for the novice—to put together a defined combination of points and, if necessary, to include meaningful body acupuncture.

In order to arrive at a detailed description of a syndrome, Chinese diagnostics relies far more intensely than modern Western medicine on the perception achieved by the five senses. This is not without influence on the structure of the patient's history.

As a first step, one should ask for the patient's **subjective perception**. Their state of well-being, case history, personal feeling of being sick, stress load, and stress tolerance should be recorded and taken into consideration.

As a **second step**, the **localization** of the disease should be determined on the basis of the patient's statements. As defined by Chinese medicine, one should clarify whether the superficial or deep layers (the *biao–li* relationship) are affected and, if necessary, which channels are involved. In Chinese ear acupuncture, the reflex zones of the auricle to be selected for therapy are those corresponding to the affected channel or the related group of functions. For example, if the large intestine channel is involved, the large intestine zone in the superior concha or the lung zone in the inferior concha (which corresponds to the linked lung channel) may be examined for irritated points and needled accordingly. Furthermore, the stomach channel, which also belongs to this axis, or its reflex zone, the stomach zone in the region of the helical crus, can be examined for irritated areas.

These channel-based concepts of the Chinese school do not correspond to the direct reflex relationships between the auricular microsystem and the inner organs or body parts. Therefore, the unverified arbitrary transfer of traditional Chinese concepts to the auricular reflex system must be critically examined.

The **third** diagnostic question relates to the **intensity** of the complaints (how severe, and for how long?) and the accompanying symptoms. The answers provide clues to the "energetic" situation, i.e., vacuity (*xu*) or repletion (*shi*). In ear acupuncture, the prevailing state leads to the choice of a particular type of stimulus and appropriate treatment intervals, as well as of complementary treatment through body acupuncture if necessary. Further clues to the classification of the syndrome as a sign of repletion or vacuity are derived, for example from the patient's speaking in a full or low voice or from the breathing pattern.

The **fourth** step of characterization describes the **type** of complaint (paroxysmal, continuing, inflammatory, traumatic?) and will influence the choice of reflex zones or points. For example, the reflex zones to be examined in cases of inflammatory and painful symptoms are different from those for diseases caused by poor posture or increased tension.

The **fifth** step, the search for the **cause** of complaints (why?), is of the utmost importance for the patient's history—as is also well known in Western medicine—otherwise any treatment will only try to cure the symptoms without achieving permanent results. In this regard, the essential and fundamental aspects must also be worked out for ear acupuncture.

External pathogenic factors (in particular, so-called foci and, above all, viral infections) often lead to stubborn neuralgia and paralytic symptoms. Other external factors include bioclimatic influences (wind, cold), which play an important role in the choice of points when looking at weather sensitivity or weather dependency.

Internal pathogenic factors (especially situations involving psychological strain and conflict) have an effect when the ability to resolve conflicts is poor. In addition, emotional traumas from long ago may be very important for the classification of symptoms, and hence for the choice of points.

Finally, one should also look into the patient's history for food incompatibilities, including real allergic reactions. In doing so, one should especially consider that food incompatibilities can induce a multitude of symptoms affecting the entire body, sometimes triggering symptoms only after a latency period of 3 days. Neglecting these aspects will make any therapeutic attempt ineffective and will promote the stigma of these patients being "imaginary" or "problem" patients. Systematic treatment of the cause is not part of the range of indication of ear acupuncture.

5.2 Therapeutic Obstacles and Special Situations

As with body acupuncture, the phenomenon of ineffective treatment can also be found with ear acupuncture. A possible reason for this may be that one is dealing with a so-called nonresponder—a rare occurrence. Another reason could be the wrong diagnosis, which is more often the case.

Apart from this, certain obstacles to therapy might play a role, and these need to be identified in the patient's history. As partially listed in Patient's History, Chapter 5.1, and also addressed under "Contraindications, Chapter 1.6," these obstacles include physical conditions such as:

- Abuse of sleeping pills or analgesic drugs.
- Chronic inflammatory processes.
- Status after otoplasty.
- Condition after cerebral or spinal cord trauma, including surgical interventions.
- Chronic fatigue (e.g., in anemia, after radiation therapy, in radiation sickness, etc.).

In addition, French/Western ear acupuncture (auriculotherapy according to Nogier) describes special types of obstacles to therapy.

For example, the so-called blockade of the first rib, signifying a shift of the first rib resulting in pressure on the stellate ganglion beneath the head of the rib, is thought to cause an imbalance between sympathetic and parasympathetic interactions, which interferes with the therapeutic outcome. Such conditions can be diagnosed using a simple manual technique. In this, pressure is evenly applied with both hands on the bend between the neck and the shoulder, in the direction of the sternum. The painful side corresponds to the blocking first rib. Among the possible causes are improper weight-bearing due to heavy lifting or unilateral physical load or overload, including as a result of sports activities.

One therapy consists of manual adjustment performed "lege artis," but this requires special chiropractic training. Another possible treatment is segment therapy, as described by Nogier. Preferential treatment is applied to the ipsilateral ear (with regard to the location of the illness).

- Locate the point of maximal irritation in the vegetative groove at the level of T1/ T2 and needle it.
- On the connecting line with point zero (82), also treat the point of maximal irritation within the zone of paravertebral muscles and ligaments (on the scapha) as this is thought to correspond to the first rib.
- Furthermore, there may also be sensitivity of the stellate ganglion point within the zone of paravertebral chain of sympathetic ganglia at the level of C7/T1.

According to the concept of auriculotherapy, another obstacle to therapy is instability of laterality, as a result of which all reflex responses in the auricular microsystem are thought to be disturbed. For diagnosis and therapy, a so-called laterality control point is presented that is located in the facial skin approximately 4 cm ventral to the midpoint of the tragus. If this point is found by using Nogier's reflex, it should be treated either with gold or silver needles depending on whether the patient is right- or left-handed.

Objective studies on this topic are at present unavailable, and therefore this procedure must be critically examined.

5.3 Diagnostic Clues through Inspection and Palpation

5.3.1 Visual Inspection

If possible, the auricle should be investigated in natural light when looking for color changes, scale formation, and red dots; a simple magnifying glass can be used if necessary. Thus, acute local inflammations resembling blackheads can be found which can be assigned to certain reflex zones. The diagnostic interpretation of visible changes on the auricle is based on the traditional knowledge of Chinese doctors on the reflex relationships between the body's surface and the internal organs (the *biao– li* relationship). Thanks to the English physician Head (1893), such reflex relationships have also become known to modern Western medicine—which makes good use of them, e.g., in the trigger point therapy. Because of the special interactions of ear somatotopy, disease-related events of the internal organs and other, more distant, body parts can express themselves as changes in the skin, blood vessels, or cartilage of the auricle.

! Caution

Do not under any circumstances needle such changed areas.

Until they subside, these hypersensitive areas should be considered for diagnosis only.

Not all signs can be taken as reflex events. For example, there are sclerotic changes in the lobule that occur in direct connection with coronary heart disease—first documented by Steinlieb (1974) and more recently been confirmed by several studies. According to these studies, a high percentage of coronary patients, compared with the healthy control group, show a sclerosed groove on the lobule running in a craniodorsal direction (a "stress groove"). However, this groove does not result from a reflex relationship of this area with the heart; rather, it can be traced back to a correlating degenerative sclerotic process of connective tissue in the lobule and, similarly, in the coronary vessels. Therefore, this phenomenon—like other similar observations in the Chinese literature—should be interpreted as defined by the "relation pathology" described by Rieker.

Normal variations in the shape of the auricle as well as malformations, which have resulted in the questionable discipline of "ear physiognomy" and all its interpretations and characteristic conclusions, are completely ineligible as criteria in ear acupuncture. These types of interpretation should be consigned to the past.

The Chinese school describes certain skin alterations that are frequently observed in the stomach zone (87); these often correlate with stomach ulcers and acute or chronic gastritis. These observations have been confirmed in my own practice, although not with the same specificity. In severe gastroduodenal affections, dotlike, whitish changes with a fuzzy reddish outline can be observed in the duodenum zone. However, it is not possible to identify the type of gastrointestinal disease as postulated in the Chinese literature. Following precise testing with the point-finder or pressure probe, an appropriate needle stimulus can then be applied at the visually conspicuous area. According to Chinese observations, obvious skin alterations also occur in the lung zone (101) during lung diseases (e.g., chronic bronchitis, emphysema, bronchial asthma); these changes can be interpreted as diagnostic clues.

Note. Conspicuous skin alterations in the area of the auricle must not be interpreted on their own as a diagnostic landmark without considering additional aspects of the patient's history or clinical condition.

5.3.2 Examination by Palpation

As a general measure for orientation and, ostensibly, as an initial step in searching for pressure points (see p. 80), it makes sense first to palpate the auricle with the thumb and index finger and examine it for conspicuously pressure-sensitive regions, nodules, etc. Using this approach, it is possible to identify the first clues to the affected zones or segments, e.g., in the projection zone of the spinal column on the antihelix and in the representation zones of the locomotor system. This is followed by a detailed examination using an acupuncture point detector, in order to demarcate the area of maximal irritation.

The patient finds this technique of preliminary examination by palpation and gentle massage very comfortable, usually even in anticipation of subsequent treatment (see also Chapter 7.5 Auricular Massage, p. 94).

6 Basic Tools and Procedures

6.1 Pressure Palpation of Points

The accurate localization of points is really just the continuation of ear palpation in a more refined manner, focusing on the point, by using an auxiliary probing device with a fine, pointed tip that is rounded to avoid injuring the skin. The tip should be roughly the size of the tip of a fine ballpoint pen; the latter may actually be used as a pressure probe once it has been emptied by writing. The **spherical filler** used by dentists (**Fig. 6.2**) is more practical and, due to its angled shape, is a very handy and inexpensive alternative. In addition, the bridge between the crank and ball may be used as a stirrup probe.

A variation of pressure palpation is the use of a **stirrup-shaped ear probe** for examining edged or convex cartilaginous structures of the auricle for tenderness or notches. It is recommended that the practitioner use the stirrup probe for exploring areas such as the antihelix, the crus of the helix, and the ascending helix. In this way, for example, the diaphragm point (82), or point zero, can be detected as a small notch in the cartilage just in front of the helical crus.

Practical Tip

The free end of a paper clip, when bent like a stirrup, may be used as an improvised pressure probe, as long as the end has been melted to form a ball.

For daily use, however, it is recommended that more sophisticated devices are employed for pressure palpation. The **telescopic pressure probe** (**Figs. 6.1 and 6.3**) features a spring-loaded tip and provides a relatively constant pressure during the examination, as long as the tip is moved within the resilient range and is not completely pushed in. It is important, however, to find a tip that is not too clumsy to use, as is often the case with these devices; the tip should measure no more than 0.3 mm in diameter. The telescopic pressure probe was originally designed by Nogier to differentiate between the postulated zones (or layers) of resonance in the skin of the ear, depending on how hard the probe was pressed against the skin (between 150 and 250 pond).

6.2 Electrical Detection of Points

Prerequisites. This neutral method of searching for points acts independently of the patient's subjective cooperation and leads to much more objective results. It is based on the fact that the irritated reflex zones or points show a reduced skin resistance (and therefore increased skin conductance), in addition to the tenderness discussed earlier. With the aid of a simple ohmmeter or potentiometer adjusted to the electrical characteristics of the skin, this parameter can be objectively assessed.

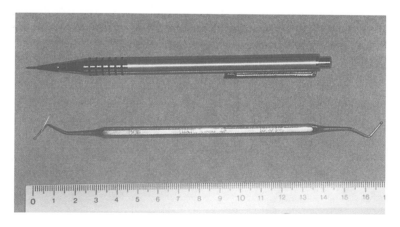

Fig. 6.1 Pressure probes: the telescopic pressure probe and the spherical filler used in dentistry.

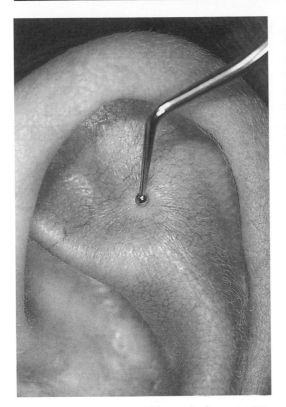

Fig. 6.2 Dental spherical filler applied at point 55.

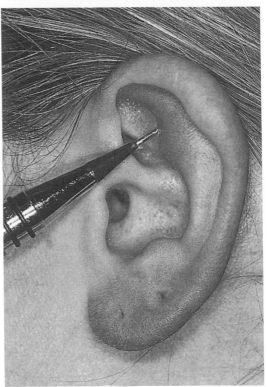

Fig. 6.3 Telescopic pressure probe applied at point 55.

According to Chinese studies (König and Wancura), the mean electrical skin resistance in healthy persons ranges from 40 to 400 kΩ. Hence, considerable individual differences exist, which means that independent of the state of health, each patient exhibits his or her own electrical skin resistance. Consequently, the measuring device needs to be adjusted to the patient's individual skin resistance prior to the examination proper. However, using fixed neutral points for this purpose, such as point zero of the French/Western school or the upper ear attachment zone according to the Chinese school, has proved unsuccessful in the past.

To calibrate the device, it makes more sense to refer to irrelevant areas of the ear, i.e., those that do not show up as irritated zones, either clinically or in the patient's history, and are not known to be representation zones as defined by ear somatotopy. This is important because different degrees of skin moisture may yield different values of skin resistance, e.g., on the scapha

or antihelix, or in deep parts of the auricle such as the inferior and superior concha. Again, this calls for individual adjustment. This addresses a major criterion that should be met by a device of this type, otherwise it will be impossible to carry out any meaningful measurement. Depending on the design of the device, individual calibration is done either automatically or manually.

While examining a suspicious skin area, an acoustic or optical signal (or both, depending on the device) will indicate when the device has detected a reduced skin resistance. When buying such an electrical point-finder, one should make sure that the individual calibration will be indicated by an appropriate signal.

Depending on the device, the required circuit with the patient can be established in different ways. With some devices, the patient must hold an electrode in his or her hand or place one hand on an integrated electrode plate. With Nogier's punctoscope, measurement takes place between a concentric electrode contained in the tip of the exploring probe and a fine rod electrode in the center of the probe; the two electrodes are insulated against each other and are telescopically cushioned. Modern exploring probes or rods are simpler and easier to handle; the circuitry is integrated into the handle, which itself serves as the contact electrode because of its metal design. In order to close the circuit, the physician must touch the auricle with the free hand, which is required anyway during the examination. Hence, these small devices are very practical and usually inexpensive.

In summary, the diagnostic device should meet at least the following **criteria**. They should:
- Be small and practical.
- Have an acoustic or optical indicator.
- Have a fine, rounded exploring tip of approximately 0.3 mm in diameter (such as a the tip of a ballpoint pen).
- Allow manual adjustment to individual differences in normal skin resistance (via an adaption button).

Examination procedure. Both pressure palpation and electrical point detection are carried out as follows: The auricle can be examined while the patient is sitting or lying, although sitting is preferred. The patient's auricle should be on a line with the eye level of the examining physician, who should also be sitting. The examiner should rest the hand holding the point-finder, as well as the free hand, by placing the lower arm on the patient's shoulder, with the ring finger and little finger placed on the mastoid or on the cheek in front of the tragus. This approach ensures that the hand is sufficiently stabilized for the pressure to be constant during the examination, and the elastic portions of the auricle to be supported. It is essential to ensure that the free hand will not apply any tension to the auricle, as this will distort its contours (as will become obvious when letting go of it) and lead to false localizations when searching for points.

The diagnostic probe is now placed perpendicular to the surface of the skin and moved slowly over the suspected zone of irritation, while keeping the pressure as constant as possible. When the tip comes across an irritated reflex point, this will be indicated by an acoustic or optical signal. So that the point can be easily located again, it must immediately be identified as a pressure point by using light pressure. When using a pressure probe, involuntary grimacing reactions may be observed on the patient's face, i.e., the patient senses the touch at the irritated point and shows this sensation by twitching slightly or by pulling a face (watch the corner of the patient's eye). In order to give the patient a chance to compare sensations, pressure palpation should be carried out from the periphery to the center in the direction of the suspected area of irritation, similar to the gradual advance toward the point of maximum discomfort when palpating a painful abdomen. Once the irritated zone has been found, the patient usually does not feel direct pain but has perceptions (electrified feeling, increased sensitivity) that are different from those felt in surrounding areas.

After pressure-marking, finding the point again by using a different localization technique, either pressure palpation or electrical point detection, will no longer be representative; pressure-marking causes a temporary microtrauma, and the reaction pattern of this trauma resembles that of an irritated point.

6.3 "Very Point" Technique

Another method of detecting points is the *very point technique*. In terms of the patient's cooperation and subjective confirmation of the results, it is of equal quality to pressure palpation, although superior to it when performed by skilled hands. The technique was developed by Gleditsch (2004) in connection with acupuncture of the mouth. Since an electrical search for points cannot be undertaken in the moist environment of the mucosa, and simple pressure palpation is not practical because of the lack of marking possibilities in the mouth, Gleditsch examined suspicious areas for sensitivity by delicate tapping with an injection needle. At the proper point of irritation, the *punctum verum* or *very point*, he regularly found a point-focal reduction of turgor, as if the needle would "fall" into the tissue. This perception of the examiner was usually confirmed by the patient grimacing or displaying an equivalent reaction. Gleditsch then applied the therapeutic injection at this "very point."

Gleditsch's delicate tapping method can be successfully used in the region of the auricle by directly using the acupuncture needle. Very fine facial needles of 0.3 µm in diameter are used, and the reflex zones in question are tapped or stroked for sensitivity. Frequently, sensitivities can be distinguished by mere gentle tangential stroking of the suspected area with the tip of the needle.

When using the very point technique, it is also important for the tapping hand and its free fingers to be supported by the patient's shoulder and cheek, respectively. Tapping with the needle should be done so gently that it does not traumatize the skin. Should microbleeding occur that is not caused by a clumsy or vigorous approach, this can be taken as a sign of local hyperemia. The affected area can no longer be used until it has healed.

To avoid perforation, it is recommended that one practices the steady tapping technique, e.g., on stretched plastic wrap. In skilled hands, this method is practical, precise, and quick. As it does not require a change of instruments, the irritated zone or point can be needled at more or less at the same time as it is detected. Although it essential to obtain feedback from the patient, the subjectivity of the procedure diminishes with increased practice and experience of the examiner, who will learn to interpret the local skin turgor as an objective result.

6.4 Vascular Autonomic Signal, Réflexe Auriculocardiac, Nogier's Reflex

The "pulse reflex," observed by Nogier in 1968, was originally named the *réflexe auriculocardiac* and was first known by this term. More recently, however, the term *vascular autonomic signal* (VAS) has come into use. Although disputed, this phenomenon serves as the essential foundation for further methods of localizing irritated reflex zones on the auricle. It is thought to be a cutaneous vascular reflex process triggered by a weak cutaneous stimulus. A gently stroking touch (e.g., with a needle) or a weak light stimulus (e.g., with a Heine's lamp) will lead to a minimal, yet palpable, shift of the pulse throughout the arterial system. If triggered via irritated points or reflex zones, this shift of the pulse is much more distinct, and thus is supposed to facilitate the accurate localization of the relevant active points.

To detect this phenomenon, the radial artery proximal to the styloid process (radial apophysis) is palpated as described by Nogier (**Fig. 6.4**). When doing this, the thumb should lie parallel

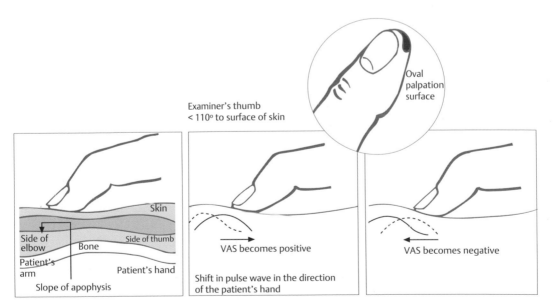

Fig. 6.4 Palpation of the vascular autonomic signal (VAS; *réflexe auriculocardiac*), adapted from Mastalier.

to the patient's lower arm, with the tip of the thumb at an angle of about 110° to the plane of the skin. This position, outlined by Nogier, will help to create an optimal supporting surface for the palpating hand. As soon as the pulse is clearly detected, the thumb pressure must be reduced to a point where the throbbing pulse is just barely palpable. If a "microstress" of the described kind is applied—such as a weak light stimulus from a Heine's lamp, or the gentle touch of an irritated ear point with the tip of a needle—a slight shift of the pulse wave is noticed, which moves toward the tip of the thumb like a "swelling" (showing the presence of a VAS), or as a "subsiding" or even disappearance (indicating the absence of a VAS).

Nogier's hypothesis states that the body's vegetative reactions affect the vascular tone via sympathetically controlled vasoconstrictors. He suggests that this then leads to a change in hemodynamic resistance, which in turn causes a shift of a stationary pulse wave in the entire vascular system. The latest studies (1996), using highly sensitive digital subtraction angiometers and undertaken by experienced auriculotherapists, have, however, been unable to establish any change in the pulse wave (Thalhammer, Haller, and Luft 1996). According to the conclusion of these authors, it is hard to believe that the palpating thumb of an experienced auriculotherapist, although highly sensitive, would detect a minimal change in the pulse wave if such a change were not being detected by the devices referred to above.

So far, there has been no well-founded study under controlled and standardized conditions that objectifies the physical postulate of a reflex reaction—e.g., by using reproducible Doppler sonography compared with measuring skin resistance. For years, advocates of this method have been holding out for the prospect of appropriate studies. In any case, the interpretation of this reflex reaction is problematic because of our incomplete understanding of the reflex process on the one hand, and the multitude of factors interfering with the test on the other. Additional speculative interpretations based on delicate subjective examination techniques do not contribute to the scientific explanation of this postulated phenomenon. With this in mind, this method is not a serious alternative or addition to the established localization techniques. The results of future research are awaited with great interest.

6.5 Needling Technique and Choice of Needles

Choice of needles. In ear acupuncture, it is a rule to needle with as little trauma as possible in order to prevent infections. Therefore, it is essential to consider certain aspects regarding the choice of needles as well as the needling technique.

Only the finest needles, with a maximum diameter of 0.3 μm, should be used; these correspond to the facial needles used in body acupuncture (**Fig. 6.5**). The needle, including its handle, should measure approximately 3 cm in total. The handle may be covered with plastic, as with disposable needles, or have a good grip provided by roughening or braiding, as with steel needles that can be repeatedly sterilized (**Fig. 6.6**).

In the case of steel needles, it should be kept in mind that the tip of the needle will become blunt after multiple uses or may be bent like a hook by improper handling or sterilization, rendering the needle useless because of an increased risk of traumatic needling. These disadvantages, including the risk of infection caused by germs

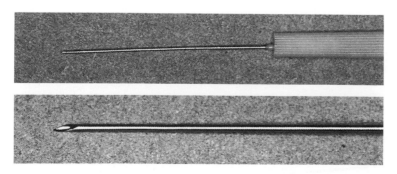

Fig. 6.5 Injection needle (bottom) compared to a facial needle used in body acupuncture.

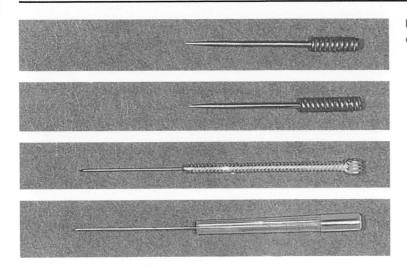

Fig. 6.6 Needles used in ear acupuncture.

remaining after improper sterilization, do not occur with disposable needles.

The use of steel needles is quite satisfactory, and today steel needles are also exclusively used in China. Arguments in favor of using silver or gold needles (originally introduced by the French acupuncturist George Soulié de Morant), especially for the ear, are usually derived from the school of auriculotherapy. They are essentially based on the postulate that the different electrical potentials of these precious metals with respect to the tissue provide a more differentiated and effective application of the stimuli. However, there is no objective confirmation of this, and any benefits are outweighed by the disadvantages: the large needle diameter (up to 1 mm) results in a wide stab wound, the increased needle weight requires a deeper stab to fix the needle, and the risk of oxidation calls for more elaborate sterilization techniques.

Needling technique. The ear should be needled perpendicularly to the skin and not too deeply. After penetrating the membrane of the perichondrium, the tip of the needle should find slight support in the cartilage. The technique of *threading* several points subcutaneously, favored by some authors, and penetration of cartilage are not recommended. There is considerable associated traumatization, which increases the risk of infection and does not act in proportion to the supposedly improved effectiveness or practicability that these techniques provide. Alternatively, the so-called *sieving*

technique may be applied by individually needling several points found in one projection zone perpendicularly to the skin, e.g., in the sciatic zone. These needled points are counted as one needle in terms of the limit of five or six needles per auricle.

We advise against the use of permanent needles of any kind. Here, too, effectiveness and risk are out of proportion to each other. In cases of complications caused by infections of the auricle (in extreme cases, perichondritis), such criteria will play a major role during forensic analysis.

Some authors prefer the *tangential stab technique* to avoid traumatizing the cartilage, with its associated increase in the risk of infection. In this technique, the tip of the needle is supposed to be passed through the perichondrium toward the cartilage, but without injuring the latter. It should be countered that, even here, traumatization of the cartilage is hardly avoidable, perhaps not so much as a result of direct traumatization, but rather through disturbing the trophism of the corresponding cartilage area, in this case originating from the perichondrium. Considering the delicate nature of the ear points, a major disadvantage of this technique lies in the relative inaccuracy of targeting the irritated zones. Thus, the approach is restricted to the inaccessible regions of the auricle, e.g., beneath the brim of the ascending helix.

There are no convincing arguments, let alone test results, for the tonifying and sedating techniques recommended by auriculotherapy, especially for those using the selective application of gold and silver needles and for the postulate that the classical rules underlying needle choice should be reversed for the auricle. The same holds true for reversing the energy-related relationships between the front and back of the ear and for the more detailed rules derived from this.

The corresponding supplying and draining techniques of the Chinese school of ear acupuncture are derived from body acupuncture and transferred to the microsystem of the auricle. There are no comprehensible arguments and far fewer verifiable studies that support such transfer onto the microsystem of the auricle. Particularly in light of the accompanying, considerable traumatization of perichondrium and cartilage on the one hand, and the lack of greater effectiveness on the other, this needling technique cannot be recommended.

7   Methods of Stimulation

The literature is full of reports on stimulation methods that are used in ear acupuncture, but not all of these can be recommended without restrictions, or have proved effective. The purpose is always to emit, increase, and prolong the therapeutic stimulus coming from the needle and to make this less painful. An objective assessment of the various methods of stimulation is only partially possible, since comparative studies and progress reports are scarce. It is relatively well documented that target-specific needle stimulation on the one hand and laser therapy on the other are equally effective. The remaining methods of stimulation have different effects in different patients; therefore, they should be selected individually and, in certain circumstances, based on practical considerations (needle phobias, a need to save time, etc.). The relatively diffuse stimulation methods—such as infiltration techniques, percutaneous stimulation according to Helmbolt, or auricular massage—are discussed here for the sake of completeness but must be critically assessed.

7.1   Needling and Electrical Stimulation

Needle stimulus. For insertion of the needle, the "very point" technique of guiding the needle using tapping and support may be applied. This method allows points to be located accurately in a calm and safe manner. The precise localization of the "active point" and the applied target-specific stimulus are decisive in obtaining good therapeutic results. It is obviously easier and at the same time more precise to carry out localization with a needle stimulus and, in some cases, by means of a laser.

Fine facial needles or ear needles, which have a maximal diameter of 0.3 mm, are inserted right in the center of the successfully located irritated point (**Fig. 7.1**). Only a few needles are used per treatment session, i.e., only the major points are needled to address the real cause of the illness. Usually, three needles per auricle are inserted; even if several irritated areas have been located, the maximum number of needles per auricle should not exceed five.

Note. The following principle applies: the therapeutic result is determined by the targeted, precisely localized needle stimulus and not by the number of needles.

The needles are left in place for at least 20 minutes but no longer than 40 minutes while the patient reclines; they can then be easily removed. With acute painful diseases (cephalalgia, neuralgia), longer periods of rest may prove practical. Experience has shown that the pain may take up to 45 minutes to subside. No additional effect has been observed with longer treatment periods. Even when there is an immediate onset of relief (i.e., immediate freedom of pain, such as the elimination of pain within seconds, as seen in neural therapy), the needles should nevertheless be left in place for at least 20 minutes.

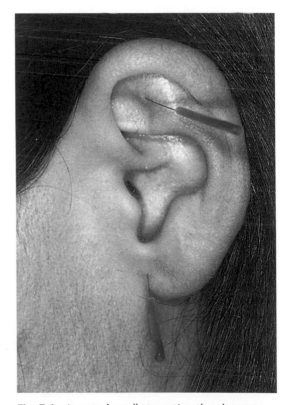

Fig. 7.1   Inserted needle targeting the *shen men* point (55).

Removal of the needles is usually easy and painless. Prematurely lost needles may be replaced if the patient has been resting for only a brief period; if this happens at a later time, it will no longer be effective. Some authors interpret the early loss of a needle as a particularly quick response to the respective needle, i.e., the needle is "set free" because of the precise targeting of another reflex point. However, there is no clinical proof for this.

The removal of needles may be carried out by an assistant. He or she should be advised that the occasional minor bleeding may be stopped by lightly pressing a pad against the bleeding spot—something the patient can usually do themself. An exception to this are those points for which bleeding acts as microphlebotomy, e.g. the allergy point (78) at the tip of the ear, where bleeding may be allowed to continue until it stops spontaneously.

Electrical stimulation. In both body acupuncture and ear acupuncture, the inserted needles may be additionally stimulated by means of a low-frequency direct current in rectangular pulses. A frequency of 10 Hz is selected for the stimulation, while the intensity of the current depends on the patient's relative sensitivity. To determine the patient's tolerance, the current is gradually increased until the patient indicates the sensation of a slightly stabbing, well-tolerated pulse. During this process, the patient should be instructed that the sensation should not reach the pain threshold and that, due to adaptation, the slightly stabbing sensation will subside during the period of rest without losing its effectiveness, which is why the current intensity should not be readjusted. The positive and negative electrodes must be applied ispilaterally, i.e., both on the same ear, and the intensity-dependent paresthesia seen during stimulation will occur at the positive electrode. Consequently, the negative electrode closing the circuit may be connected to a needle that does not need to be stimulated.

In ear acupuncture, electrical stimulation is not as important as it is in body acupuncture. It is recommended only for chronically recurrent pain conditions, and even then only at intervals. This restriction applies because, during electrical stimulation of the ear points, there is a risk that the applied stimulus will be too strong and will not be able to self-regulate. As a result, the symptoms may get worse.

7.2 Infiltration of Points and Zones

As in neural therapy, irritated points or zones of the auricle may be infiltrated, or wealed, by the targeted injection of a local anesthetic, such as licodaine or classically procaine (the so-called "wet needle" technique). The flooding of a disturbed ear zone frequently creates a large wheal immediately beneath the skin. The practitioner must cautiously assess if this method is justified when weighing the considerable traumatization (lifting of the perichondrium) against the undocumented advantage of the allegedly quicker pain relief. From the author's point of view, this method of stimulation is not recommended.

Helmbold's percutaneous regulation therapy of is based on a similar principle. In this, the irritated zones of the auricle are either swabbed with a 2% tetracaine/glycerine solution or massaged with an ion-balancing ointment. This approach has the advantage that it is free of pain and complications, and that it can be combined with a targeted massage of points or zones. Its effectiveness is, however, questionable. The method may be tried in vegetatively sensitive patients, particularly in children, and may also serve as the starting point for future treatment with needles.

7.3 Use of the Soft Laser

In the microsystem of the auricle, soft laser irradiation using a helium–neon laser or infrared laser as a method of stimulation has proved to be an effective alternative to conventional stimulation with needles, for several reasons. Especially in pain-sensitive patients and in children, the laser has proved advantageous as it can be applied without any pain or trauma. Particularly in such patients, the threshold of anxiety or inhibition toward acupuncture is difficult to overcome, no matter whether ear acupuncture or body acupuncture is to be applied; frequently, treatment is only tolerated when carried out with a laser. The disadvantages of laser treatment in body acupuncture—that working with a multitude of points is very time-consuming, and that the laser ray does not always penetrate deeply enough to reach certain acupuncture points, not even with powerful laser equipment—do not apply to ear acupuncture. The reflex zones of the auricle are superficially located so that even soft lasers are effective. Application of the laser stimulus to individual irritated points or zones, with the number of points ranging only between three and five, is kept within reasonable limits and does not require too much time. The procedure is similar to the application of a needle stimulus: after finding the irritated point, the laser is directed to the center of the point in the form of a stroking stimulus for a period of 20 to 30 seconds After the treatment session, the patient should be allowed to rest for about 20 minutes.

The use of soft laser involves a certain risk that should not be underestimated—its potential to cause damaging retinal flash burns. Although such damage is only possible when radiation from class 3b laser equipment is directed at the eyes, both the therapist and the patient should wear protective glasses. The entrance to the treatment room must carry a warning sign. Apart from this risk, the practitioner should make sure when buying a soft laser unit that the device has been tested by the safety standards authorities and approved as defined by the regulations for medical devices. Whether the purchase of a laser unit is appropriate cannot be decided in terms of its higher effectiveness compared to conventional needle therapy or with specific syndromes. The decision should depend on the specific demands arising, e.g., when dealing with a large group of particular patients or with many children.

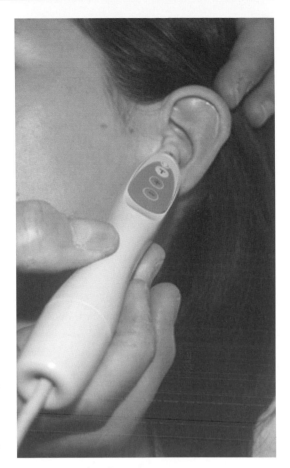

Fig. 7.2 Modern laser devices.

7.4 The Use of Laser in Ear Acupuncture

H.-J. Weise

7.4.1 Introduction

As early as 1917, Einstein predicted the principle of the laser as a stimulated emission of light, and Prokhorov and Basov completed the theoretical and physical principles in 1954. The term LASER (light amplification by stimulated [or induced] emission of radiation) was used for the first time in 1958 by Schalow and Townes, but it was only in 1960 that Mainman succeeded in putting a rubin laser into operation.

The subsequent vigorous developments in this field produced different types of laser, depending on the active material used: gas, semiconductor, and solid-state lasers. The special properties of light emitted by a laser gave rise to a multitude of possible uses in science and technology. Apart from various applications in medicine (e.g., neurosurgery, endoscopy), lasers have also been available for acupuncture (especially ear acupuncture) since the early 1970s. Since then, various devices with different technical designs have been developed (**Fig. 7.2**).

7.4.2 Physical Principles

The light from an electric lamp consists of individual electromagnetic waves, each of which oscillates at a different wavelength (color) and travels in a different direction. This erratic nature is explained by the way light originates, with photons being created independently of one another when electrons jump from a higher to a lower level of energy.

Lasers, on the other hand, have the following properties:

- **Monochromatic light:** The laser emits electromagnetic radiation of a single wavelength. Thus, unlike natural light, the emerging laser beam is very pure.
- **Coherence:** The peaks and troughs of energy distribution within the beam are perfectly in step with each other. Thus, a fixed spatial and temporal relationship exists between the phases, with all rays in the laser beam oscillating in the same cycle.
- **Minor divergence:** The resulting electromagnetic radiation is characterized by almost perfect parallelism and distinct bundling of the emitted light, thus making the realization of high-energy densities possible.

The material of which the laser is made (gas, semiconductor, solid) is present at the lowest energy level of atoms or molecules, or the basic state. Bombardment with light of a suitable wavelength (e.g., from a flashbulb) elevates the atoms to a higher level of energy, or an excited state. This process is called optical pumping. Each atom then returns to the basic state while emitting a photon. The resulting electromagnetic waves oscillate exactly in the same phase. They are amplified between two mirrors, one of which is semitranslucent. Due to this arrangement, only those waves which oscillate along the proper axis can emerge from the device.

7.4.3　Biological Principles

The soft lasers used in acupuncture are lasers with a low-density output. They are helium–neon lasers emitting red light with a wavelength of 632 nm, and semiconductor lasers (also called diode lasers) with a wavelength between 680 and 904 nm in the infrared region. Soft lasers are limited per definition to an output of no more than 50 mW, and hence are atraumatic. The aim of the weak radiation is to affect different biological phenomena.

In the laboratory, specific laser effects have been observed in cell cultures, such as effects on the synthesis of DNA and adenosine 5′-triphosphate (ATP). The effect on ATP was studied by Warnke (1987) in yeast, in which the rate of synthesis and the glucose turnover were optimal at a radiation dose of 10 mJ. There is

probably a light-sensitive enzyme complex in the mitochondria that is affected by laser light. However, the biostimulatory effect seems to occur only within a narrow range of emission parameters in terms of the wavelength, dose, and pulse rate of the laser. A prerequisite for any effect to take place is absorption of the laser light within the tissue. This absorption depends on the composition of the tissue (water content, pigment). In practical terms, absorption at wavelengths higher than 750 nm depends only on the presence of melanin, while scatter in the 600 to 750 nm range of the spectrum plays a bigger role. This also determines the depth of penetration; it is approximately 2 mm for helium–neon lasers and approximately 5 mm for infrared lasers (Birngruber 1984). It is important with both laser types that enough therapeutically effective absorption takes place in the auricle.

A prerequisite for optimal biostimulation is a precise knowledge of the laser's output capacity (or diode's pulse rate, respectively) and the exposure time used. The decisive factor is the product of the laser output (in mW) and duration of exposure (in seconds), representing the energy (in Joules) applied to the tissue. In ear acupuncture, the radiation dose (i.e., the energy applied per ear point) should be 1 J/cm^2.

▶ **Formulas:**
Energy = laser output × exposure time.
Radiation dose = energy/square unit. ◀

▶ **Measuring Units:**

Energy:	Joule = Watt-second (Ws)
Output:	Milliwatt (mW) = 0.001 W
Time:	second (s)
Square unit:	square centimeter (cm^2)
Radiation dose:	Joule/cm^2
Exposure time:	second (s)/cm^2 ◀

7.4.4　Clinical Use

Using a soft laser in ear acupuncture (**Fig. 7.3**) has the following advantages over classical needle acupuncture:

1. The laser beam is painless. Therefore, it is well suited to the treatment of children and sensitive patients.
2. The laser beam has no traumatic side effects and is aseptic.

3. Laser treatment saves time: approximately 100 seconds per point is equivalent to a total treatment period of 4 to 6 minutes per patient.
4. The laser is easy to use, so the treatment procedure can be learned within a short period of time.

The following descriptions are examples of some indications in the pediatric field.

7.4.5 Treatment Examples

Headaches

In children, headaches and particularly migraines are not yet characterized by the typical unilateral manifestation, i.e. associated with the gallbladder, but rather by disturbed stomach functions. Accordingly, the following points are selected (**Fig. 7.4**):

- *Shen men* point (55).
- Jerome point (29 b).
- Sensory line–occiput point (29).
- Sun point (35) and forehead point (33).
- Solar plexus zone.

Radiation is carried out with a 10 mW laser for 100 seconds per point on both ears. Treatment

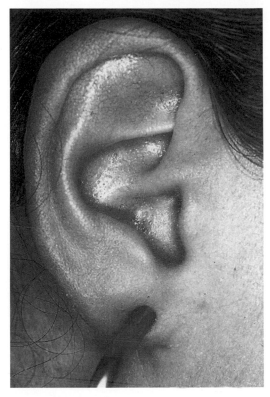

Fig. 7.3 Laser application in ear acupuncture.

Table 7.1 Exposure time in seconds

		Laser output in mW			
		10	20	25	30
Radiation dose	**0.1**	10	5		
in J/cm²	**0.2**	20	10	8	7
	0.3	30	15	12	10
	0.5	50	25	20	17
	0.8	80	40	32	27
	1	100	50	40	33
	1.5	150	75	60	50
	2	200	100	80	67
	3	300	150	120	100
	4	400	200	160	133
	5	500	250	200	167
	6	600	300	240	200
	7	700	350	280	233
	8	800	400	320	267
	9	900	450	360	300
	10	1000	500	400	333

Example: To achieve a radiation dose of 1 J/cm² with a soft laser output of 10 mW, the exposure time per ear point should be 100 seconds.

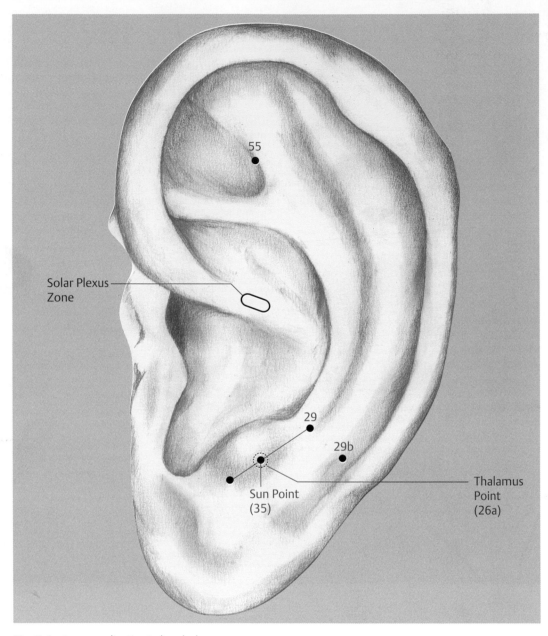

Fig. 7.4 Laser application in headaches.

takes place twice a week over a period of 1 month. If clinically indicated, another treatment series may follow after a break of 2 to 4 weeks. The therapeutic results should be recorded in a headache diary, which should be kept by the child, starting from the age of 7 years. If the response is insufficient, intolerance of food should be considered and the diet changed accordingly.

Allergic Rhinitis

As the incidence of allergic diseases is increasing, hay fever is often the first step toward the development of a disease. Here, primarily in the acute phase, a swift alleviation of symptoms can be expected by means of laser acupuncture of the auricle. The following points are preferentially treated (**Fig. 7.5**):

- Allergy point (78).
- Inner nose point (16).
- *Shen men* point (55).

- ACTH point (13).
- Occiput point (29).
- Forehead point (33).

In the advanced phase, the vegetative points should be included in the therapy. We know from experience that the treatment is particularly effective when carried out as prophylaxis,

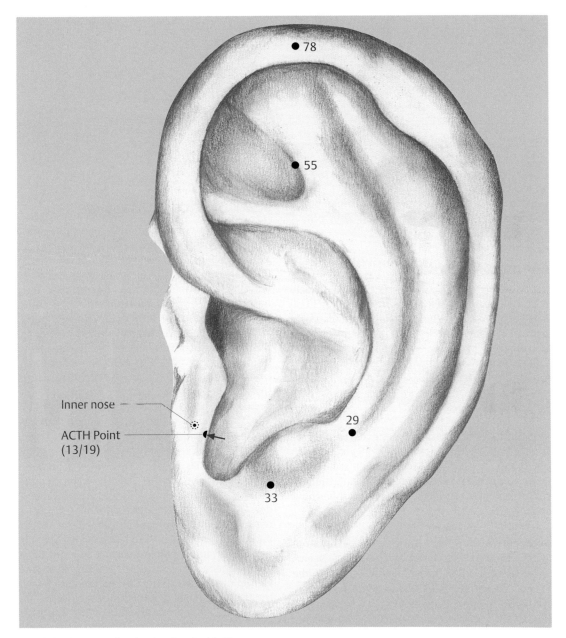

Fig. 7.5 Laser application in allergic rhinitis.

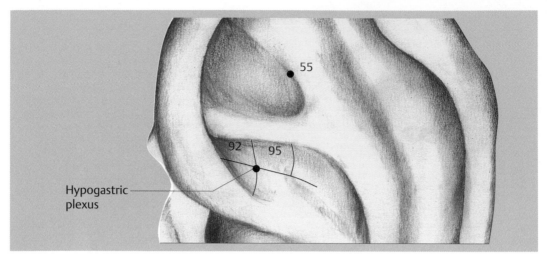

Fig. 7.6 Laser application in enuresis.

i.e., prior to exposure to the allergens. A response to the therapy often becomes clear after only 1 to 2 weeks.

Enuresis

In the case of children who do not spontaneously become continent before the first day of school, it is recommended that, as well as the classical body acupuncture (laser), the less common laser acupuncture of the auricle should be tried. The following points are important here (**Fig. 7.6**):
- Urinary bladder zone (92).
- Kidney zone (95).
- Hypogastric plexus point.

The duration of treatment depends on the response and should not exceed 4 to 6 weeks, with one or two sessions per week being planned.
If the condition is resistant to treatment, therapy should include primarily psychological learning strategies.

Note. As we know from comparative clinical studies, the clinical effectiveness of the soft laser seems to be less distinct than that of needles. Yet, in the case of children and also for appropriate indications, the soft laser complements the therapeutic repertoire of ear acupuncture. Demarcation of the range of indications depends on additional clinical studies.

7.5 Auricular Massage

Similar to body acupuncture, the therapeutic stimulation of irritated points or zones can also be achieved in ear somatotopy by means of a targeted pulsating pressure or massage. In addition, the whole body can be given a soothing harmonizing stimulus by stimulating the entire microsystem through systematic massage of the auricle. The latter is called auricular massage; this should be distinguished, with regard to its direction of action as well as its handling, from the direct stimulation of individual points through pressure massage.

Auricular massage (according to Lange 1985) (**Fig. 7.7**) is carried out without an auxiliary instrument, i.e., just using thumb and index finger. Due to the patient's active involvement, auricular massage has proved effective as a therapy-supporting measure, particularly when treating problems with concentration and sleeping disorders. After appropriate instruction on the proper regime, the massage may be carried out by the patients themselves. When massaging the ear, it is important to hold the auricle in a pinchlike grip between the index finger and thumb so that the tip of the thumb lies behind the auricle and the tip of the index finger is able to perform light massaging, circular movements on the front side of the auricle. The pressure of the massage should not be painful but rather perceived as pleasant.

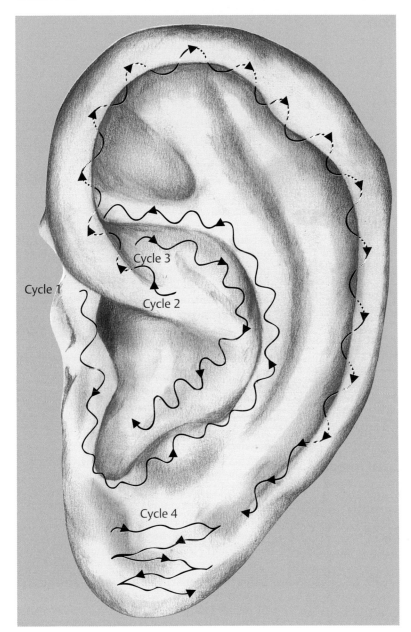

Fig. 7.7 Direction of auricular massage (according to Lange 1985).

Generally, focal massage of irritated ear points as defined by acupressure can only be performed with the help of rod- or probelike devices such as the ones used for detecting tenderness. This specific form of stimulation can be used when other possibilities for stimulation are not available or are not tolerated by the patient. Focal self-treatment by the patient is usually not practical, apart from two exceptions: kinetosis in order to support the treatment, and cases of pre-examination anxiety or stage fright. In such instances, the patient is instructed to massage the respective zones in the region of the postantitragal fossa or crus of the helix as required during the intervals between treatment. Self-treatment should be carried out carefully and with changing pressure from the fingernail.

7.6 Microphlebotomy

This type of therapeutic stimulation is included in the discussion despite its rather limited scope of indications. It has proved effective as an auxiliary measure in allergic disorders such as pollinosis and urticaria, and is also used in neuralgia, e.g., trigeminal neuralgia. Microphlebotomy may be used either alone in the directly indicated zone or as part of a combination therapy involving several points. One or several facial needles are sufficient for the punctures. To avoid unnecessary traumatization, cruder instruments (such as lancets) are not recommended. In the region of the well-vascularized lobule, it is even possible to pierce the tissue like a sieve with several needles (e.g., in the trigeminal zone). After an appropriate period of time, the needles are simultaneously removed; the resulting bleeding is not stopped but allowed to drip onto a cotton swab. In the region of the ear cartilage (e.g., at the tip of the ear: the allergy point), a quick stab with the needle from the inside or outside is usually sufficient to induce the appropriate bleeding.

Microphlebotomy of the auricle should only be used in connection with a pool of points appropriate for the particular syndrome. Its therapeutic stimulus is insufficient when used on its own and at any location.

7.7 Methods of Continuous Stimulation

General remarks. When using permanent needles or ear clamps to provide continuous stimulation of the irritated reflex zone over a longer period of time, both the risks and the therapeutic advantages must be very carefully assessed. As acupuncture, including ear acupuncture, constitutes an "intervention of choice," i.e., it is not an essential therapeutic measure, possible risks matter much more, especially when it is not obvious that there will be additional specific therapeutic results. For the various methods aiming at continuous stimulation (such as permanent needles, pellet plasters, or ear clamps), there is no evidence, either from comparative studies or from empirical observations, with regard to achieving improved effectiveness that would justify the disadvantages.

The major risk of permanent needles and pellet plasters is their subperichondrial incorporation into the cartilaginous parts of the tissue. This process starts with a mechanically induced, initially localized, inflammatory reaction and is followed by infection and tissue necrosis. The latter facilitates the entrance of foreign objects, especially when the patient is advised to massage the permanent needle or pellet plaster with a small magnet or with the tip of a finger to stimulate the point. If such a course of complications is recognized early enough, the foreign object can be removed without consequences. In more advanced states, however, when the adhesive band that keeps the needle or pellet in place is removed, the necrotic skin of the perichondrium, undermined by pus, will be seen to come away as it adheres to the plaster together with the needle or pellet. At this stage, there is a great risk that perichondritis will develop. In addition, it can be observed that after a prolonged, uncontrolled period of applying the pellet pressure at one site, and as a result of the massage, the small pellet can be pushed through the pressure-damaged tissue between the perichondrium and the cartilage, ending up underneath intact areas of skin that are clearly distant from the original site of application.

The ear clamps predominantly used by the Chinese school may lead to pressure-induced disturbances in local blood flow, with the danger of skin necrosis, although this is relatively rare. Patients must be informed accordingly of the risk of such complications, as well as of their legal rights. Foreign objects applied to the ear must be checked at short intervals (daily) for inflammatory reactions. In view of the potential problems, the application of this continuous stimulation method at the auricle is not recommended by the author.

Permanent needles (Fig. 7.8, Fig. 7.9). The popular types of permanent needles currently available on the market vary considerably in their shape and mode of application. The most traumatizing, and therefore least recommendable, permanent needle has a hook at its tip, which anchors itself in the cartilage after the needle has been pressed in with the aid of a guiding probe (**Fig. 7.11**). A small magnet inside the handle of the plastic probe is periodically used by the patient to stimulate the needle (**Fig. 7.12**). Another type of permanent needle is fixed to a small adhesive plaster; it has a circular overlay surface with the tip of the needle protruding from its center.

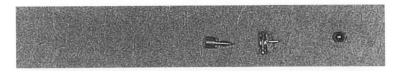

Fig. 7.8 Commercially available permanent needles.

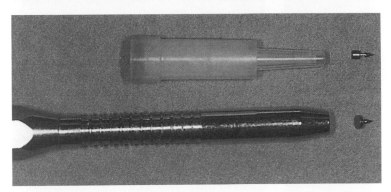

Fig. 7.9 Applicators for permanent needles.

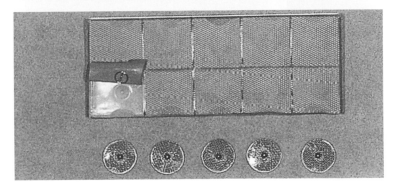

Fig. 7.10 Pellet plasters.

The small adhesive plaster and the wide overlay surface are supposed to ensure a firm fit. Tissue traumatization is much less severe; nevertheless, the above-mentioned possibility of complications still exists.

Pellet plasters (Fig. 7.10). This method was designed with the idea of exerting a constant pressure on the irritated zone. The chromium-plated small steel pellet, or seed, is fixed onto an adhesive plaster and stuck onto the point to be treated. The patient must be advised to lightly and repeatedly press the pellet. Applying the pellet to the specific point is not easy and also not precise.

Ear clamps. This method also serves for focal pressure stimulation. The clamp is applied in such a way that the tip of its overlay adheres to the reflex zone to be treated. Because they are very conspicuous, such clamps are not well accepted in the West and are therefore hardly ever used.

Magnetic plasters. Fixation of a small magnetic plaster onto the irritated reflex zones aims to induce a continuous therapeutic stimulus. There are no risks associated with this method; however, we cannot confirm its effectiveness, either through our own observations or on the basis of available studies.

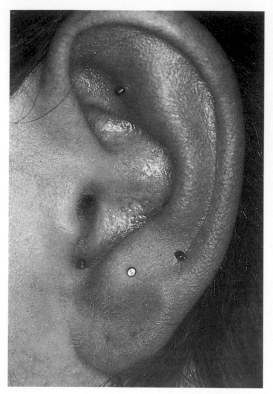

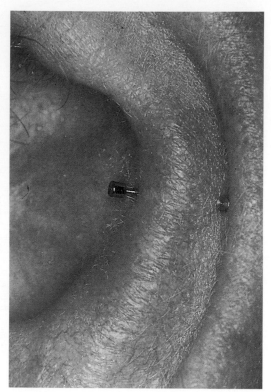

Fig. 7.11 Applied permanent needle with barb (Jerome, sun [35], *shen men*, and endocrine system points).

Fig. 7.12 Close-up view of a permanent needle in situ.

8   Practical Approach

It is important especially for the beginner that the practical approach is structured in accordance with a certain basic scheme, whereby the sequence of individual steps may be designed according to the therapist's own practical considerations. It is advisable that the beginner sets up separate appointments: one for the patient's history and a physical examination, if necessary, and another one for the actual ear acupuncture treatment. This will guarantee that there is enough time to draw conclusions, look up details, and draw up a regimen of points to be treated. At the actual treatment appointment, the therapeutically meaningful zones are then systematically searched for according to the chosen regimen.

8.1   Preparation and Positioning of the Patient

Preparation. Patient preparation involves informing the patient about the possibility of experiencing pain during needle insertion and about the kind and strength of the pain. Furthermore, it is advisable to inform the patient of the disposable needle material that will be used and to explain the search for points in general terms. In addition, the patient must remove all ear ornaments and, if necessary, clear interfering hair away from the ears. These preparatory measures may be taken care of by the nurse, including the necessary disinfection of the auricle.

The physician then briefly explains the procedure in plain language to the patient and, most importantly, points out that the symptoms tend to improve after four or five treatments. Otherwise the indication needs to be reviewed and the patient must consent to continuation of the treatment. It is also helpful to get the patients' cooperation in so far as they will inform the physician at the next treatment session, preferably without being asked, of any changes in their condition or symptoms so that therapeutic measures may be taken quickly and flexibly way by adjusting the combination of points.

For the whole of the treatment series, the patient should avoid narcotics, such as sleeping pills and alcohol, in the 12 hours preceding the treatment. It is advisable that the patient is not exposed to situations of physical stress, such as sauna or strenuous sports, during the 2 to 3 hours following treatment.

Positioning the patient. Examination and needling of the auricle can be performed with the patient either sitting or lying. Unless clues in the patient's history or a state of vegetative instability favor the lying position, sitting is generally preferred because it provides better access to the ear points. If required by the treatment regimen, laterality may be clarified at the beginning to identify which auricle should primarily be treated.

Even after brief practical experience, the physician will be familiar with all these steps. This will prevent him or her from making the patient feel uneasy as a result of incomplete information or improvised changes in the combination of points, which could disturb the course of treatment.

Bedding. After treatment, the patient should be left in a relaxed lying position for 20 to 45 minutes. The room should be sufficiently warm or the patient covered with a blanket to avoid even the slightest hypothermia, as this would interfere with complete relaxation. Unfortunately, these seemingly straightforward rules are often not observed in practice, or they are neglected due to insufficient engagement on the part of the physician or nurse. This may lead to unfavorable accompanying symptoms and may cause the patient to abandon the treatment at a critical phase.

8.2   Choice of Primary Therapeutic Access

From the patient's history and the general physical examination, the attending physician will frequently have already arrived at concrete ideas on which zones and points may be treated most successfully. It is advisable to complement this approach by a systematic examination process. This will include selecting the primary therapeutic access according to the syndrome, i.e., searching for the most irritated, and hence therapeutically most favorable, zone of the auricle and giving it preferential treatment. This is done best by repeating the following steps each time:

Step 1: Segment therapy.

Step 2: Choice of analgesic or anti-inflammatory points.

Step 3: Choice of psychotropic and vegetative points.

Step 4: Choice of supplementary points.

8.2.1 Segment Therapy or Choice of Correspondence Points

Segment Therapy

- In diseases of the locomotor system and in segmental neuralgia, segment therapy (ear geometry, according to Nogier) is the first choice, complemented by a choice of suitable correspondence points (e.g., joint points). First, the vegetative groove (zone of origin of sympathetic nuclei) in the scapha beneath the helical brim is examined to locate irritated points depending on the clinically conspicuous segment; if appropriate, this is then needled.
- The imaginary line of treatment drawn by connecting these points with point zero is then examined for more irritated points.
- Needling of the irritated points in the region of the zone of paravertebral muscles and ligaments should take priority.
- In cases of neuralgia or causalgia, it is more advantageous to search for sensitive points in the zone of the spinal cord, namely, in the region of its zone of sensory tracts.
- In chronically recurrent diseases (e.g., activated arthrosis, chronically recurrent lumbago), it is also highly advantageous to choose the latter zone as the primary therapeutic access.

Choice of Suitable Points of Correspondence

This applies to diseases of the locomotive system as well as cases of, e.g., organic disease or allergies.

- First, the irritated points corresponding to the diseased organs and the points modulating the immune system are located.
- This does not mean that organ diseases, for example, cannot be treated with segment therapy; however, the latter step is the second line of treatment. For example, when cholecystitis is assumed, the irritated gallbladder zone of the right ear must be needled first in combination with point 55. If the symptoms are not sufficiently alleviated, the disturbed segment of the upper abdomen may then be included in the treatment.

8.2.2 Choice of Analgesic or Anti-inflammatory Points

- In conditions of pain that are not organ-specific (such as cephalalgia or nonspecific neuralgia), the primary therapeutic access lies in the selection of sensitive analgesic or anti-inflammatory points.
- In most cases (e.g., general headache syndrome), the clinician should selected analgesically acting points in the region of the sensory line, the *shen men* point and, in extreme cases, also the thalamus point.

8.2.3 Choice of Psychotropic and Vegetative Points

- In case of mental illness or for treating addictions, the so-called psychotropic points and vegetative points are initially more important.
- If there are more than three or four irritated points per auricle, preferences must again be established depending on clues in the patient's history. The remaining points are recorded and marked with a felt-tip pen if they are sensitive, and then needled in a second session, making alternating treatment sessions at short intervals necessary.
- Frequently, the "extinction phenomenon" occurs during such this approach, whereby after needling the primarily preferred points, the secondarily preferred points are no longer found to be irritated.

> **! Caution**
>
> Remove felt-tip pen markings prior to needling (as there is a risk of a tattooing effect)!

8.3 Choice of Supplementary Points

The choice of supplementary points is made after needling the primary therapeutic access points. Depending on the syndrome, other points that could provide therapeutic support are examined for their state of irritation. For example, if there is gastritis as an organic disease, the organ points of the stomach and the solar plexus zone are chosen as the primary access points, but certain psychotropic points and vegetative points will definitely be included as supplementary points.

After any acute organic symptoms have subsided, treatment preferences may be completely reversed: previously supplementary points (in this case, the mental and vegetative balancing points) may gain importance, while the correspondence or organ points may become less important and finally will no longer be found to be irritated.

This procedure may of course also be followed when treating diseases of the locomotor system, e.g., lumbago–sciatica syndrome. As well as the psychotropically or vegetatively effective points mentioned above, the following supplementary points may also be considered: the muscle-relaxing Jerome point, and the *shen men* and ACTH points because of their analgesic and anti-inflammatory effects.

In cases of arthritic pain in the region of the knee joint, the two knee points (in the region of the triangular fossa and superior antihelical crus) are most important. Supplementary points are selected depending on whether the symptom complex can be assigned primarily to inflammation, a pain process, or a radiation of pain. Accordingly, supplementary points may be included individually or in combination.

Frequently, only the selection of supplementary points and their interaction with the primary therapeutic access points (correspondence point or segment therapy) will bring about the decisive therapeutic breakthrough.

8.4 Choice of Stimulation Method

Inserting a **fine needle** into the irritated point has certainly become the most popular method of auricular stimulation. So far, this type of stimulation has been unsurpassed in its practicability and effectiveness and has not been replaced by any other method of ear stimulation. Hence, needling is the treatment method of choice. All other forms of stimulus must be viewed as therapeutic supplements or less effective substitutes whenever the needle-stimulation method cannot be applied. Generally, electrical stimulation of the inserted needle has an enhancing effect, especially in neuralgia and causalgia, as well as in recurrent colicky pain conditions in the intestinal region (diverticulosis, spastic colitis, etc.). Microphlebotomy presents itself as a supplement to needle treatment, particularly for allergies and cephalalgia.

In hypersensitive or extremely anxious patients, the stimulation methods discussed earlier are an alternative to needle treatment, albeit an imperfect one. Initially, the targeted pressure massage of points (acupressure) is one possibility for the less well-equipped physician; it may be further developed by means of the pellet pressure method. However, for reasons already discussed, the latter requires stringent control on the part of the physician.

Point stimulation by means of a **soft laser** is more costly and less effective than the needle method. In all cases where the patient is unable to keep appointments for treatment at suitable intervals (e.g., because of prolonged travel), self-treatment by targeted **auricular massage** may be recommended, provided the projection zones to be treated can be easily located.

8.5 Strength of Stimulus, Treatment Intervals, and Duration of Sessions

Strength of stimulus. The French/Western school of ear acupuncture (auriculotherapy) calls for the differential use of gold and silver needles with regard to stimulus intensity: the drainage (= reducing) method requires strong stimulation, whereas the supplying (= reinforcing) method requires a weak stimulus.

The proponents of this school of thought use silver needles for drainage and gold needles for supplying in body acupuncture as well. As already discussed in connection with the choice of needles, puncturing different points of the tissue results in different electrical potentials, from which the respective replenishing or draining effect is inferred.

Without any explicit reasoning, auriculotherapy takes the view that the rules for choosing the needle type are reversed on the auricle, so that gold needles should be used for reducing and silver needles for reinforcing. Interestingly, only the terms *drainage* and *supplying* are borrowed from Chinese medicine and applied to particular syndromes. In neither Chinese body acupuncture nor Chinese ear acupuncture does the choice of metal have this meaning, let alone this range of applications. Furthermore, auriculotherapy talks about opposing "energetic relationships" on the front and back of the auricle. Consequently, on the back of the ear, gold needles are supposed to be used for "supplying" and silver needles for "drainage," again in analogy with body acupuncture.

According to the concept of auriculotherapy, mediation of the desired intensity of the stimulus depends on employing gold or silver as the material, whereas steel is neutral. Needles made of platinum or molybdenum are also in use, although, once again, their postulated special effect cannot be confirmed empirically.

In Chinese ear acupuncture, by contrast, the strength of the stimulus is not determined by the differential choice of needle types. Here, the reinforcing and draining techniques used are the same as in Chinese body acupuncture. The latter identifies three kinds of stimulus intensity, which, in a modified form, are supposed also to play a role in ear acupuncture.

The *ti dao fa* of ear acupuncture (the draining, reducing measure) corresponds to the famous *xie fa* of body acupuncture (as a strong stimulus); the *eao fa* of ear acupuncture (the supplying, replenishing measure) corresponds to the *bu fa* of body acupuncture (as a weak stimulus). The *nian zhuan fa* in ear acupuncture (as a medium-strength stimulus) corresponds to the third classical strength, i.e., the combination of *xie fa* and *bu fa*.

8.5.1 Drainage

Drainage in ear acupuncture (*ti dao fa*) is achieved by repeated minor lifting and lowering of the inserted needle for 1 to 2 minutes, while slightly rotating the needle. This strength of the stimulus is primarily indicated in states of *yang* or *yang* repletion, i.e., in acutely severe and painful diseases.

For **medium-strength stimulation**, i.e., for combining drainage and replenishing (*nian zhuan fa*), the needle is moved by rotating it back and forth for 1 to 2 minutes, emphasizing the clockwise direction. This strength of the stimulus is applied particularly in chronic and chronically recurrent symptoms or syndromes.

8.5.2 Supplementation

Supplementation in ear acupuncture (*eao fa*) is achieved by merely inserting the needle and leaving it without further manipulation. This type of stimulus is indicated in all states of *yin* or *yin* vacuity as defined by Chinese medicine,

i.e., primarily in chronic syndromes and conditions of pain (e.g., *yin* pain with the following characteristics: pain at night and while resting that improves with movement). Furthermore, it is advisable to choose this strength of the stimulus when warranted by the patient's constitution, i.e., particularly in weak or chronically ill patients, elderly individuals, and children.

Hence, in Chinese ear acupuncture, the strength of the stimulus is chosen depending on the syndrome, as defined by Traditional Chinese Medicine. For this purpose, patients and their illness should be assessed according to the classical eight guiding principles: vacuity/repletion, *yin/ yang*, heat/cold, interior/exterior.

The drainage and reinforcing techniques of Chinese ear acupuncture require relevant training and skills, especially the forms of *nian zhuan fa* and *ti dao fa*. If handling are clumsy, the ear cartilage may be considerably traumatized or even pierced, which will increase the risk of infection. For this reason, it is up to the physician to assess the need for this technique in relation to its effectiveness. As in the case with auriculotherapy, critical reservation is advisable, because here too there are still no convincing comparative studies or empirical results with regard to improved effectiveness over simple needle stimulation.

If we assume that ear acupuncture is based on a microsystem that reflects the entire body and in which direct and fairly short reflex pathways to the corresponding organ are clearly available, it is doubtful whether the laws of body acupuncture can be applied to ear acupuncture in a meaningful way, particularly since the organ projections are not analogous to the functional pathways (channels) defined by Chinese medicine. However, this does not exclude the consideration of diagnostic clues obtained according to traditional rules when choosing ear points. Unfortunately, we have only recommendations by individual authors regarding the effectiveness of the three different stimulus intensities; we have no insight into the original Chinese studies.

▶ Far more important than the choice of stimulus intensity is the choice of stimulus location. According to the current state of practical experience and in recognition of the available information from both Chinese ear acupuncture and French/Western auriculotherapy, the precise localization of the needle, rather than its manipulation, is the decisive factor. ◀

Treatment intervals. In Chinese ear acupuncture, the intervals between individual treatments depend on processes of Chinese medicine on the one hand (e.g., on the patient's constitution), and vary according to the type of syndrome on the other. Fairly short treatment intervals (twice a week or every 2 days) are indicated for *yang* repletion conditions, while longer intervals (i.e., once per week or every 2 weeks) are indicated in states of *yin* vacuity.

In Western auriculotherapy, the treatment intervals depend on the patient's needs:

- The patient is treated again when symptoms reappear or have not subsided sufficiently.
- The usual shortest interval is 1 to 2 days, but can be less where points other than those used for the previous or initial treatment are selected.
- The treatment intervals are gradually prolonged, depending on the patient's condition. The aim is to have intervals of 7 to 10 days.
- After the patient is free of symptoms, treatment is repeated once or twice, and the patient is advised to return for a new round of treatment if the symptoms recur, even if this is weeks or months later. This is likely to happen repeatedly, particularly with chronic illnesses.

Chronically ill patients return after 3 to 6 months, and a type of restorative treatment of about five sessions at intervals of 1 week apart will return them to their desired freedom from symptoms.

Duration of session. The needles are usually kept in place for 20 to 45 minutes. In old and very weak patients, the needles may be removed during the initial sessions after 10 minutes. The period of time is then gradually increased during subsequent sessions, depending on the patient's reaction. In severe pain conditions, the needles may be kept in place for a longer period, in individual cases perhaps for 45 to 60 minutes.

Practical Tip

A series of basic treatments should generally include approximately 10 sessions, and the patient must be informed that an alleviation of symptoms is frequently noticed after about five or six treatments. If the patient fails to respond, it may make sense to continue the treatment by mutual agreement, although the prospects are now less promising.

8.6 Combination with Other Methods of Stimulation

There are numerous possibilities for using ear acupuncture in combination with other therapeutic methods. However, beware of polypragmasy: the selection should be based on indication and syndrome in the same way as when ear acupuncture is used as monotherapy.

The use of ear acupuncture with its immediate painkilling effect has been tried and tested in the acute phases of recurrent chronic disorders such as migraine, as has including body acupuncture in more refractory cases, preferably during the treatment intervals. The combination of ear and body acupuncture is recommended for the treatment of difficult chronic syndromes. In chronic rheumatoid arthritis, for example, body acupuncture is used primarily and ear acupuncture is included as a supplementary measure, especially when acute symptoms appear. In such cases, irritated zones are usually found in the corresponding area of the auricle, offering the opportunity for therapeutic support. Acute pain can be alleviated in this way, even if the underlying illness cannot be permanently controlled with ear acupuncture alone.

Because of the reflex connections, ear acupuncture may also be used for follow-up. In syndromes not belonging to the primary range of indications for ear acupuncture, a reduction in initial irritation of the corresponding reflex zones can be interpreted as a sign of successful body acupuncture, independent of the course and often even prior to the onset of any subjective improvement in symptoms.

Treatment and follow-up take place during the same session. First, the auricle is examined as usual for irritated zones, which are then marked with a water-soluble felt-tip pen. Optimal body acupuncture is then carried out. Subsequently, the previously active zones are reassessed—they are often found to be less irritated or even silent. This "extinction phenomenon" may occur only after a series of treatments and is useful in that it indicates that the practitioner is proceeding correctly. Neural therapy presents another good opportunity for combination in acutely painful diseases. Although both methods compete with each other as far as the indication is concerned, their combination represents an improved therapy for disturbed areas (scars, foci). In these cases, neural therapy should be used primarily, and persistently irritated zones of the auricles should be considered for supplementary treatment. In acute neuralgia, such as headache syndromes, the method of choice should depend on the patient's preference or dislike—the decision will usually be in favor of ear acupuncture. Neural therapy will still be a sensible supplementary measure if there are residual symptoms.

> **Practical Tip**
>
> The therapist should always prefer the method that has provided the best results for the indication in question, in order to be able to apply another supplementary method if the symptoms remain or show insufficient improvement.

For example, the cervicobrachial syndrome can be superbly treated by acupuncture of the mouth according to Gleditsch and is the method of choice. In cases of needle phobia or patient hypersensitivity, it makes sense to stabilize the therapeutic outcome by switching to ear acupuncture after one or two sessions. This will not interfere with the success of mouth acupuncture, which may be readily reapplied after such an interruption.

In addition, ear acupuncture has proved effective for the preparation or initiation of physical treatment measures in chiropractic and kinesiological treatment. This approach has the advantage, among others, that the site of therapy lies outside the body areas involved in these measures, so that both treatments can be carried out in parallel. Ear acupuncture has also proved successful as a parallel treatment to conventional medical therapies. For example, one can take advantage of the analgesic and anti-inflammatory effects of the corresponding ear points following surgical interventions on the locomotor system. Through accompanying ear acupuncture, possible incompatibilities or allergic reactions can be avoided and medications saved. This also applies to bronchial asthma, in which the dosage of conventional medication can frequently be reduced as a result of parallel treatment with ear acupuncture.

These examples demonstrate that, although the combination of ear acupuncture with other procedures and indications has its limitations, multiple possibilities are open for exploration. Its direct mechanism of action is so clear and defined that ear acupuncture has become an ideal component of combination treatment.

9 Established Indications

The indications presented in this chapter are also dealt with in the corresponding chapters elsewhere in this book and can, with the aid of ear or body acupuncture, be successfully treated by a medical specialist or general practitioner. The detailed description of these indications facilitates familiarization with therapeutic procedures and, after giving the various aspects proper and critical consideration, should help the practitioner to set up an individualized therapy plan.

It should be pointed out however, that diseases must be checked by a medical specialist if necessary, and the patient must be informed about conventional medical options.

9.1 Diseases of the Eye

If there is any risk of acute loss of sight, the treatment of eye diseases with alternative methods is naturally out of the question. This certainly applies, for example, when retinal detachment is suspected in cases of acute glaucoma or in temporal arteritis (giant cell arteritis). However, tentative recognition of such diseases of the eye lies within the medical scope of the ear acupuncturist. Prior diagnosis by a specialist is, therefore, usually not required. If a specific disease is suspected, the patient is referred to an ophthalmologist. Needless to say, in cases with a doubtful diagnosis, it is always advisable to seek a second opinion from a specialist prior to starting any acupuncture treatment, because the responsibility always lies with the treating physician regardless of his or her specialty area.

Ear acupuncture is a beneficial approach in all acute and inflammatory diseases of the outer eye (e.g., hordeolum, conjunctivitis, blepharitis). The Chinese school describes first of all the eye point (8) located in the center of the lobule as the **primary** therapeutic access; in addition to the above indications, it also lists glaucoma, optic atrophy, and retinitis. In practice, however, the eye point (8) on the lobule has only proved effective with inflammatory eye diseases. In diseases of the inner eye, the eye points 24 a and 24 b at the caudal edge of the intertragic notch are more important; they too are derived from the Chinese school. Monitoring and care by an eye specialist is essential, especially when treating glaucoma.

Even in severe conditions such as optic atrophy and macular degeneration, use of ear acupuncture at the eye points 24 a and 24 b has proved helpful. It must be noted, however, that ear acupuncture may never result in healing or complete restoration—it can only achieve a distinct delay in the progression or persistence of the condition. From that point of view, the patient's subjective description should not be taken exclusively into account, not least because improved findings are frequently superimposed with a concomitant, objective improvement in the patient's general well-being; the specialist should also regularly document the progress of the disease.

After the primary selection of these specific eye points (corresponding points), **supplementary** treatment by means of segment therapy should be considered in chronic conditions. The vegetative groove (zone of origin of sympathetic nuclei, see **Fig. 3.22**) should be examined at the level of the upper cervical spine, as well as the zone of paravertebral chain of sympathetic ganglia (see **Fig. 3.17**), namely, the superior and middle cervical ganglion points.

With diseases of the inner eye, i.e., those affecting the sensory organ, it is also advisable to examine the antitragus in the region of the sensory line (points 29, 35, 33) for irritations (**Fig. 9.1**).

Supplementary points are inferred by the findings. Depending on the condition, different points should be considered, for example, the *shen men* point (55) and the ACTH point (13) in eye diseases with inflammatory tendencies. If an allergic condition predominates, the allergy point (78) at the tip of the ear must also be searched for and needled from the inside, if possible. In such cases, the thymus gland point (26 a), located in the antihelical wall at the level of C7/T1, will often also prove sensitive and may be included in the therapy.

It is also possible to treat the above noninflammatory eye diseases as defined by Chinese medicine, which assigns them to the liver (LI). Consequently, the liver zone (97) (see **Fig. 3.28**)

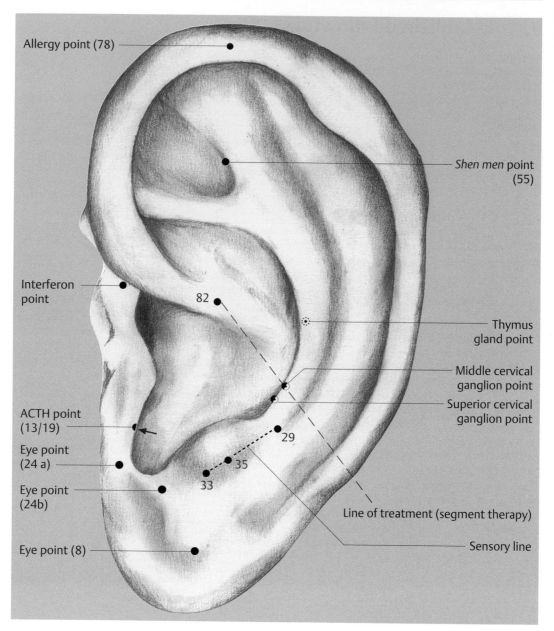

Fig. 9.1 Pool of points for diseases of the eye.

of the auricle may be examined for irritation and included in the treatment.

The following two treatment examples are intended to clarify the basic procedure and facilitate the first therapeutic steps. The first example shows a quick and fair response to ear acupuncture, while the second one usually shows improvement only after prolonged, continuous therapy.

9.1.1 Allergic Conjunctivitis

In contrast to infectious conjunctivitis, which must be treated with antibiotics, acute allergic conjunctivitis can be treated well with ear acupuncture, which opens up a real alternative to the therapies of conventional medicine. Obviously, antiallergic agents and antihistamines are available. However, patients often prefer treatment by (ear) acupuncture, either because of drug intolerance or because of a general aversion to allopathic drugs.

One must here distinguish between *acute* treatment, which is restricted to the selection of a few points, and *prophylactic* treatment, which lasts for approximately 4 weeks and is performed in good time prior to the expected allergic exposure. For prophylactic treatment, therapeutically differing supplementary points are required during the course of treatment.

When treating *acute conjunctivitis*, the eye point (8) at the center of the lobule must be located. In addition, the allergy point (78) must be found and needled in such a way that it causes microphlebotomy. This treatment can be repeated daily. If sensitive, the interferon point in the supratragic notch can be added. In addition, the *shen men* point (55) can be examined for sensitivity. As a rule, it is enough to select the allergy point (78), *shen men* point (55), and eye point (8). The sensation of a foreign object will subside within a few hours, whereas hyperemia of the conjunctiva will take 1 to 2 days to subside.

9.1.2 Optic Atrophy

This severe syndrome, occurring frequently in connection with multiple sclerosis, is currently treated in conventional medicine over a relatively long period of time and with only moderate results.

In those cases where corticoid therapy is not tolerated or is rejected by the patient in the long term, auricular stimulation therapy can be recommended. A response to therapy is manifested by delayed progression or stagnation of the disease compared with the pretreatment phase.

Initially, 5 to 10 treatments are set up, if possible at daily intervals. Later, when the symptoms recede, treatment should take place weekly. Prior to this, in order not to have to rely only on the patient's subjective feelings, the attending eye specialist should document the objective state of the eyes, carrying out an update approximately 6 to 10 weeks into the treatment. If a tendency

toward improvement is observed, continuation of treatment makes sense and treatment intervals may be extended to 2 or 3 weeks. If the findings worsen after about 6 weeks, a return to weekly intervals is indicated.

To justify the continuation or repetition of a series of ear acupuncture sessions, the findings obtained by the eye specialist after 3 months should clearly show a tendency toward improvement. If this is confirmed by the patient subjectively, a good prognosis may be expected.

> **Practical Tip**
>
> Terminate the treatment if neither subjective nor objective improvements can be observed after the first round of approximately 10 sessions.

The following ear points may be considered for the **primary** basic regimen and may be supplemented individually, depending on the patient's response and condition. First, the eye points 24 a and 24 b on the lower cartilaginous edge of the intertragic notch and, furthermore, the ACTH point (13) at the start of the endocrine zone (22) are searched for; the *shen men* point (55) is usually sensitive, too. These areas should be found on both sides and then needled.

The primary therapeutic approach is **supplemented** by points located on the sensory line. However, points in the zone of paravertebral chain of sympathetic ganglia often prove sensitive, too, especially the superior and middle cervical ganglion points at the C2/C3 level, just before the transition of the antitragal wall into the plain of the concha (**Fig. 9.1**). Since patients with this severe, dangerous syndrome are subjected to considerable suffering accompanied by emotional instability, the psychotropic points should also be examined for sensitivity and included as supplementary points if the maximum of four or five needles per auricle has not yet been reached.

To stabilize the achieved delay or stagnation in the course of the disease, a series of approximately six treatments should be repeated every 6, or even every 3, months.

A similar approach may be taken in case of *macular degeneration*. The sensory line is emphasized in this syndrome. Once again, the *shen men* point (55) as well as points in the zone of paraverbral chain of sympathetic ganglia may be used as supplementary points. The sensitive areas may be found within this zone but are mostly found just next to the ganglion points proper. If verifiable, the area of the vegetative point II (34) is a beneficial addition. Various points can be found here (sieving technique).

9.2 Diseases of Ear, Nose, and Throat

9.2.1 Globus Sensation

This syndrome is also called "globus hystericus." The sensation of having a lump in the throat is usually a typical psychosomatic disorder with vegetative symptoms and is frequently accompanied by myogelosis in connection with cervical syndrome. Therefore, it is recommended that more be found out about such symptoms, both in the patient's history and during the clinical examination. This will help in putting together an individual set of points.

In case of conspicuous findings concerning the cervical spine and a corresponding history supplied by the patient, the **primary** therapeutic access should be the segmental approach (formerly **ear geometry**). For this purpose, the vegetative groove is first searched for irritated points, and the segment is narrowed down by connecting those points with point zero (diaphragm point) (82) to form an imaginary line of treatment. More irritated points are usually found along this line, e.g., in the zone of paravertebral muscles and ligaments, which is located in the scapha and antihelical wall.

When searching for **supplementary** reflex zones, the following zones should be considered if globus sensation is viewed as an *organ-related syndrome*: the larynx/pharynx point (15) (see **Fig. 3.3**) and esophagus zone (85) (see **Fig. 3.26**). They are projected as a narrow band in the inferior concha bordering on the ascending helix. The solar plexus zone on the crus of helix should be examined too.

With respect to underlying *vegetative disturbances*, of course, vegetative point I (51) on the inferior antihelical crus and vegetative point II (34) on the inside of the antitragus should be considered. Based on the Chinese school's interpretation that generalized vegetative disorders result from vacuity (*xu*) of spleen (*Pi*) and liver

(*gan*), the Chinese school often includes the corresponding points, the liver zone (97) and spleen zone (98) (see **Fig. 3.28**), of the auricle. Treatment takes place every 2 to 3 days. A therapeutic success should already be evident after five or six treatments; as a rule, therapy may be terminated after a cycle of approximately 10 sessions.

9.2.2 Laryngitis

Laryngitis requires different therapeutic approaches, depending on whether it is the acute, inflammatory type or the chronic type of manifestation.

In the acute type caused by infection or excessive strain, symptoms usually quickly subside. Here, ear acupuncture is only indicated when improvement is not as rapid as expected or if improvement is continuingly absent.

Among the acute types, the most frequent indication is recurrent laryngitis due to excessive strain. This affects the patient time and again because of stress at work; the suffering caused is similar to that seen with the chronic type and may require treatment by ear acupuncture. If speech therapy has already been initiated, although not yet completed, it should be continued during the treatment series.

In *acute laryngitis*, the following points are recommended as the **primary** basic regimen:
- Larynx/pharynx point (15).
- *SHEN men* point (55).
- Trachea zone (103).

In cases of infection this should be **supplemented** by the apex of tragus point (12) and, if appropriate, the interferon point (see **Fig. 3.2**). If there is an underlying allergic component, the allergy point (78) and the ACTH point (13) should be included. If caused by excessive strain of the vocal cords as a result of faulty speech technique or prolonged strain, the following psychotropic points should be considered as well: frustration point, PT1 (formerly antiaggression point), PT3 (formerly antidepression point). In most cases, vegetative point I (51) and vegetative point II (34) are also found to be quite irritated.

According to the concept of Chinese medicine, the voice is affected by the *qi* of the lungs. Hence, the lung zone (101) can be searched for sensitive points (sieving technique).

Note. In cases of *chronic laryngitis*, one should consider that this might initially be a warning sign for laryngeal cancer. Hence, this possibility must definitely be excluded by laryngoscopy prior to the start of ear acupuncture. Once again, treatment of the laryngitis is carried out according to the **primary** basic regimen; for the chronic type, however, the apex of tragus point (12) is omitted in favor of the ACTH point.

The individual **supplementary** points used depend on the possible causes and contributing factors, similar to acute laryngitis caused by excessive strain. For chronic laryngitis, the difference in treatment lies in the larger treatment intervals (once per week) but, unfortunately, also in a slower improvement and lower chances of success. Therefore, combination with **body acupuncture** is absolutely recommended here. The symptoms are usually interpreted as a disease of vacuity (*xu*); hence, the following body acupuncture points should be considered: CV-22 and CV-23 as well as ST-9.

Frequently, there is an underlying chronic infection of the paranasal sinuses or bronchi. This should be clarified prior to treatment and, if necessary, treated further by different therapeutic methods.

9.2.3 Meniere's Disease

This syndrome is characterized by impaired hearing in the range of low-pitched sounds that is associated with noise in the ear, paroxysmal rotatory vertigo, and concomitant vegetative symptoms, such as nausea or vomiting. The cause of the disease is unknown; it therefore constitutes a considerable therapeutic problem in Western medicine as well. The therapeutic results obtained with ear acupuncture, as well as in combination with body acupuncture, are generally not very good. Nevertheless, very good results can occasionally achieve be, which justifies an attempt to treat the disease with ear acupuncture.

Apart from the **primary** basic combination, the selection of a set of therapeutic points is individualized to the patient, depending on the individual triggers. The primary basic idea is to search first for points in the area of the sensory line (points 29, 35, 33). Next, it makes sense to examine vegetative point I and vegetative point II for their sensitivity. In this syndrome, the kinetosis

point (29 a) and a point in the solar plexus zone may also be irritated and should be included in the set of points. Inclusion of the latter two points may be decisive because of their vegetative harmonizing effect, and thus may contribute to fundamental stabilization beyond the purely symptomatic effect.

The **supplementary** points include the *shen men* point (55), vegetative point II (34), and stellate ganglion point (in the zone of paravertebral chain of sympathetic ganglia).

The factors triggering the attacks of vertigo need to be thoroughly established while taking the patient's history, because they play an important role in the choice of points. The triggers are not always known to the patient; therefore, this essential aspect is often missing when considering the set of points to be treated. Common triggers are (in the order of frequency): hypersensitivity to changes in the weather, psychosocial overload, tension caused by faulty posture, and hydrops of the inner ear. As an example, the following ear points may be searched for sensitivity:

- Weather point on the ascending helix.
- Psychotropic points in the order of their most likely sensitivity, namely, PT1 (antiaggression point) and PT3 (antidepression point).
- PT2 (anxiety/worry point).
- If sensitive, the oppression point (83) in the solar plexus zone (crus of helix).
- Von Steinburg's vertigo line.

Because conditions of cervical tension often develop in connection with a prolonged faulty posture resulting from physical overload, the therapeutic approach of segment therapy (formerly **ear geometry**) should be considered in cases of vertigo. Accordingly, the point corresponding to the affected segment is searched for in the vegetative groove and needled if it is sensitive. Obviously, the **primary** regimen should also include the Jerome point (29 b). In cases of hydrops of the inner ear, this treatment is **supplemented** by the inner ear point (9) and ACTH point (13).

Chinese medicine classifies Meniere's disease with its attacks of rotatory vertigo as a disease related to wind (*feng*). Accordingly, it is recommended that the liver zone (97) be included in the treatment. Combination with **body acupuncture** is possible, e.g., through the lateral *yang* channels, triple burner (TB) and gallbladder (GB).

Note. For all the possible sets of points presented here, the maximum number of needles should not exceed more than four or five per ear.

9.2.4 Pollinosis

The sharp rise in allergic diseases (including pollinosis) in recent years is undoubtedly related to the increasing inability of the human immune system to cope with environmental pollution (air, food, water) and its inadequate reaction to natural substances previously tolerated, depending on an individual's constitution. The harmonizing effect of acupuncture can be put to good use, both in acute cases and as a preventive measure. In the treatment of *acute cases*, like that of allergic conjunctivitis, depending on the main symptoms, the correspondence points of the eye (8) and inner nose (16) are needled first, followed by the allergy point (78) on the tip of the ear, if necessary from the inside. When removing the needle, the spontaneous bleeding is allowed to stop on its own (microphlebotomy). The allergy point may also be punctured from above; this usually does not result in spontaneous bleeding. The *shen men* point (55) should also be included because of its component of antiphlogistic action, as should the ACTH point (13) if it is sensitive. If asthma is a contributing factor, irritated points in the region of the lung zone (101) should be considered. In the *acute phase*, sessions take should place twice a week, or daily if required, and are continued weekly or biweekly following stabilization. The selection of points should be adjusted to the individual course and symptoms. The individual set of points will become more and more distinct and should be adhered to during the subsequent treatment period, starting with the fourth or fifth session.

After the pollen season has come to an end, *prophylactic treatment* for the following year is worthwhile. The prophylactic approach for hay fever treatment differs from the acute treatment only with respect to the timing of the start and course of treatment. However, it should be considered that certain points, which are clearly reactive during the acute phase, cannot be detected during the pollen-free period. Hence, they cannot be included in the treatment at this point. These points are the eye point (8), inner nose point (16)

and lung zone (101). Needless to say, the sensitivity of these points varies from person to person and is not always uniformly expressed. In case of persistent sensitivity, these points should certainly be included in the prophylactic treatment.

During the prophylactic phase of treatment, it is recommended that the interferon point on the supratragic notch and the thymus gland point be selected, according to their sensitivity. Furthermore, combination with **body acupuncture** is recommended. In Chinese medicine, weakness in the defense *qi* is assumed, and possibly weakness of the kidney yang. This results in vacuity (*xu*), which underlies hay fever and allergic bronchial asthma as a possible contributing factor. The nose—interpreted according to Chinese school as the opener of the lung (*fei*)—provides clues to possible disturbances along the lung channel, so treatment points should be selected along the lung (LU) and large intestine (LI) channels. The following body acupoints have proved effective: LI-20, LI-4, and LU-11. Treatment takes place twice a week during the first 4 to 6 weeks; thereafter, it is switched to weekly treatment intervals. In total, 15 to 20 sessions are required per year; for prophylaxis, this treatment is repeated for 2 to 3 subsequent years, depending on the intensity of the seasonal complaints.

Small children should be treated the same way, but with laser rather than needles.

9.2.5 Forms of Rotary Vertigo

Rotatory (systematic) vertigo and other conditions of vertigo are among the most varied and most frequent complaints in general practice. In order to facilitate meaningful and successful treatment by means of ear acupuncture, thorough diagnostic clarification is a must, even more than with other symptoms because of the multitude of possible organic and functional causes. Within the bounds of the rather vague term *vertigo*, only those forms of vertigo may be considered for ear acupuncture treatment which have been clearly diagnosed but cannot be treated by conventional medical means and respond well to ear acupuncture. These include, e.g., sensations of dizziness classified as *vestibular vertigo* and *vertebral vertigo*. According to recent findings, the latter may be interpreted as a myofascial syndrome. These forms must be strictly distinguished from *asystematic vertigo*, i.e., diffuse cerebral dizziness. The latter is characterized by a feeling of rotation or vacuity in the head that is associated with drowsiness and things turning black in front of the eyes; this is caused by insufficient cerebral blood flow.

The Drs von Steinburg (ear, nose, and throat specialists in Munich, Germany) have documented significant therapeutic results within the framework of a thoroughly conducted clinical study. Among the 100 patients whose data were recorded for analysis, a complete improvement of symptoms was found in 74%, a good improvement in 15%, relapse in 9%, and no effect in 2%. The ear points used in this study were located on the "vertigo line" discussed above (**Fig. 9.2**).

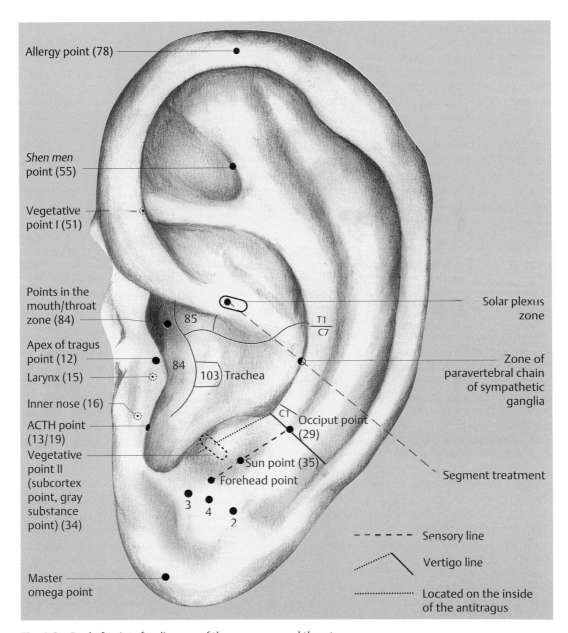

Fig. 9.2　Pool of points for diseases of the ear, nose, and throat.

On the auricle, additional **primary** therapeutic access is provided when searching for points at the C1/C2 level and in the zone of sympathetic trunk (zone of paravertebral chain of sympathetic nuclei, stellate ganglion point; see **Fig. 3.17**) and also in the vegetative groove according to Lange (zone of origin of sympathetic nuclei). This set of points can possibly be expanded by applying **ear geometry**.

To **supplement** this approach, points on the antitragus may be examined. These centrally acting points are often sensitive in conditions of vertigo and hence may be used therapeutically. Of significance is the sun point (35) on the outside of the antitragal base; this is listed primarily as an important point for headache. As the central point on the sensory line, according to Nogier, it is also very effective in vertigo, especially in combination with forehead point (33) and occiput point (29). Just above the occiput point (29) lies point 29 a, which is indicated in *kinetosis*, i.e., vertigo and nausea (motion sickness). Frequently, this point is also sensitive in other forms of vertigo. In addition, vegetative point II (34) should be considered.

Further therapeutic access is provided by points or zones corresponding to the inner ear/labyrinth. The "acoustic state point," which the Chinese school refers to as the apex of tragus point (12), is located slightly inside the tip of the tragus and is primarily indicated in painful and feverish conditions caused by infections. However, it may also be sensitive in forms of vertigo associated with symptoms resembling tinnitus and hence in need of treatment. Furthermore, the inner ear point (9) (see **Fig. 3.9**) is another region that is supposed to be effective in *vestibular vertigo*.

In a simplistic way, vertigo may be understood as a symptom resulting from a disturbance in the relationship between body and space, which depends on optimal interactions between the vestibular, visual, and deep sensibility systems. Hence, the eye points 24 a and 24 b (see **Fig. 3.4**) may be indicated as well. The system of deep sensibility is functionally best represented in the thalamus point (26 a) (see **Fig. 3.6**).

Since the vestibular nuclei are closely related in space and function to switches in the autonomic nervous system, the body–space relationship can be influenced in a stabilizing way by means of vegetative points I and II and also by the (vegetative) heart zone (100) and cardiac plexus point.

Visual interaction of the three systems mentioned is controlled by the cerebrum through diverse visual centers in the occiput, temples, and forehead, as well as through vestibulocortical pathways. This may explain the psychopathological relationships in the genesis of symptoms of vertigo, an example being *vertigo caused by heights*.

Depending on their sensitivity, the psychotropic points offer the opportunity for ear acupuncture to exert a harmonizing and stabilizing effect. These points include primarily PT1 (formerly the antiaggression point), PT2 (formerly the anxiety/worry point), the frustration point (see **Fig. 4.5**) and if applicable the Jerome point (29 b) (see **Fig. 4.4**).

According to the Chinese concept, attacks of *rotatory vertigo* are classified as wind (*feng*) diseases and are treated as an outside (*biao*) disease via the lateral *yang* channels of the triple burner ([TB] and gallbladder (GB), as well as the liver channel (LI). When transferring this concept to the auricle, the liver zone (97), gallbladder zone (96), and triple burner zone (104) should be searched for sensitivities (see also 2nd step of medical history.

One of the most important diseases involving the vestibular system is insufficiency of the basilar artery. This syndrome is also called *vertebrobasilar circulatory disorder, cervicovascular vertigo*, or *postural vertigo*. Depending on its severity, the dominant diagnostic sign is either rotary vertigo lasting for seconds, rotatory vertigo combined with disturbed vision (nephelopia), noise in the ear and hyperacusis, or, in mild cases, rotatory vertigo that depends on head posture and unsteadiness associated with pain in the shoulder and neck.

In these cases, **primary** therapy starts with the cervical spine segment; i.e., sensitive points on the segmental treatment line are needled, starting with the reflex points in the cervical spine zone and the corresponding points on the back of the auricle. In addition, all of the previously mentioned points have proved effective as **supplementary** points: the kinetosis point (29 a), inner ear point (9), vegetative point I (51), and vegetative point II (34). (See the treatment examples for Vestibular Vertigo, p. 174.)

9.2.6 Tinnitus

This very burdensome symptom is a more or less intense sensation of noise in the ears, which can vary considerably in terms of its character and time of appearance. Conventional medicine lists many different causes of this symptom, some of which (e.g., infections, foreign bodies, inflammation of the auditory meatus or middle ear) can be relatively easily eliminated. Acupuncture treatment should only be started after an ear, nose, and throat (ENT) specialist has excluded such causes by. Needless to say, it is a doctor's responsibility to diagnose possible systemic diseases, e.g., severe generalized infections or possible injuries.

In principle, ringing in the ears in its essential form is as difficult to treat with ear acupuncture as it is with conventional medical methods. This should be openly admitted to the patient, who often has high hopes, especially with regard to lasting success.

Experience has shown that this symptom will often cause considerable mental sequelae, if it has not done so already. Treatment is therefore carried out either to bring about a temporary alleviation or with the aim of making the ear noises disappear for several days. During these symptom-free periods, the patient is then able to recover physically and emotionally, if necessary. In this way, depressive or suicidal developments may be avoided.

The following reflex zones or points have proved successful: the points of the sensory line, such as occiput point (29), sun point (35), forehead point (33) and *shen men* point (55).

In addition, the ganglia points of the zone of paravertebral chain of sympathetic ganglia at the C2 to C7 level should be examined for irritation.

According to the Chinese view, the phenomenon of tinnitus is associated with disturbances along the liver (*gan*) or kidney (*shen*) channels. In case of repletion (*shi*), the liver zone (97) should be considered; in case of vacuity (*xu*), treatment of the kidney zone (95) is more important.

In addition, it is recommended that vegetative zones (vegetative points I and II) and the psychotropic points on the lobule be examined for sensitivity. The master omega point in the ventral lower third of the lobule should also be considered.

The first 10 treatments should be performed twice weekly. The point selection should be reconsidered after five or six treatments if there is no improvement. If success is achieved, which often already shows itself after the first treatment even though it may be short-lived, the treatment may be repeated regularly every 2 to 3 weeks, with similar results. As already mentioned, this will help the patient's overall stabilization.

9.2.7 Sinusitis

Both the acute and chronic forms of this syndrome can be treated successfully. In the general practitioner's ordinary everyday practice, patients with this condition usually come for treatment with ear or body acupuncture only once they are in the chronic or chronically recurrent phase. As a rule, the patient has unsuccessfully passed through several attempts of "established" therapies by specialists (such as fenestration, permanent drainage, adenotomy, and treatment with antibiotics, as well as physical therapy). Disturbed bacterial flora in the intestine resulting from antibiotic treatment and common malnutrition, as well as the common chronic hyperplasia of the nasal mucosa that results from the continuous use of decongestant nose drops, contribute significantly to the chronicity of the process. In view of this, exclusive treatment with ear or body acupuncture is often not enough, especially with chronic sinusitis. Therapeutic microbial support of the gut, in the sense of *symbiotic management*, is usually required and may be supplemented by local care of the nasal mucosa with panthenol, 0.9% NaCl spray or its equivalent.

In both *acute* and *chronic* forms of sinusitis, a general therapeutic concept can prove successful which, unlike with other syndromes, does not really depend on the patient's individual characteristics. This concept includes combination with certain **body acupuncture** points and/or, in the *acute phase*, supplementary treatment by selective **mouth acupuncture** (according to Gleditsch) combined with Adler's selected pressure points on the neck at the level of C6/C7. The **primary** therapeutic point combination for ear acupuncture consists of the following points, which should be needled on both ears: inner nose point (16), forehead point (33), ACTH point (13), and lung zone (101).

Supplementary points—second-choice reflex points that are used alternately with the primary points with short treatment intervals (less than 2 to 3 days), particularly in severe frontal pain—comprise the following reflex zones: the *shen men* point (55), occiput point (29), and vegetative point II (34). In contrast to the primary points mentioned above, these are not always found to be irritated. However, they should be included in the examination and documentation of points during the first treatment, even if they will not be used right away. Depending on their recurrent sensitivity, these points may be used for assessing the course of disease or as supplementary points.

As standard points for combination with **body acupuncture**, the following body acupoints have proved successful: LI-4 and LI-20 as well as BL-2 and BL-10. In children, they should be treated with a laser.

In ear acupuncture, the treatments for acute and chronic sinusitis differ not so much in terms of the selection of points, but rather with respect to the treatment intervals and choice of body acupoints that are suitable to be used in combination. In the *chronic* form of sinusitis, treatment intervals of at least 1 week should be chosen. Suitable body acupoints for combination are first of all local points, namely, LI-20 and BL-2. On the average, 10 to 20 treatments are required, initially twice a week, and later at weekly intervals. By contrast, *acute* sinusitis requires 5 to 10 treatments that must be carried out daily in the acute phase. The effectiveness of the method has been convincingly documented in a dissertation by Wimmer (1984) at the ENT outpatient clinic in Munich, Germany.

9.3 Diseases of the Respiratory System (Fig. 9.3)

9.3.1 Bronchial Asthma

Bronchial asthma is discussed here as representative of a series of diseases of the respiratory system that are characterized by dyspnea as the leading symptom. In most cases, patients with this syndrome arrive for acupuncture treatment only after the condition has become chronic and a concomitant intolerance to conventional medication has developed. At this stage, the patient's expectations are no longer focused on healing but on an alleviation of symptoms or on a bearable life without medication. From the medical point of view, it must be emphasized that curing asthma by means of acupuncture is achieved only in very rare cases; hence, exaggerated expectations should not be encouraged.

Regarding the selection of points, it is helpful to differentiate each clinical case of bronchial asthma according to its trigger mechanisms and concomitant symptoms, as this will help to uncover decisive clues to the combination of points for treatment. The therapist should not be upset when this approach leads to deviations from the standard set of points. Specifications such as those outlined in this book are for orientation only and should not tempt the practitioner into treating the syndrome blindly according to a preset combination of points.

For **primary** therapeutic access, it is advisable to search initially for irritated points by means of the disturbed segment ("segmental treatment line"). For this purpose, the vegetative groove (zone of origin of sympathetic nuclei) is examined at the level of the cervical/thoracic spine. The line of treatment is then established by connecting the irritated points with point zero (diaphragm point) (82), which is usually not sensitive and hence does not need to be treated. In most cases, more irritated points will be found along this line of treatment in the region of the lung zone (101), the zone of paravertebral chain of sympathetic ganglia, and the zone of paravertebral muscles and ligaments.

The following **supplementary** points may be used, depending on the individual situation: the *shen men* point (55), asthma point (31), and occiput point (29), as well as the lung zone (101) and trachea zone (103). vegetative points I (51) and II (34) and the (vegetative) heart zone (100) should also be considered according to symptomatic clues.

Depending on the trigger mechanisms, such as the weather, emotional stress, and allergic factors, the corresponding points should also be examined for possible irritation: the weather point (vegetative point), psychotropic points such as PT1 (formerly the antiaggression point), the frustration point or PT2 (formerly the anxiety/worry point), and PT3 (formerly the antidepression point). If there is an underlying allergic process, the following points are usually found to

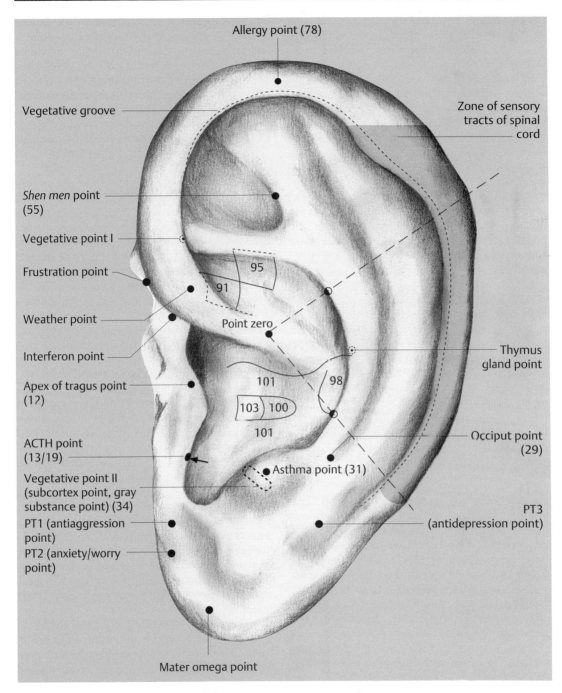

Fig. 9.3 Pool of points for diseases of the respiratory system.

be sensitive to pressure: the allergy point (78), ACTH point (13), and adrenal gland point located in the zone of nervous control points of endocrine glands (in the ant-helical wall at the T12 level). In cases of recurrent infectious exacerbations of a chronic asthmoid disease, which may be accompanied by high fever, it is preferable to include the following points in the treatment: the apex of tragus (12), interferon point, vegetative point II (34), and *shen men* point (55).

According to the Chinese concept, all lung diseases, and therefore also asthmoid disease processes, are caused by *Yang* Vacuity in the area of lung (*fei*) and spleen (*pi*). This illness may erupt under the influence of cold and dampness and under excessive strain. Accordingly, Chinese ear acupuncture recommends including the large intestine zone (91), spleen zone (98), and kidney zone (95) in the treatment, depending on the state of their irritation, in order to strengthen the *qi*.

In very rare cases, asking their physician for acupuncture treatment is the asthma patient's first therapeutic choice. As they are usually already undergoing drug therapy, treatment with acupuncture is supposed to facilitate, among other things, a discontinuation or reduction of medication.

Note. Do not simply discontinue medication involving sympathomimetics or corticoids and replace them with acupuncture.

On the contrary, two, three, or even four acupuncture sessions should be carried out under continuous medication according to the criteria described earlier, and objective tests of assessment should be included for follow-up, such as peak flow measurements and, at certain intervals, additional pulmonary function tests. In the initiation/discontinuation phase, it has proved successful to carry out the acupuncture sessions twice a week at intervals of about 3 days. Under the cover of acupuncture, a slowly progressive reduction in medication can be attempted, beginning with the systemic corticosteroid, while bronchiospasmolytics (both local and systemic ones) are initially maintained at the usual dosage. Only after reaching low doses of corticosteroid medication (the Cushing's threshold dose) or after complete discontinuation of the corticoid, can a reduction

of any additional medication take place. During this phase, treatment may initially take place at weekly intervals; depending on the individual course of the condition and after its stabilization, treatment may proceed at longer intervals.

With this kind of chronic disease, patients return of their own accord for further treatment at intervals of 3 to 6 months, even after minor changes in their symptoms, in order to be stabilized by a new series of about five sessions.

9.3.2 Chronic Bronchitis

Chronic bronchitis and chronically recurrent bronchitis may have various underlying causes. These should clearly be identified within the scope of the patient's history and the clinical symptoms, in order to aim for an elimination or at least reduction of these possible causes in collaboration with the patient. Without such a cause-oriented approach, ear acupuncture would be limited to the alleviation or subjective improvement of symptoms and could not stop the progression of the chronic process.

Possible causes include, for example, chronic nicotine abuse. In this case, treatment of the addiction must come first. Chronically recurrent bronchitis may also be caused by susceptibility to infections or by strain on the respiratory system as a result of today's ubiquitous air pollution, especially in population centers and industrial belts. In these situations, it makes sense to strive for a systematic strengthening of the immune system (e.g., by means of *symbiotic management*) prior to, or in parallel with, a series of ear acupuncture treatments. Total avoidance of exposure may not be possible, but easing of exposure (e.g., by a prolonged recreational vacation in an area with clean air) will help in creating a favorable basis for reflex therapy by means of ear acupuncture.

If clues to a contributory allergic process surface, these may call for important therapeutic measures introduced in parallel. In addition, allergy-related reflex zones on the auricle have to be included in the set of points.

As a **primary** combination of points, irritated points in the lung zone (101) and bronchopulmonary plexus point should be searched for. This also includes the anti-inflammatory *shen men* point (55), as well as the ACTH point (13) and the adrenal gland point (nervous control point in the antihelical wall at the T12 level). In addition, vegetative points I (51) and II (34) should be considered.

The following points should be considered as **supplementary** points: the interferon point in the supratragic notch on the one hand, to utilize its immune-enhancing effect, and on the other hand, the allergy point (78) on the tip of the ear in combination with the antiallergic thymus gland point (antihelical wall).

As defined by the Chinese school, chronic or chronically recurrent bronchitis is assumed to be caused by vacuity resulting from a *yin* vacuity (*xu*) of the lung; therefore, additional needling of the spleen zone (98) and kidney zone (95) will strengthen the *qi*.

As with bronchial asthma, chronic or chronically recurrent bronchitis requires a prolonged treatment period of approximately 6 months. In view of the continuing diathesis and risk of relapses, repeated treatment at longer intervals (approximately every 6 to 9 months) is recommended.

9.4 Diseases of the Cardiovascular System (Fig. 9.4)

9.4.1 Hypertension, Hypotension

With respect to circulatory regulation, it should be stated here that, in contrast to widely held views and corresponding references in the literature, it is unfortunately impossible to raise or lower the blood pressure by selective ear acupuncture independently of the prevailing blood pressure conditions. Names such as "high blood pressure point" or "blood pressure lowering point" are, therefore, misleading, and statements concerning the special effects of gold and silver needles are also entirely unfounded, both practically and theoretically. It is assumed, however, that an acupuncture stimulus applied to a specific reflex zone on the auricle triggers an entire complex of regulatory actions at the nervous and humoral levels that aims for restoration of the respective disturbed functional system. Based on this assumption, the effect of ear acupuncture on circulatory regulation may still be utilized, to the patient's benefit, although it cannot specifically aim at normalizing blood pressure

levels. This explains why most of the points considered for the treatment of hypertension and hypotension are identical. Depending on the cause and accompanying symptoms, different supplementary points are included in each case.

Note. It should be kept in mind that in cases of pronounced *hypertension*, which is difficult to treat by means of ear acupuncture, a precise diagnosis of the syndrome is compulsory, and the patient has to be informed about the primary required measures of basic therapy that are available using conventional medicine.

Important contributing factors (such as overweight, persistent emotional stress, lack of exercise, and abuse of coffee, tea, cigarettes, etc.) should be taken into consideration when treating hypertension.

As **primary** therapeutic points, the following are available: the reflex zone of the adrenal gland, i.e., the ACTH point (13) (formerly the antihypertension point, 19), heart zone (100), and occiput point (29).

As **supplementary** points, the following points should be examined for their state of irritation, depending on the patient's predominant symptoms: thalamus point (26 a), vegetative point II (34), and sun point (35). It also makes sense to use vegetative point I (51) and omega point II.

The *antihypertension groove (105 m)* on the back of the auricle should also be mentioned as this is supposed to be effective according to Chinese specifications. Furthermore, the psychotropic points of PT1 (formerly antiaggression point) and the master omega point should be taken into consideration.

According to the Chinese concept, the symptoms of hypertension (such as dizziness, headaches, and reddening of the face) are interpreted as a sign of increased liver *yang*. Therefore, Chinese ear acupuncture attempts "drainage" by needling the liver zone (97). Furthermore, acupuncture treatment should distinguish between vacuity (*xu*) and repletion (*shi*): in the state of repletion, for example, needling of the *shen men* point (55) is preferred.

As in the case of bronchial asthma, it is also possible to combine treatment of hypertension by ear acupuncture with conventional drug therapy, or to needle with the aim of reducing

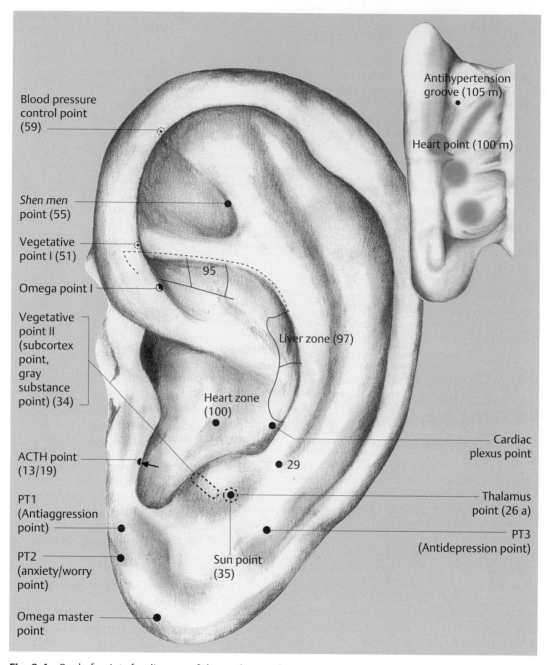

Blood pressure control point (59)

Antihypertension groove (105 m)

Heart point (100 m)

Shen men point (55)

Vegetative point I (51)

95

Omega point I

Vegetative point II (subcortex point, gray substance point) (34)

Liver zone (97)

Heart zone (100)

ACTH point (13/19)

Cardiac plexus point

29

PT1 (Antiaggression point)

Thalamus point (26 a)

PT3 (Antidepression point)

PT2 (anxiety/worry point)

Sun point (35)

Omega master point

Fig. 9.4 Pool of points for diseases of the cardiovascular system.

medication. Here too, depending on the severity and course of the disease, the aim is to prescribe medication according to the effectiveness of the ear acupuncture performed and to correspondingly adjust the treatment intervals as well as the sets of points.

During the first treatment for hypertension, acupuncture is carried out twice a week; sustained lowering of blood pressure can already be achieved after a series of about 10 sessions. If the treatment is effective, the accompanying general symptoms (such as dizziness, headache, and insomnia) already subside after one or, at the latest, five or six sessions. Repeated treatments are usually required at intervals of about 6 months, or continuous treatment at larger intervals of 2 to 3 weeks.

Practical Tip

The treatment of *hypotension* is less difficult than that of hypertension. The reflex zones affecting the circulatory system that are known to be relevant in hypertension are also examined here for sensitivity: the heart zone (100), ACTH point (13), occiput point (29), and thalamus point (26 a). The sympathicotonic points vegetative point I (51) and vegetative point II (34) serve as individual supplementary points.

The **Chinese school** describes an additional point in the middle of the ear, the oppression point /"bifurcation point" (83), which is located in the solar plexus zone defined by Nogier's auriculotherapy, and lies close to point zero (the diaphragm point) (82). To what extent these points can be distinguished according to their location remains to be explored in more detail in individual studies. Nevertheless, in case of hypotonic dysregulation, it is sensible to search for irritated points in the solar plexus zone.

Approximately three to six sessions are usually enough for prolonged stabilization of low blood pressure. In individual cases, a single follow-up treatment is warranted after a long interval, i.e., about 3 months.

The **Chinese school** also describes a *blood pressure raising groove*, located on the back of the ear, approximately in the middle third of the antihelical groove.

Once again, it should be pointed out that the specified reflex zones do not allow the blood pressure to be raised or lowered the blood pressure in a direct, calculated way when blood pressure is normal. Similarly, existing high blood pressure cannot be raised further. Hence, there is no risk of inducing a hypertensive crisis by using points that are not indicated; the worst-case scenario would be an absence of the hoped-for effect. However, in the course of such ineffective treatment, as in all cases of untreated hypertension, dysfunctional blood pressure regulation may result. Simple follow-up by means of routinely documented results of blood pressure measurements should always accompany the therapy.

9.4.2 Paroxysmal Tachycardia

It goes without saying that prior to acupuncture treatment of this symptom, any severe cardiac irregularities must be ruled out by long-term electrocardiogram (ECG) surveillance. Patients usually seek out acupuncture when conventional medical measures—from recommending drinking some water during the attack to administrating a low-dose β blocker—have failed or are unacceptable to the patient. **Primary** treatment by ear acupuncture relies on the vegetative and heart-specific reflex zones already discussed.

Most important is the heart zone (100) in combination with the cardiac plexus point (at the C2/C3 level in the inferior concha at the transition to the antihelical wall); vegetative points I (51) and II (34) should be considered too. Furthermore, the solar plexus zone, or the oppression point (bifurcation point) (83) according to the Chinese school, should be examined for sensitivity. According to the Chinese concept, these symptoms develop with vacuity (*xu*), e.g., after a severe and weakening illness. Furthermore, predisposition to paroxysmal tachycardia may develop in connection with mental disease, such as a depressed mood and depression. Therefore, the Chinese school uses—apart from heart zone (100)—the following points to promote the circulation of *qi* and blood (*xue*): small intestine zone (89) and, as a sedative component, occiput (29) and vegetative point II (34).

It has proved successful to possibly include the following psychotropic points: PT2 (formerly anxiety/worry point), PT3 (formerly antidepression point), and PT1 (formerly antiaggression point). Before considering more extensive sets of points, it is worth trying to needle—as the only irritated reflex zone during an attack—the oppression point (bifurcation point) (83) in the solar plexus zone, in order to achieve a lower pulse rate. This may be followed by further treatment using additional combinations, e.g., heart zone (100) and cardiac plexus point, and also by including the solar plexus zone.

The treatment interval is 2 to 3 days and is extended to weekly intervals once the situation has stabilized. Usually, five to 10 sessions are sufficient.

9.5 Diseases of the Gastrointestinal Tract (Fig. 9.5)

9.5.1 Chronically Recurrent Gastritis

When selecting the primary points for treating acute and chronically recurrent gastritis, identical reflex zones may be found to be irritated. In the case of *acute gastritis*, symptoms experienced during the spontaneous course of this disease can be clearly alleviated or even eliminated using these points. As a result, burdensome medication can be avoided. This fact is only of marginal interest, however, since patients rarely turn to acupuncture treatment at the beginning of their illness.

The physician is far more often confronted with *chronically recurrent gastritis* and a request for acupuncture treatment as a substitute for repeated and more or less successful drug therapy. Also in this situation, the patient may be subjected to ear acupuncture with good prospects for success, provided a diagnosis (esophageal diaphragmatic hernia, *Helicobacter pylori*) has been established.

The **primary** set of points, which is also very effective in acute gastritis, is found within the reflex zones of stomach and duodenum, which should be examined for irritated points. It will help first to find a line of treatment according to the tried and tested principle of segment therapy (formerly **ear geometry**). Along this line, sensitive points can then be identified specifically within the region of the stomach zone (87) and duodenum zone (88), as well as in the zone of

paravertebral chain of sympathetic ganglia. Any points found in the vegetative groove (zone of origin of sympathetic nuclei) are also needled, in addition to point zero (diaphragm point) (82), which in this case will certainly be irritated.

When painful spastic symptoms associated with nausea or vomiting dominate the acute phase, it is advisable to include retro-point zero (112 m) in the central posterior sulcus. The *shen men* point (55) can be included if it is sensitive, because of its analgesic and anti-inflammatory effects.

However, it should be remembered that no more than four or five needles per ear should be used.

If more than five active points are present, a selection is made according to the patient's actual condition, while the remaining points are documented and used in alternating second treatments arranged at short intervals. The therapist should not become confused if some of these points are no longer sensitive by the second session. This may signal a therapeutic effect that often appears in parallel to a subjective improvement in the patient's condition or may even precede it. Hence, these normalized points are of no further use.

As **supplementary** points, vegetative points I (51) and II (34) may be included in the treatment. Especially in chronically recurrent gastritis accompanied by repeatedly occurring duodenal or stomach ulcers, all of the following psychotropic points should be examined for sensitivity: frustration point, PT1, PT2, and PT3. In contrast to the points of primary therapy, these points play a major role during symptom-free periods. If necessary, the occiput point (29) and Jerome point (29 b) are included as well.

According to **Chinese** specifications, the spleen zone (98) and lung zone (101) may also be sensitive. In severe cases, omega point I and omega point II are often useful.

By necessity, treatment intervals are shorter: 2 to 3 days, depending on the state of the acute phase. They are then increased, particularly with repeated treatments. Treatment intervals of 7 to 10 days have proved successful.

We know from experience that stabilization has taken place once the familiar relapses occur in a weakened form, if at all. After four or five sessions beyond this stage, treatment can be regarded as complete. When new, although mostly

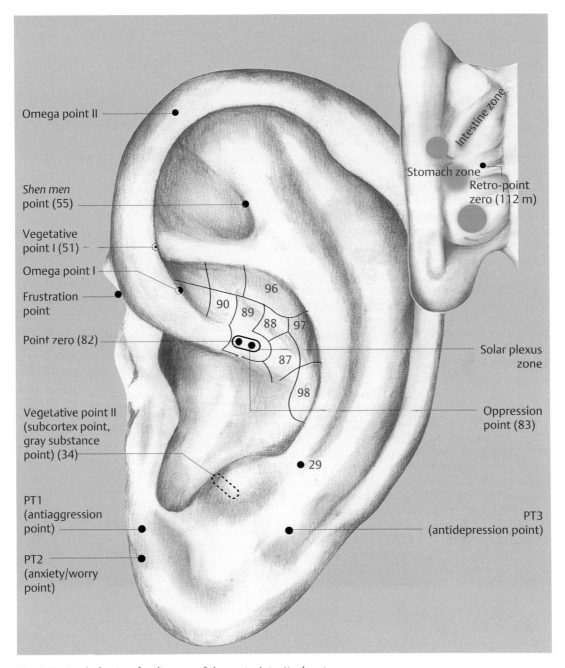

Omega point II

Shen men
point (55)

Vegetative
point I (51)

Omega point I

Frustration
point

Point zero (82)

Vegetative point II
(subcortex point,
gray substance
point) (34)

PT1
(antiaggression
point)

PT2
(anxiety/worry
point)

Intestine zone

Stomach zone
Retro-point
zero (112 m)

96

90

89

88

97

87

98

Solar plexus
zone

Oppression
point (83)

29

PT3
(antidepression point)

Fig. 9.5 Pool of points for diseases of the gastrointestinal system.

weakened, relapses occur after a long period of time, they can be quickly controlled in two or three sessions.

Note. With this syndrome, it is important to cope with the underlying psychosomatic process in a competent way; otherwise relapses are unavoidable.

9.5.2 Acute Enterocolitis

This syndrome, which usually appears swiftly and takes a dramatic course, is relatively easy to manage by ear acupuncture, so that the otherwise obligatory drug therapy can be avoided. However, especially in the most frequent type (enterocolitis caused by infection), it is essential to take temporary nutritional measures and to ensure that liquid and electrolytes are sufficiently replenished. The excruciating, spastic abdominal pain and the increased stool frequency, which usually make the spontaneous course of this illness very hard for the patient to endure, are quickly alleviated by means of ear needling.

For **primary** therapy, the following reflex zones are systematically searched for irritated points: large intestine zone–small intestine zone (sigmoid) (91, 90), jejunum (89), and also the rectum zone (81). Next, point zero (diaphragm point) (82) is examined. This is part of the primary therapeutic set of points because of its excellent spasmolytic effect on the smooth muscles of the intestine. To enhance the spasmolytic effect, retro-point zero (112 m) should definitely be included in the treatment. If the stomach is involved as well, which is often the case, the stomach zone (87) and solar plexus zone should certainly also be included. Corresponding to the most affected section of the intestine, a cluster of irritated points will be found in the respective reflex zone. In that case, several needles per reflex zone are inserted next to one another (the sieving technique)—these count as one needle. We advise against the often-promoted threading technique in view of the considerable traumatization discussed earlier and the associated risk of infection. Additional alleviation of pain is achieved through the *shen men* point (55).

The following **supplementary** points have proved helpful: vegetative point I (51), Jerome point (29 b), and sometimes also vegetative point II (34).

The Chinese school recommends needling the spleen zone (98) and lung zone (101) due to vacuity (*xu*) of the spleen (*pi*). In the region of the lung zone (101), two or three irritated points are often found next to one another, in particular close to the antitragus.

As a rule, one or two sessions over 2 to 3 days are enough for treating this condition. When symptoms recur or 2 days of persistent diarrhea

have already passed prior to starting the treatment, a microbiological examination of the stools should be arranged.

In patients who have just returned from tropical countries, the possibility of parasitic diseases should be considered to ensure that a more serious condition is be overlooked due to the masking of symptoms as a result of acupuncture.

9.5.3 Chronic Obstipation

Chronic obstipation has many different causes and, without doubt, represents a medical puzzle. Patients frequently treat their problem as a taboo subject or are left on their own after extensive diagnostic clarification; this often leads to the abuse of laxatives and progression of the problem. Nevertheless, these patients can often be helped by ear and/or body acupuncture. In addition to clarifying the symptoms with respect to underlying organic changes (polyps, malignancies), it is important to exclude a relatively rare form of obstipation, called delayed transit, in which acupuncture treatment will not be successful. Apart from this special case, attempts at treatment using ear acupuncture are always promising.

As in cases of enterocolitis, the following **primary** therapeutic reflex zones of the intestine should be examined for irritated points: large intestine zone, small intestine zone (90, 91), and rectum zone (81). Vegetative point I (51) may in addition be needled. It also makes sense to include the following sedative and relaxing points in the treatment too: Jerome point (29 b) and occiput point (29), but also PT1 and the master omega point, if they are sensitive.

As an accompanying measure, the patients are encouraged to reassess their dietary habits, namely by integrating a high-fiber diet and plenty of fluids into their food consumption patterns. The aim should also be use the protective effects of acupuncture to free the patient from the often compulsive scheduling of bowel movements.

Initially, treatment is carried out twice a week; after four sessions, an attempt is made to reduce this to weekly intervals.

After a series of 10 sessions, patients usually have regular bowel movements. Booster treatment after 6 to 12 months is necessary in some patients, although this usually involves only two or three sessions. In persistent cases, especially following the abuse of laxatives, longer treatment periods are required, and it also makes sense to combine ear acupuncture with **body acupuncture**. In this context, the established point combination according to Kampik should be mentioned. Using the *shu/mu* technique, body acupoints BL-25 and ST-25 are bilaterally needled and electrically stimulated. In cases of delayed transit as a form of constipation, a comparative study carried out at the Chirurgische Universitätsklinik Innenstadt in Munich, Germany, has, however, reported that this technique does not produce the desired results.

9.5.4 Singultus Point (Hiccup Point)

Patients with singultus will come for acupuncture treatment only when the hiccup persists, when it occurs against the backdrop of painful injuries, if it appears following surgery on the thoracoabdominal region, or if it is recurrent. It is even possible to eliminate singultus by ear acupuncture when it suddenly occurs during surgery.

It is usually sufficient to needle, on both ears, point zero (diaphragm point, singultus point) (82) in the solar plexus zone—the hiccup will stop within a few minutes. In persistent cases, it is recommended that the effect be enhanced by including retro-point zero (bifurcation point of the vagus nerve, 112 m) in the central posterior sulcus at the back of the ear.

In chronically recurrent singultus, further irritated points should be searched for in the solar plexus zone, the vegetative groove (zone of origin of sympathetic nuclei), and also the zone of paravertebral chain of sympathetic ganglia, along the imaginary line of treatment according to Nogier's **ear geometry**.

For **supplementary** treatment, it makes sense to utilize vegetative points I (51) and II (34) during symptom-free periods.

During surgery, singultus can usually be interrupted by a single stimulation of point zero (diaphragm point) (82). In persistent chronic forms of hiccup, this result is usually achieved with two or three treatments. However, experience shows that four or five sessions at weekly intervals may be required for stabilization and to guarantee a lasting effect. The regimen is similar in chronically recurring hiccups. Here, too, longer periods of treatment must be anticipated, and selection of the points described should be based on each patient's clinical symptoms and medical history.

9.5.5 Cholecystitis, Cholelithiasis

In cases of cholecystitis and cholelithiasis, patients come for acupuncture because they want to delay impending surgery or because of mounting intolerance to that which have so far been helpful in mitigating their symptoms. Rarely is a physician asked for ear or body acupuncture treatment because of an acute biliary colic.

Nevertheless, an established selection of points should be mentioned for such a case: First of all, the thalamus point (26 a) and *shen men* point (55) are needled for immediate pain relief. The spasmolytic effect of point zero (diaphragm point) (82) and retro-point zero (112 m) is also utilized. The affected segment is determined through the vegetative groove. Along the imaginary line of treatment between point zero (82) and the irritated point in the vegetative groove, further irritated zones are usually encountered on the antihelix, corresponding to the abdomen point (43) of the Chinese school, and also in the pancreas/gallbladder zone (96) and liver zone (97). In *chronic cholecystitis*, which is most often caused by cholelithiasis, this set of points is combined with **supplementary** points, such as the ACTH point (13), adrenal gland point (nervous control point in the antihelical wall, at the T12 level), and vegetative point I (51).

Patients are treated over a period of 6 to 8 weeks. During this time, sessions are arranged initially at intervals of 2 to 3 days until the complaint has been eliminated. Thereafter, treatment is carried out weekly. The combination of points varies during the subsequent course of treatment, depending on individual conditions.

Note. Be sure to inform the patient about the surgical measures that might become necessary, and also about the possibility of the less stressful approaches of endoscopic cholecystectomy and lithotripsy.

This information should be given prior to starting therapy, but it makes sense to come back to this topic during the treatment series. In this way, no time will be lost, and the patient can still continue with ear acupuncture treatment.

9.6 Gynecological Disorders (Fig. 9.6)

9.6.1 Menstruation Disorders

Menstruation disorders appear in various forms and should be treated accordingly with different sets of points.

Practical Tip

The most frequent syndrome, dysmenorrhea, can be influenced fairly well by ear acupuncture. Yet it also applies here that a preset combination of points will bring only moderate success. Therefore, the selection of points should be based on individual factors.

The **primary** choice of points forms the foundation for treatment. It includes first the uterus point (58) in the triangular fossa beneath the ascending helix, the ovary point (23) of the endocrine zone (22) in the intertragic notch, and the hypogastric/urogenital plexus point in the superior concha.

In severe conditions of pain, retro-point zero (112 m) and possibly the thalamus point (26 a) should be considered as **supplementary** points; they are used predominantly in the *acute* phase.

Individual reflex zones selected according to the patient's medical history and clinical condition play a role in both prophylaxis and treatment between the menstrual periods. Approximately 3 weeks prior to the expected onset of menstruation, treatment is started with two sessions per week. Depending on the irritated reflex zones, different sets of points may be appropriate for individual sessions. In the week prior to the expected onset of menstruation, returning to the basic set of points has proved successful. During prophylaxis or treatment between the periods, the following points are examined for irritation: vegetative points I (51) and II (34) as well as the psychotropic points—the frustration point and PT1 to PT4. It goes without saying that only some of these points may be found to be sensitive, depending on the patient's individual situation, such as her life circumstances, her emotional state, the symptom characteristics, prodromes, etc.

In addition, segment therapy should be considered. Therefore, with the help of the vegetative groove and the often irritated point zero, additional albeit less well-defined points will be found on this corresponding treatment line.

According to Chinese considerations, treatment of the symptoms of dysmenorrhea should differ depending on whether there is repletion (*shi*) or vacuity (*xu*). In cases of repletion, the symptoms of which are usually caused by emotional excitement (e.g., depression, anger) or exogenous influences (e.g., hypothermia, cold), the treatment includes the liver zone (97) and kidney zone (95).

In case of vacuity, which develops from vacuity in either the blood (*xue*) or qi and/or from disturbance of the conception vessel (CV, *ren mai*), combination with **body acupuncture** is recommended (e.g., SP-6 and CV-6). In addition, the spleen zone (98) and stomach zone (87) should be examined for sensitivity.

Practical Tip

In cases of *amenorrhea,* only secondary amenorrhea responds well to treatment with ear acupuncture. Primarily, the following points are treated: uterus point (58), ovary point (23), and vegetative point II (34). The reflex zone of vegetative point I (51) has also proved successful. If the patient's history provides clues to psychogenic components, irritations are often found among the psychotropic points, such as the frustration point, PT1, and PT3.

Treatment takes place at weekly intervals. After 8 to 10 sessions, menstruation can be expected to commence.

In Chinese medicine, treatment is based either on symptoms of vacuity resulting from qi vacuity and kidney (*shen*) vacuity, in which case the kidney zone (95) is included in the treatment, or on circulatory disturbance resulting from dysfunction of the liver (*gan*), in which case inclusion of the liver zone (97) and spleen zone (98) is recommended.

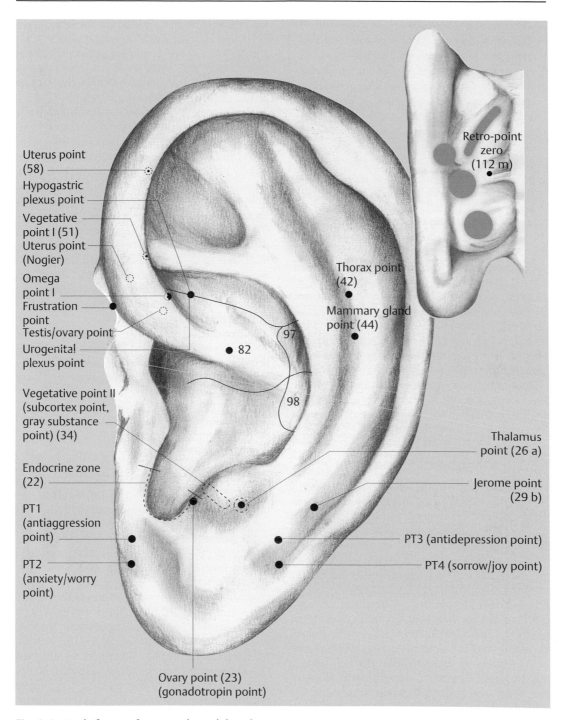

Fig. 9.6 Pool of points for gynecological disorders.

125

> **Practical Tip**
>
> The syndrome of *metrorrhagia,* a form of dysmenorrhea, is primarily approached using the same selection of points that are applicable to dysmenorrhea. During the course of treatment, however, a distinct set of points will predominate, depending on the sensitivity of various points. The most important points are the uterus point (58), uterus zone (according to Nogier), ACTH point (13), and testicle/ovary point (23) in the endocrine zone (22), and also the adrenal gland point (nervous control point in the antihelical wall) and point zero (82).

As a rule, acupuncture is carried out for prophylaxis or between the periods. Treatment may start immediately at the end of a prolonged or profuse menstruation. After initial treatment of two sessions per week, treatment changes to weekly intervals. After 5 to 10 sessions, menstruation will begin to normalize. Treatment should continue for five additional sessions, provided the reflex zones continue to be sensitive.

According to experiences in Chinese medicine, the following reflex zones are also used in treating metrorrhagia: the spleen zone (98), vegetative point II (34), and liver zone (97).

9.6.2 Menopausal Syndrome

Because this syndrome is accompanied by a multitude of symptoms, it is important to focus on the predominant symptoms described by the patient. These include hot flashes, intermittent profuse sweating, insomnia, increased emotional sensitivity, defined vertigo, and functional heart complaints. These agonizing, rather vegetative disturbances often do not subside despite conventional hormone replacement therapy (HRT). If the woman also has osteoporosis that needs to be treated, hormonal substitution should if possible continue during acupuncture, or be modified only in consultation with a gynecologist. In other cases, discontinuation of hormone treatment during ear acupuncture is optional, depending on the course of treatment; discontinuation should take place in agreement with the patient and her gynecologist.

The selection of points for **primary** therapy focuses on the sex-specific points, such as testicle/ovary point (23), uterus point (58), or uterus zone

(according to Nogier), and on the *shen men* point (55). Also important are vegetative points I (51) and II (34), as well as the vegetative/functional heart zone (100). With the heart zone (100) in mind it is helpful to also examine the cardiac plexus point for sensitivity.

The following points may be sensitive and can be used for **supplementary** treatment: occiput point (29), PT1, the frustration point, and vegetative point II (34). Initially treating this syndrome at intervals of 2 days in a series of 10 sessions has proved successful. Different sets of points will be indicated from session to session, depending on the sensitivity of the points and the result of the follow-up. Once improvement has been achieved, treatments at weekly intervals should be aspired to.

According to the Chinese medicine concept, which assigns the activity of female hormones primarily to the liver (*gan*) and kidney (*shen*), the liver zone (97) and kidney zone (95) are included in the treatment as well.

When certain presenting symptoms predominate in the syndrome, establishing priorities with respect to the reflex zones to be selected becomes important. In cases of insomnia associated with irritability and functional heart complaint, this applies to the following points: heart zone (100), Jerome point (29 b), occiput point (29), and also the TSH point in the endocrine zone (22).

9.6.3 Insufficient Lactation

This disorder of the female mammary gland can be treated quite well in most cases with a few ear needles in only two or three sessions.

For **primary** therapy, the prolactin point (according to Nogier) takes precedence. According to the Chinese school, this is located close to the acoustic meatus in the lower part of the inferior concha, almost as part of the endocrine zone (22). The mammary gland point (44) at the level of T5 (in the zone of nervous control points of endocrine glands) has also proved successful. It is often found along the line of treatment established by **ear geometry** according to Nogier. Other sensitive points found in the region of vegetative groove, scapha, and antihelix, e.g., thorax point (42) or mammary gland point (44), are points derived from the Chinese school. They can be reliably found by means of the segmental approach.

As **supplementary** points, vegetative points I (51) and II (34) may be included in the treatment if they are sensitive. Sessions may take place daily and with alternating sets of points.

9.6.4 Mastitis

This syndrome results from congestion in the milk ducts of the mammary gland and usually occurs at the beginning of the breast-feeding period, but also later during this stage. Usually, the majority of mothers strictly refuse to take medication during this period, which frequently leads to the application of ear acupuncture. Using this therapy, severe pain and inflammatory processes can be quickly alleviated or even eliminated. In case of a feverish general reaction accompanied by the onset of putrid processes and a risk of abscess formation, it is inevitable to combine ear acupuncture with antibiotics. However, we cannot report such a course of events from personal experience.

For quick relief of pain, the following points serve as **primary** therapeutic access: the *shen men* point (55), occiput point (29), and thalamus point (26 a). The segmental approach has proved successful as well. The following points derived from the Chinese school can be easily found along the line of treatment established between point zero (82) and the sensitive point found in the vegetative groove: the thorax point (42), mammary gland point (44), and liver zone (97). In the same way, the mammary gland point (according to Nogier) can be searched for sensitivity at the Th5 level in the zone of nervous control points of endocrine glands.

If vegetative point II (34) and ACTH point (13) in the endocrine zone (22) are found to be irritated, they may be used for **supplementary** treatment.

The other commonly used practical measures, such as emptying the ducts by intensive pumping (only, of course, after alleviation of the pain) and alcohol dressings, are not affected by ear acupuncture.

9.6.5 Perinatal Pain Management, Facilitation of Delivery

For perinatal pain relief and ease of delivery, the following points may be needled at the onset of delivery between uterine contractions: the thalamus point (26 a), point zero (diaphragm point) (82), *shen men* point (55), vegetative point I (51), and Jerome point (29 b).

Additional irritated points may be found in the lumbar spine zone (40) and sciatica zone (52). In most cases, the hypogastric plexus point (in the superior concha) is also found to be sensitive and may be used for relaxation during delivery.

> **— Practical Tip —**
>
> The same approach is possible in combination with the induction of labor; if induction becomes necessary, primarily the uterus point (58) and uterus zone (according to Nogier) are included. According to Chinese school, both the urinary bladder zone (92) and vegetative point II (34) have also proved successful during induction of labor. It should be pointed out that, depending on their sensitivity, no more than three or four of the possible points listed should be needled.

Needling takes place on both ears and possibly already when the contractions are still weak but regular. The needles remain in place during delivery and may be stimulated by repeated gentle rotation.

9.6.6 Ear Acupuncture in Obstetrics

C. Schulte-Uebbing

Pschyrembel's motto—that one "must know as much as possible in order to do as little as possible"—also applies to obstetric acupuncture Besides, there are no "forbidden ear points" but only false indications. Under no circumstances should first experience with ear acupuncture be gained by treating pregnant women.

Note. As a rule, as few points as possible should be needled in pregnant women.
Ear zones densely innervated by the vagus nerve are to be avoided.

Neither powerful techniques nor techniques inducing pain sensation should be used during pregnancy. Everything that might be perceived as uncomfortable by the pregnant woman must be avoided; with premature contractions, for example, only gentle needling should be carried out. Only those individuals who have completed basic courses in acupuncture and subsequently have been able to acquire the necessary knowledge and skills—and, in particular, dexterity—are suitable to meet the requirements of acupuncture for pregnant patients. Ideally, acupuncture on pregnant women should initially always take place under the guidance of a specialist.

Obstetric Indications for Adjuvant Ear Acupuncture

- Bleeding during early and late pregnancy.
- Diseases related to pregnancy: emesis, hyperemesis, EPH (edema, proteinuria, hypertension) gestosis.
- Diseases unrelated to pregnancy.
- General infections during pregnancy.
- Imminent premature birth: premature rupture of membranes, preterm labor, cervical insufficiency, placental insufficiency.
- Preparation for labor and delivery.
- Induction of labor—with a mature cervix or immature cervix.
- Pain relief in labor and delivery.
- Dystocia: reduced, increased, or irregular uterine contractions.
- Postpartum: bleeding due to laceration, atony, placental retention.
- Puerperium: disturbed involution, puerperal mastitis, problems with breastfeeding.
- Mental problems during pregnancy, delivery, and puerperium.

Bleeding During Pregnancy

Bleeding in the First Trimester
This must be clarified using a proper list of differential diagnoses.

Imminent Abortion
- In cases of **imminent abortion**, adjuvant ear acupuncture (in addition to immobilization and, if necessary, progesterone medication) proves helpful, using the following:
  - Uterus point (58).
  - Uterus point according to Nogier.
  - Vegetative point II (34).
  - ACTH point (adrenal gland point) (13).
  - Ovary point (23).
  - And, if necessary, adrenal gland point (in the antihelical wall) and
  - Point zero (82).

Condition Following Recurrent Miscarriage
- In conditions following **recurrent miscarriage**, immunostimulating and psychotropic points are found to be irritated, namely:
  - Interferon point.
  - ACTH point (adrenal gland point) (13).
  - Thymus gland point.
  - Vegetative point I (51).
  - Vegetative point II (34).
  - The psychotropic points: frustration point, PT1 to PT4.

Bleeding in the Second and Third Trimesters
These are complications of pregnancy that must always be taken seriously as they may become a threat to both mother and child. Possible causes should be immediately clarified by differential diagnosis. The conventional therapy then depends on the particular cause.

In cases of **mild bleeding prior to week 37 of pregnancy** (e.g., a deep position of the placenta, partial placenta previa, indications for tocolysis and cerclage) and in cases of **heavy bleeding** (e.g., the onset of cervical opening), compression treatment is indicated.

- This is supplemented by needling of the following points:
  - Uterus point (58).
  - Uterus point according to Nogier.
  - ACTH point (adrenal gland point) (13).
  - Ovary point (gonadotropin point) (23).
  - Vegetative point II (34).
  - Endocrine zone (22).

If **fetal (umbilical) bleeding** is suspected, further therapy depends on the extent of the blood loss; cesarean section is indicated in most cases.

Practical Tip

From the point of view of Chinese medicine, heavy fetal (umbilical) bleeding leads to maternal and fetal symptoms of vacuity with vacuity in the *qi* of the kidney and spleen and concurrent liver dysfunction. Therefore, the following points should be needled: the kidney zone (95), liver zone (97), and spleen zone (98).

To enhance the effect on these, some Chinese schools suggest needling the following reflex points on the back of the ear: the kidney point (95 m), liver point (97 m), and spleen point (98 m).

Imminent Premature Birth

It goes without saying that the conventional therapy in line with well-known criteria has priority.
- Needling of the following ear points is recommended as an accompanying measure:
  - Uterus point (58).
  - Uterus point according to Nogier.
  - ACTH point (adrenal gland point) (13).
  - Ovary point (23).

Practical Tip

As premature birth results from rising liver *yang* in connection with *QI* weakness in the kidney and spleen, the following reflex zones should be examined using the "very point technique" (see p. 82): the kidney zone (95), liver zone (97), and spleen zone (98).

Vegetative problems such as **anxiety, worry, agitation**, and **nervousness** are often found in these patients, not least because of hospitalization and intensive care.
- We recommend the use of the following ear points:
  - Vegetative point I (51).
  - Vegetative point II (34).
  - Frustration point.
  - Heart zone (100).
  - Jerome point (29 b).
- If there is **pain**:
  - Sciatica zone (52)—using the sieving technique.
  - Thalamus point (26 a).
  - Analgesia point according to Nogier.
  - *Shen men* point (55).
  - Master omega point.
  - Omega II.

Complications of Pregnancy

In cases of relatively **mild hyperemesis gravidarum**, the metabolism is eased by changing the diet: frequent and small meals, food that is low in protein and salt, and vitamin supplementation, particularly with vitamin B.

In case of more **serious hyperemesis gravidarum**, which is associated with insufficient intake of food and liquid, acidosis, vitamin B deficiency, polyneuropathy, muscle weakness, rising bilirubin values, and increasing dehydration, admission to the hospital and intervention with infusion therapy is required.
- The **following** ear points are suitable in all cases of **hyperemesis**:
  - Point zero (82).
  - Jerome point (29 b).
- If the patient's history reveals **anxiety, worry,** and **ambivalence**, the following ear points should be needled, depending on their irritation:
  - PT1 to PT4.

Practical Tip

In order to compensate for the repletion in the stomach and liver channels, some Chinese schools (e.g., in Tianjin) also use the stomach zone (87), liver zone (97), and spleen zone (98).

EPH-gestosis (Fig. 9.7)

This syndrome is per definition associated with edema, proteinuria, and hypertension; it requires stress management and, if necessary, sedation, hypotensive medication, and possibly admission to the hospital.
- The following points are needled if **hypertension** is present:
  - Blood pressure control point (59).
  - Points in the antihypertension groove (105 m).
  - For treatment of **proteinuria**, good results were achieved in the TCM clinic in Tianjin by needling the following points: kidney zone (95), triple burner zone (104).
- In cases of **mental problems**—which, as we know from experience, are associated with most cases of EPH-gestosis—the autonomic system is imbalanced:
  - Vegetative point I (51).
  - Vegetative point II (34).
  - PT1 to PT4.
- In cases of **pain** during EPH-gestosis, the following points are used:
  - Sciatica zone (52) (using the sieving technique).
  - Thalamus point (26 a).
  - Analgesia point .
  - *Shen men* point (55).

With pre-existing **systemic diseases**, see the corresponding indications.

Addiction during Pregnancy

- If the pregnant woman is addicted to alcohol, nicotine, or other drugs, needling is carried out according to the National Acupuncture Detoxification Association (NADA) protocol (see **Fig. 9.16**), among others:
  - Vegetative point I (51) (in the United States of America: sympathetic point).
  - Kidney zone (95).
  - Liver zone (97).
  - Lung zone (101).
  - *Shen men* point (55).

See also Treatment of Addictions, page 156.

Infections during Pregnancy

- To support passive or active immunization, the following **immunomodulatory** points are very useful:
  - Thymus gland point.
  - Interferon point.
  - Allergy point (78).
  - ACTH point (adrenal gland point) (13).

┌─ *Practical Tip* ──────────────
│ The School of Chinese Medicine in Tianjin rec-
│ ommends using the following points in case
│ of vacuity of defense *qi* and kidney *yang*: the
│ spleen zone (98), liver zone (97), and kidney
│ zone (95).
└────────────────────────

- Most infections during pregnancy are associated with **mental and vegetative symptoms**; hence, it makes sense to needle the following points if they are sensitive:
  - Vegetative point I (51).
  - Vegetative point II (34).
  - Psychotropic points: frustration point and PT1 to PT4.

Premature Rupture of Membranes, Habitual Forms

The prevention of renewed premature rupture of membranes may be supported by ear acupuncture.
- After late abortions and early deliveries, and in cervical insufficiency, premature labor, multiple pregnancies, colpitis, and cervicitis, the following points may be used:
  - Uterus point (58).
  - Uterus point according to Nogier.

- Ovary point (23).
- Hypogastric plexus point.
- If the indications listed are associated with **mental symptoms** (nervousness, anxiety, worry, depressive mood, aggressiveness), psychotropic points are needled and, if necessary, also vegetative points:
  - Vegetative point I (51).
  - Vegetative point II (34).
  - Heart zone (100).
  - Jerome point (29 b) for muscle relaxation.
  - Frustration point, PT1 to PT4.

Pain

Pain Prior to Week 36 of Pregnancy

- As well as using causal conventional therapy, the corresponding and analgesic points may be needled as an accompanying measure:
  - Sciatica zone (52) (using the sieving technique).
  - Thalamus point (26 a).
  - Analgesia point according to Nogier.
  - *Shen men* point (55).
  - Occiput (29).
  - Jerome point (29 b).

Severe Attacks of Pain

- The following points may be included:
  - Omega point I.
  - Master omega point.
  - PT1 to PT4.

Colicky Pain

- In cases of dystocia, as well as in renal colic during pregnancy, it makes sense to include the following points because of their spasmolytic effect:
  - Point zero (82).
  - Retro-point zero (112 m).

Preparation for Labor and Delivery, after Week 36 of Pregnancy

- According to "Straubinger's scheme", the following points are recommended:
  - Uterus point (58).
  - ACTH point (adrenal gland point) (13).
  - Kidney zone (95).
  - Liver zone (97).
  - Spleen (98).

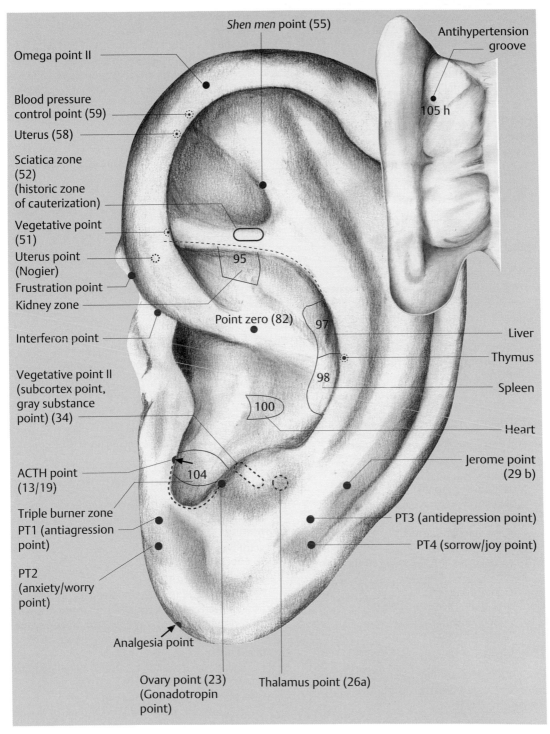

Fig. 9.7 Pool of points for EPH-gestosis.

- The following points prove helpful in case of **anxiety**, **worry**, **agitation**, and **nervousness**:
  - Vegetative point I (51).
  - Vegetative point II (34).
  - Jerome point (29 b).
  - Frustration point, PT1 to PT4.

Induction of Labor

- When further waiting is contraindicated or when the body's natural mechanisms of inducing labor do not start on their own, the following ear points are needled in support of conventional measures (**Fig. 9.8**):
  - Uterus point (58).
  - Uterus point according to Nogier.
  - ACTH point (adrenal gland point) (13).
  - Ovary point (23).
  - Hypogastric plexus point.
- The corresponding **vegetatively relaxing psychotropic points** have a harmonizing effect on the induction of labor (the "very point" technique):
  - Vegetative point I (51).
  - Vegetative point II (34).
  - Frustration point, PT1 to PT4.
  - Heart zone (100).
  - Jerome point (29 b).

Analgesia in Labor and Delivery

- The following points prove helpful (**Fig. 9.9**):
  - Sciatica zone (52) (using the sieving technique).
  - Thalamus point (26 a).
  - Analgesia point according to Nogier.
  - *Shen men* point (55).
  - Master omega point.
  - Omega point II.
- To compensate for *qi* vacuity in the kidney and spleen:
  - Kidney zone (95).
  - Liver zone (97).
  - Spleen zone (98).

Dystocia

Difficult childbirth may be treated with ear acupuncture once a precise differential diagnosis has been carried out.

Postpartum Period

- The following points have proved helpful in case of **bleeding due to laceration, abnormal placental detachment, postpartum hemorrhage, atony**, etc.:
  - Uterus point (58).
  - Uterus point according to Nogier.
  - ACTH point (adrenal gland point) (13).
  - Ovary point (23).
  - Kidney zone (95).
  - Liver zone (97).
  - Spleen zone (98).

Note. Particularly in cases of **bleeding due to laceration**, surgical intervention can be effectively supported by ear acupuncture if needling takes place during or immediately after complete emptying of the uterus. Experience has shown that the above-mentioned points are also effective in preventing abnormal placental detachment, e.g., in detachment anomalies resulting from previous deliveries. It has been observed time and again in the delivery room that the conventional medical therapy for a **retained placenta** can be rendered much more effective by ear acupuncture applied in advance.

- If manual **placental detachment** is considered, it should be preceded by needling of the following ear points:
  - Uterus point (58).
  - Uterus point according to Nogier.
  - Ovary point (23).
  - ACTH point (adrenal gland point) (13).

Puerperium (Fig. 9.10)

Adjuvant or preventively, two childbed conditions, puerperal mastitis and postpartum depression, can be successfully treated with ear acupuncture.

Puerperal mastitis

Acupuncture should be carried out as soon as possible for prophylactic treatment in multipara with previous mastitis and as a therapeutic measure in the puerperium for women with an onset of mastitis.

- The following ear points are also suitable to alleviate the **inflammation**:
  - Mammary gland point (44).
  - Mammary gland point according to Nogier (see **Fig. 3.16**).
  - Thorax point (42).
  - Liver zone (97).

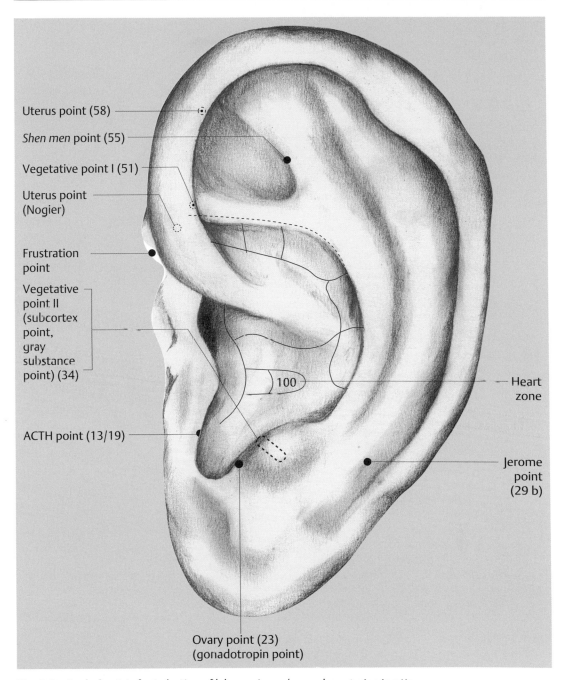

Uterus point (58)

Shen men point (55)

Vegetative point I (51)

Uterus point
(Nogier)

Frustration
point

Vegetative
point II
(subcortex
point,
gray
substance
point) (34)

ACTH point (13/19)

100

Heart
zone

Jerome
point
(29 b)

Ovary point (23)
(gonadotropin point)

Fig. 9.8 Pool of points for induction of labor: primary/secondary uterine inertia.

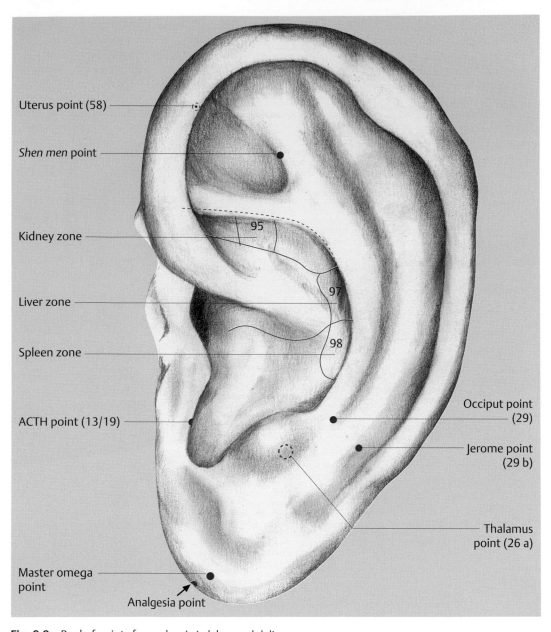

Fig. 9.9 Pool of points for analgesia in labor and delivery.

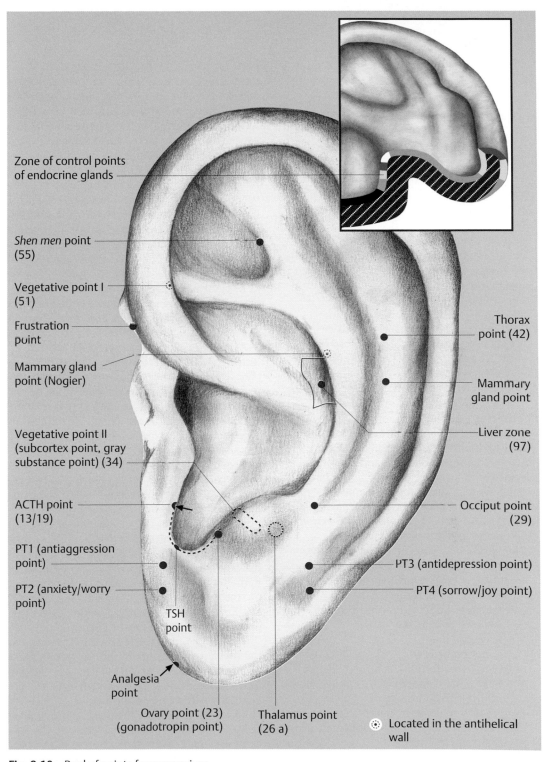

Zone of control points of endocrine glands

Shen men point (55)

Vegetative point I (51)

Frustration point

Mammary gland point (Nogier)

Vegetative point II (subcortex point, gray substance point) (34)

ACTH point (13/19)

PT1 (antiaggression point)

PT2 (anxiety/worry point)

TSH point

Analgesia point

Ovary point (23) (gonadotropin point)

Thalamus point (26 a)

Thorax point (42)

Mammary gland point

Liver zone (97)

Occiput point (29)

PT3 (antidepression point)

PT4 (sorrow/joy point)

⊛ Located in the antihelical wall

Fig. 9.10 Pool of points for puerperium.

- In cases of **severe pain** associated with **extensive mastitis**, we recommend the following points:
  - Thalamus point (26 a).
  - Analgesia point.
  - Occiput point (29).
  - *Shen men* point (55).

Practical Tip

The segmental approach has also proved successful in the treatment of puerperal mastitis. The line of treatment runs between the point zero (82) and the sensitive point found in the vegetative groove. The points indicated by the Chinese school are found here as well: the mammary point (44), thorax point (42), and liver zone (97). Nogier's mammary gland point in the zone of nervous control points of endocrine glands can be detected without difficulty using the segmental approach.

- The following points have proved helpful, if irritated:
  - ACTH point (adrenal gland point) (13).
  - Ovary point (23).
  - Vegetative point II (34).

Postpartum depression

The hormonal changes during puerperium can lead to serious mental problems, which are usually of a depressive nature and may manifest themselves in a variety of symptoms. About 50% of all puerpera suffer from a depressive mood ("the blues"), 15% fall ill with "postpartum neurosis," and 0.1 to 0.3% fall ill with the extremely problematic "postpartum psychosis."

- The following vegetative and psychotropic points are primarily used for the **prophylactic treatment** of postpartum depression:
  - Vegetative point I (51).
  - Vegetative point II (subcortex point, gray substance point) (34).
  - Frustration point.
  - Occiput point (29).
  - PT1 to PT4.
  - omega point II, master omega point, point R (according to Bourdiol).
- As mental problems in puerperium are usually the **result of hormonal changes**, endocrine points are also indicated:
  - Ovary point (gonadotropin point) (23).
  - Endocrine zone (22).

- ACTH point (adrenal gland point) (13).
- TSH point (thyroid gland point).

9.6.7 Infertility

We know from experience that the causes of male and female infertility are complex and that many aspects are still unexplained by science. As a result, most patients seek out acupuncture treatment only after a thorough diagnostic clarification and exhaustion of all conventional therapies. Possible causes have often been found in men, e.g., insufficient mobility and vitality of the spermatozoa, or low serum levels of luteinizing hormone, follicle-stimulating hormone, and testosterone. Distinct causes are far less often found in women, and in many cases acupuncture treatment can be carried out successfully even if infertility seems to result from hormonal imbalance.

It is usually sufficient to treat patients by either ear or body acupuncture. Only in difficult cases (e.g., verified severe hormonal imbalance) does it make sense to combine ear and body acupuncture.

As **primary** therapeutic access in cases of infertility, ear acupuncture has a range of points to choose from. All of these must be selected according to individual parameters, depending on the patient, and should be needled only if they are sensitive. First, the uterus point (58) and uterus zone (according to Nogier) should be mentioned, but also the ovary/testis point (according to Nogier) and ovary point (gonadotropin point) (23). Furthermore, it makes sense to search for less defined points in the endocrine zone (22), starting from the TSH point and proceeding in the direction of the concha. Frequently, the ACTH point (13) at the ventral end of the endocrine zone (22) and the adrenal gland point (nervous control point in the antihelical wall) may be included in the set of points. The hypogastric plexus point (in the superior concha) should be especially emphasized among the points of first choice, because it is sensitive in most cases.

Vegetative points I (51) and II (34), as well as the psychotropic points of the frustration point and antiaggression point (PT1) may be helpful for **supplementary** treatment, provided they are indicated by the patient's history.

According to Chinese medicine, hormonal activity in the human body is assigned to the kidney (*shen*) and liver (*gan*); therefore, the liver zone (97) and kidney zone (95) are included in the treatment, depending on their sensitivity.

Initially, a series of 10 treatments is carried out daily or every second day, if possible. Depending on their sensitivity, two or three points per ear are selected and needled alternately with other points found to be similarly sensitive.

Based on the idea that kidney vacuity may be the root of the problem, combination with the following **body acupuncture** points should be considered in order to strengthen the kidney: KI-3, BL-23 and, if necessary ST-26.

9.6.8 Loss of Libido

Sexual problems such as loss of libido and impotence result from complex psychovegetative processes. It goes without saying that they cannot be approached simply by ear or body acupuncture. These therapies have a purely supportive, but sometimes also initiating, effect, which prepares the patient to willingly undergo the required treatment through psychotherapy or sex therapy.

As the **primary** set of points, the most important libido points are the Bosch point on the ascending helix (external genitals point according to Nogier), ovary/testis point (according to Nogier), and hypogastric plexus point. For **supplementary** treatment, the zone of paravertebral chain of sympathetic ganglia at the lumbosacral level should be searched for irritated points. Again, these may possibly be combined with vegetative points I (51) and II (34), as well as the psychotropic reflex zones PT1 to PT4 and the frustration point.

Treatment is initially carried out twice a week and then once a week; five or six sessions will be required before any improvement is noticed. A total of approximately 10 to 15 treatments should be carried out.

9.7 Urinary Tract Disorders (Fig. 9.11)

9.7.1 Nocturnal Enuresis

This condition mainly affects children and, in rarer cases, also adolescents or adults. It usually has a psychosomatic background. Nevertheless, successful therapy can often be achieved by ear acupuncture alone. Younger patients should be exclusively treated with a laser stimulus rather than by needling.

Occasionally, it is recommended that the treatment be accompanied by psychotherapy. The following reflex zones are treated **primarily**: the urinary bladder zone (92) as well as hypogastric plexus point, thalamus point (26 a), and occiput point (29). Furthermore, the urethra point (80) and kidney zone (95) should be considered.

The following points should be taken into consideration as **supplementary** points: vegetative point I (51), vegetative point II (34), and the psychotropic points.

Two or three points are treated initially every 2 days, and the maximum number of points should not be greater than five. After 3 to 4 days of treatment, the frequency is changed to two sessions per week. If therapy is successful, it can be terminated after 10 sessions; in severe cases, it should be extended. If the results are less than optimal, a second treatment series may become necessary.

9.7.2 Irritable Bladder

Irritable bladder is rarely caused by pathological changes of the bladder itself. However, there is no reason why it should be described as purely psychogenic. It is conceivable that it results from hyperactive dysfunction of the terminal section of the urinary tract. Experience shows that, in cases of irritable bladder, only the organ-related reflex zones, such as the urinary bladder zone (92), urethra point (80), and hypogastric plexus point, and possibly complementing vegetative or psychotropic points, are found to be irritated.

According to the concept of Chinese medicine, this condition is due to vacuity of kidney *qi* (*shen*); therefore, strengthening of the kidney *qi* is achieved through the kidney zone (95). Once again, vegetative point II (34) and vegetative point I (34) may be needled.

It is recommended that treatment initially be carried out every day or every second day, changing to two sessions per week upon improvement. As a rule, treatment can be successfully terminated after a series of 10 to 12 sessions.

9.7.3 Urinary Incontinence

This condition, which is fairly common and does not only occur in old people, usually becomes a reason for treatment by body or ear acupuncture only after extensive urological diagnostic clarification and ineffective drug therapy. Urinary

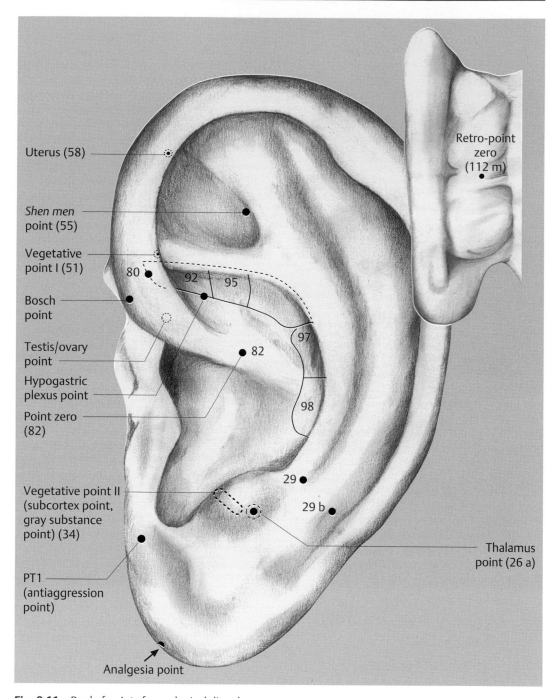

Fig. 9.11 Pool of points for urological disorders.

incontinence is frequently associated with rectal incontinence, thus leading to considerable social restrictions. Patients are subject to extensive suffering, as they cannot help losing some urine or stool when coughing, sneezing, or experiencing other involuntary abdominal pressure.

The **primary** therapeutic access in ear acupuncture lies predominantly in the organ-related reflex zones, such as the urinary bladder zone (92), urethra point (80), and hypogastric plexus point. In most cases, the point zero (diaphragm point) (82) is also sensitive. Its tonifying effect on the intestinal smooth muscles is relevant in this case and may be enhanced by including retro-point zero (112 m) on the back of the ear.

According to the concept of Chinese medicine, the disorder is caused by vacuity of kidney *qi*, particularly in older people. Therefore, it is important to strengthen this *qi* by including the kidney zone (95). The following points are included as **supplementary** points: the liver zone (97), spleen zone (98), and uterus point (58), if they are sensitive. In our own experience, it including vegetative points I (51) and II (34) in the treatment has proved successful.

Treatment begins with intervals of 2 days and then changes to two sessions per week once the symptoms start to improve. Only two or three points per session are needled, alternating with other points from session to session. Improvement of symptoms may be expected after a series of six to eight sessions. Although complete freedom from symptoms is achieved only in rare cases, a tolerable situation can be brought about through repeated treatments planned over a long period of time. By extending the treatment intervals step by step, the question of how to achieve long-term, treatment-independent freedom from symptoms should be explored. Pointing this out is important because many patients return for treatment too early, even before any further deterioration of their condition.

9.7.4　Urinary Retention

Treatment of urinary retention by ear acupuncture competes with conventional medical measures, ranging from spasmolytic medication to emergency catheterization and suprapubic bladder puncture. Treatment with ear acupuncture is usually taken into consideration only in the initial phase. The use of acupuncture in the

extreme case of *acute urinary retention*, whatever the cause may be, is indicated only in an emergency when it is impossible to relieve the bladder by catheterization or bladder puncture within a reasonable time. With this in mind, the description below deals only with *non-acute urinary retention*, e.g., in postoperative or posttraumatic situations, although the same reflex zones are indicated for acute cases.

For **primary** treatment, the hypogastric plexus point and point zero (82) with its spasmolytic effect are selected. The corresponding areas of the urinary bladder zone (92), kidney zone (95), and urethra point (80) may be added. Furthermore, it has proved helpful to enhance the effect of point zero (82) by including retro-point zero (112 m). Experience has shown that it is also helpful to make use of the relaxing properties of the occiput point (29) and Jerome point (29 b). Two or three points are needled bilaterally and stimulated at intervals of 15 minutes by rotating the needle. This means that the needles remain in place longer than usual, i.e., up to 60 minutes. The effect usually takes place within 1 hour after termination of acupuncture, if not, the procedure may be repeated with a different set of points. It is, however, advisable to also treat or combine alternately with the established points of **body acupuncture**: BL-32, SP-9, and also CV-4 and CV-6.

This alternating approach can especially be used in *recurrent urinary retention*. Different sets of points may be used for ear acupuncture, as long as the points are found to be irritated. The method is very effective especially in the postoperative state; it is recommended that the patient already be informed prior to surgery about the possibility of acupuncture treatment to avoid urinary retention, so that preventive ear acupuncture may be started in the recovery room. During recovery, only two or three sensitive points are usually found, namely, in the region of the organ-related reflex zones, such as urinary bladder zone (92) or hypogastric plexus point, as well as vegetative points such as vegetative points I (51) and II (34).

9.7.5　Renal and Ureteral Colic

As a rule, colic of the kidney and ureter have to be treated with drugs according to standard medical principles. Nevertheless, the possibility of efficient treatment by ear acupuncture should be introduced here. Apart from the fact that a causal therapy, such as lithiasis or infection, is absolutely essential, it is possible to reduce the frequency of colics by acupuncture and to keep the pain of the colic itself tolerable for the patient.

Note. On principle, in such conditions of pain (not just with colics), the needles must remain in place longer than usual, even up to several hours. If the pain increases, the needle stimulus should be intensified by gentle rotation of the needle.

In the acute phase, the following **primary** points are important: the kidney zone (95) and urinary bladder zone (92), and also the spasmolytic point zero (diaphragm point) (82) and its counterpart retro-point zero or bifurcation point (112 m). Particularly worth mentioning for this phase are the anesthetic points of the thalamus point (26 a), analgesia point, hypogastric plexus point, and vegetative point II (34).

These **supplementary** points may also be considered: vegetative point I (51), the *shen men* point (55), and the ACTH point (13). They play an important role particularly in preventive and intermediate treatment.

Another route of therapeutic access is provided by segment therapy. In cases of kidney or ureteral colic, an irritated reflex zone is often found in the cranial part of the vegetative groove, approximately at the level of the darwinian tubercle. Although this zone by itself is in need of treatment, it also forms a line of treatment together with point zero (82). On this line, other less well-defined but very effective points may be found. Needling of these points may also be helpful during the acute treatment, especially if there is referred pain.

With this method, in place of or complementing spasmolytic medication, it is also possible to promote the spontaneous passage of stones by treating regularly every 2 days and using alternating sets of points.

9.8 Diseases of the Locomotor System (Fig. 9.12)

Diseases of the locomotor system (and also the conditions listed in the chapter on neurological disorders) can effectively be treated by ear acupuncture. However, here it should especially be pointed out that a focal process or area disturbance can interfere with the effect of acupuncture. Such foci and area disturbances can repeatedly or persistently lead to functional disturbances in all regulatory systems, not just the auricular system. These systems then become unstable, and reactions to minor stimuli become abnormal, i.e., exaggerated. For the locomotor system, this means unnecessary hyperactivity of the neuromuscular system in the form of pseudoradicular myospasms and pain syndromes, which are far more intense in a body unburdened with toxins.

In such cases, both ear and body acupuncture—when used strictly in the symptom-oriented way as part of a point regimen—will achieve at best only temporary relief of the symptoms. Even local or minor general stimuli may lead to a reappearance of symptoms because the therapy does not address the underlying cause of the regulatory disturbance. Hence, it is a very important aspect of ear acupuncture treatment to consider also the possibility of focal processes and to arrange for a removal of septic foci (if this is possible), or at least to treat the disturbed area with neural therapy.

Information on a possible area disturbance is usually found in the patient's history but also as hyperactive reflex zones on the auricle, which may be considered as diagnostic clues.

9.8.1 Cervical Syndrome

The cervical syndrome is characterized by various pain conditions that share a common localization, predominantly in the neck region and radiating into the shoulder, arm, and suboccipital-occipital region. It can have many different causes, most of them of a functional nature (e.g., the result of chronically bad posture). They range from *degenerative changes* in the spinal column to the classic *whiplash injury* and acute *muscular torticollis*. Accordingly, relatively uniform sets of points are selected for the relief of acute pain, whereas individually different points are selected for prophylaxis and intermediate treatment. Provided the appropriate preconditions and opportunities exist, **manual therapy** may be preferred or used in combination with ear acupuncture.

Within the framework of ear acupuncture, segment therapy as part of Nogier's **ear geometry** has proved to be an elegant and very successful

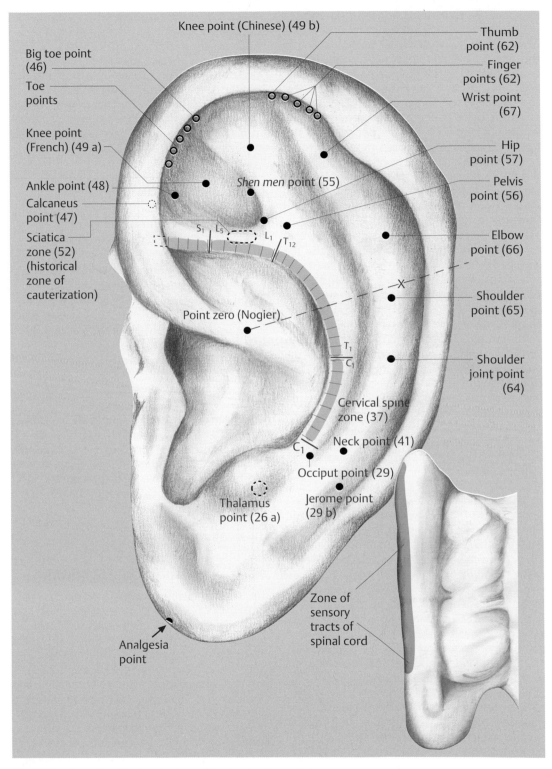

Knee point (Chinese) (49 b)

Thumb point (62)

Big toe point (46)

Finger points (62)

Toe points

Wrist point (67)

Knee point (French) (49 a)

Hip point (57)

Shen men point (55)

Ankle point (48)

Pelvis point (56)

Calcaneus point (47)

Elbow point (66)

Sciatica zone (52) (historical zone of cauterization)

S_1 L_5 L_1 T_{12}

X

Shoulder point (65)

Point zero (Nogier)

T_1
C_1

Shoulder joint point (64)

Cervical spine zone (37)

Neck point (41)

C_1

Occiput point (29)

Thalamus point (26 a)

Jerome point (29 b)

Zone of sensory tracts of spinal cord

Analgesia point

Fig. 9.12 Pool of points for diseases of the locomotor system.

approach for painful conditions in the cervical region. The vegetative groove is first searched for irritated points at the C1 to C7 level. While doing this, the Jerome point (29 b) will also be found to be sensitive. Its muscle-relaxing, and hence analgesic, effect turns it into a standard point for diseases of the locomotor system. By connecting one or two irritated points in the vegetative groove with point zero (82) (which is not irritated), different segmental assignments corresponding to the symptoms can be made. The neck point (41) and cervical spine zone (37) described by the Chinese school, both located in the zone of paravertebral muscles and ligaments, are frequently found along the imaginary segmental line of treatment.

Furthermore, the *shen men* point (55) and, especially with suboccipital symptoms, also the occiput point (29) are usually sensitive. In severe conditions of pain in this area (e.g., after whiplash or in acute torticollis), the thalamus point (26 a) should definitely be included. When examining the line of segmental treatment, special attention should also be paid to the zone of paravertebral chain of sympathetic ganglia (at the transition of the antihelix to the inferior concha). Here, irritations may be detected that cannot always be assigned to the familiar localizations, such as the superior, middle, and inferior cervical ganglion points (the latter also called stellate ganglion point). In addition, sensitive points are frequently found in the projection zone of the sensory part of the zone of spinal cord (on the helical brim). In view of a possible vegetative and psychosomatic component, vegetative points I (51) and II (34) and psychotropic areas PT2 and PT1 and the frustration point are recommended as **supplementary** points. Last but not least is the projection zone of the neck muscles on the back of the ear antihelical sulcus.

According to the concept of Chinese medicine, treatment depends on which of the channels is affected. Increasing pain while inclining or reclining the head corresponds to *tai yang*, the pair of the bladder/small intestine channels (BL/SI); hence, bladder zone (92) and small intestine zone (89) should be needled as well.

If pain increases while turning the head to the right or left, the condition is assigned to *shao yang*, the pair of the gallbladder/triple burner channels (GB/TB). In this case, treatment includes the gallbladder zone (96) and liver zone (97) depending on their sensitivity. Experience has

shown that, in the case of cervical syndrome, the segmental approach is most successful, as symptoms subside quickly within 2 to 3 days.

If necessary, *acute* treatment can be performed daily or every 2 days. It is recommended that the needles be left in place beyond the usual 30 minutes, as needed. After four or five sessions, a tolerable condition will be achieved, and treatments can be reduced to once a week until the symptoms have finally subsided.

Practical Tip

Two sessions per week have proved successful in *chronically recurrent* processes; this can be reduced to one treatment per week if the response is good. Repeated treatment series of 10 to 15 sessions each are required; these should be carried out in combination with specific **kinesitherapy** for correcting, e.g., bad posture (e.g., the Rolfing, Feldenkrais, or similar methods). Experience has shown that ear acupuncture can actually help make kinesitherapies or conventional physiotherapeutic exercises possible in the first place because it is so effective.

Combination with **body acupuncture** has proved helpful in cases of severe chronicity. If the *tai yang* axis, the pair of the bladder/small intestine channels (BL/SI), is affected, treatment includes the body acupoints BL-2, BL-10, and BL-60, as well as SI-3. If the *shao yang* axis, the pair of the gallbladder/triple burner channels (GB/TB), is affected, the following acupoints may be treated: GB-20, GB-42, and TB-15.

9.8.2 Cervicobrachial Syndrome

The cervicobrachial syndrome may have many causes; in cases of severe chronicity, these lead to lasting changes in the muscles and ligament system, possibly with participation of the joints in the area of the shoulder girdle. The primary causes are cervical pseudoradicular irritation, cervical disk prolapse, and posttraumatic and postoperative irritation. Such syndromes may also result from humeroscapular periarthritis. Differentiation of this syndrome according to ventral, lateral, or dorsal pain in the shoulder (as we know it from body acupuncture) does not play a role in choosing the points for ear acupuncture.

Once again, the **primary** approach takes advantage of the established segment therapy. Here, one or two sensitive points are found in the vegetative groove, at approximately the C6 to T8 level. Along the segmental line of treatment established through the connection with point zero (82), irritated points are usually found in the zone of paravertebral muscles and ligaments, and these may correspond to the master points of the Chinese school, such as the shoulder point (65) and shoulder joint point (64). Naturally, with certain identified causes (e.g., cervical disk prolapse), the zone of intervertebral disks (located beneath the antihelical edge toward the concha) should also be considered. Additional essential points can be found in the zone of spinal cord (with its sensory parts on the helix) and further points in the projection zone of the shoulder muscles on the back of the auricle.

Important points in this connection are also the occiput point (29) and Jerome point (29 b) and, with its analgesic and anti-inflammatory effect, as well the *shen men* point (55). With respect to *acute* traumatic processes (e.g., shoulder joint dislocation), one should recall the strong, general anesthetic effect of the thalamus point (26 a) in combination with the analgesia point. In such acute situations, it is possible to bring about sufficient pain relief during repositioning by needling the *shen men* point (55), occiput point (29), and Jerome point (29 b), as well as the thalamus point (26 a) and analgesia point. After successful repositioning, acupuncture may be continued during the follow-up treatment using the segmental approach described above.

The same procedure is carried out following relief from acute pain in the shoulder. During follow-up treatment and during the intermediate treatment of *chronic* shoulder–hand syndrome, the recommendation is to use individual sets of points including the segmental approach, depending on the response. The thalamus point (26 a) and analgesia point are usually no longer detectable, while in the combined point selection the ACTH point/adrenal gland point (13) remains relevant.

According to the concept of Chinese medicine, it is important to consider—as discussed above under Cervical Syndrome—the main localization of pain together with the resulting channel pair. In case of *ventral* pain in the shoulder, for example, mainly the pair of the lung/spleen channels (LU/SP) is affected, and hence the lung zone (101) as well as spleen zone (98) should be examined for sensitivity. With *lateral* pain in the shoulder, the pairs of the stomach/large intestine channels (ST/ LI) and of the gallbladder/triple burner channels (GB/TB) predominate according to the classic understanding. Therefore, the stomach zone (87) and large intestine zone (90) as well as the pancreas/gallbladder zone (96) are supposed to exhibit sensitive points.

In cases of *dorsal* pain in the shoulder, the pair of the bladder/small intestine channels (BL/SI) is affected. Hence, the bladder zone (92) and small intestine zone (89) should be included according to the Chinese school.

In addition to these assignments, treatment of the above conditions is also combined with **body acupuncture**, especially if they run difficult or chronic courses; the corresponding points are selected according to the affected channels. Depending on the acute or chronic state of the symptoms, treatment distinguishes between distal points and local points. For example, with ventral pain in the shoulder, one should consider including body acupoint LU-2 as a local point, whereas LU-5 or SP 9, as well as ST-38, may be included as distal points. In combination treatment of lateral pain in the shoulder, acupoints LI-15 and TB-14 are available as local points, while ST-36 and ST-38, as well as GB-34, are distal points.

Finally, for dorsal pain in the shoulder, the acupoints SI-9, SI-11, and SI-12 are local points, and BL-60, SI-3, and ST-38 are distal points.

Treatment intervals are 1 to 2 days in the *acute* phase, and approximately five sessions should be planned. After the symptoms have improved, this may be reduced to two sessions per week and finally to one session per week. Depending on the severity, a total of 10 to 14 sessions may be required.

In *chronic* processes, treatment starts with two sessions per week, and this may be reduced to one session per week, depending on the course of the condition. Two series of 10 sessions each are usually required, with a treatment-free interval of 1 to 2 weeks.

9.8.3 Lumbago, Lumbago–Sciatica Syndrome

Considering that ear acupuncture was rediscovered due to the observation of scars derived from cauterization in the sciatica zone (52) in Algerian immigrants, lumbago and lumbago–sciatica syndrome are the classical indications of this therapy. These syndromes may have many different causes, which should prompt the physician to establish a detailed diagnosis. The possible causes include gynecological, urological, and intestinal diseases, which may affect the lumbar region through reflexes. It goes without saying that, apart from these, degenerative diseases of the spinal column, bad posture, arthrodesis, and psychosomatic processes should be considered as well.

The lumbago–sciatica syndrome is often associated with the protrusion or prolapse of an intervertebral disk. Accordingly, it may exist with or without loss of neurological function. Conventional measures usually predominate so that, even in severe cases, patient, if they so desire, can be treated with ear acupuncture or a combination of ear and body acupuncture, after giving them proper information on possible conventional therapeutic measures, such as surgical interventions if the symptoms get worse.

With regard to the choice of points, ear acupuncture does not distinguish between lumbago and lumbago–sciatica syndrome. Selection from the points available is made according to their sensitivity. However, it is important to compile a number of points first, depending on the patient's history and clinical symptoms, before examining them systematically for sensitivity.

Following the repeatedly described approach of segment therapy, the practitioner may try the segmental assignment of symptoms with this syndrome, first clinically and then through the corresponding reflex zones on the auricle. However, the latter is not done primarily through the vegetative groove, for experience has shown that this zone is not representative enough in the region past the thoracolumbar transition. Instead, first the sensitive points in the zone of paravertebral muscles and ligaments close to the inferior antihelical crus are located to establish the segmental line of treatment. Here, the sciatica zone (52) and also the area beyond the L5 to S1 transition must be considered. These points are then connected to the point zero (82) (which are not irritated) to form the line of treatment. Additional useful points may be found also along this line in the triangular fossa, on the superior antihelical crus, possibly in the vegetative groove and in the area of the helical brim.

If several sensitive points in the sciatica zone (52) require needling, this should preferably be carried out by the "sieving" technique rather than by subcutaneous threading of L1 to L5, as recommended by the Chinese school. Experience has shown that needling only the sciatica zone (52), as suggested by the Chinese school, has not proved successful.

In the acute phase, the following analgesic points are treated first: the *shen men* point (55), thalamus point (26 a), and analgesia point (at the ventral edge of the lobule, at the level of the master omega point), and the muscle-relaxing Jerome point (29 b).

During the phase of subsiding symptoms or during chronic processes, the following **supplementary** points are included: the ACTH point (13) and adrenal gland point (the nervous control point in the antihelical wall), as well as vegetative points I (51) and II (34). In this phase, the thalamus point (26 a) is usually no longer detectable. Frequently, the following psychotropic points are sensitive: PT1 (antiaggression point), PT2 (anxiety/worry point), PT3 (antidepression point), and PT4 (sorrow/ joy point). In addition, both the master omega point and omega point II may play a vital role during this phase.

First, the ipsilateral auricle with regard to the site of symptoms is searched for sensitivities and needled. Only afterwards can the contralateral side be treated. After treatment on the ipsilateral auricle, the irritated points are found to be less distinct on the contralateral auricle and do not always correspond to the ipsilateral points. This is normal and, in terms of an extinction phenomenon, may suggest a choice of points.

Once the acute symptoms have subsided, physical exercise should be introduced in the form of specific physiotherapy and backstroke swimming in order to strengthen the paravertebral muscles.

9.8.4 Knee Pain

This nonspecific symptom may have many different causes and requires thorough diagnostic clarification. If caused by underlying structural alterations in the knee joint that are definitely in need of surgical therapy, ear acupuncture may only make sense as an adjuvant to analgesic and antiphlogistic therapy. This applies especially to the postoperative phase of mobilization so that analgesic and antiphlogistic drugs can be spared and the possible side effects associated with them avoided.

Ear acupuncture has turned out to be very successful in chronically recurrent gonarthrosis during both acute episodes and symptom-free periods.

The **primary** points for treatment of *acute knee pain* are initially selected independently of the cause, no matter whether the cause is arthrosis, trauma, or the postoperative situation. The following points predominate: the two knee points (49 a, 49 b), *shen men* point (55), and Jerome point (29 b). Frequently, the ACTH point (13) is also found to be sensitive during this phase.

With the objective of alleviating pain as soon as possible, three or four of the points listed are selected for the first treatment. The thalamus point (26 a) and analgesia point are rarely sensitive. Whenever possible, treatment is carried out daily with alternating sets of points selected from the points listed above until the pain substantially subsides. During follow-up treatment and intermediate treatment, the ACTH point (13) and one of the two knee points (depending on the underlying cause of the pain) become more important. One knee point (49 a) is usually found to be sensitive in cases of arthrosis, while the other knee point (49 b) is more often detected in case involving distortion of the joint and postoperative conditions in which only the capsule and ligaments are affected.

Practical Tip

In the *acute phase* of a painful disorder of the knee joint, both knee points are detectable; hence, both are needled independent of the cause.

During follow-up and intermediate treatment, the zone of paravertebral muscles and ligaments should definitely be examined for sensitive reflex zones of the lower extremity (e.g., the Thigh POINT in the area of scapha or superior antihelical crus). Treatment begins primarily on the ipsilateral auricle; depending on the sensitivity of the **supplementary** points, it may then be continued on the contralateral auricle.

In cases of *chronic knee pain*, combination with **body acupuncture** should be considered from the outset as much better results can be obtained this way. Note that, with regard to the selection of points, body acupuncture—unlike ear acupuncture—distinguishes between lateral, dorsal, and medial knee pain. For example, body acupoints ST-35 and ST-36 as well as GB-34 are considered for lateral knee pain, whereas acupoints SP-9 and LI-8 are for medial knee pain. These are exclusively local points that can be combined well with ear acupuncture, especially in chronic cases.

In cases of response to the therapy, it is recommended that the patient be encouraged to do specific nonstraining body exercises, e.g., bicycling. Until such time that the atrophic quadriceps muscle of the thigh is sufficiently strengthened, the thigh point (on the superior antihelical crus) will be be easily detected; hence, it should be needled on both ears.

9.8.5 Coxalgia

Criteria similar to those described for knee pain also apply to coxalgia. Particularly in cases of pain in the hip, diagnostic clarification requires special attention as there is an increased risk that severe, albeit rare, causes may be masked or not treated properly because of the anesthetic effect of ear or body acupuncture. Such causes of coxalgia include, e.g., adolescent coxa vara (slipped upper femoral epiphysis) and coxitis.

Following a thorough diagnostic clarification, coxalgia can be successfully treated by means of the auricular microsystem, using different sets of points.

Two approaches should be considered as the **primary** therapeutic access: the segmental therapeutic approach and the use of reflex zones. Segmental diagnosis and therapy have proved successful in cases when none of the corresponding reflex zones is responsive. This does not necessarily apply to coxalgia because the reflex zones hip point (hip joint point) (57) and lumbar spine zone (40) are well defined and easy to find. The area of the vegetative groove almost cranial to the thoracolumbar transition is possibly not sufficiently reliable for finding the corresponding line of treatment by means of an irritated point. It is possible to proceed by means of the correlating hip point (hip joint point) (57), as well as possibly irritated points found in the area of the thigh point (at the beginning of the superior antihelical crus) and in the sciatica zone (52) (on the inferior antihelical crus). If irritated points are detected in these reflex zones, treatment can be carried out in combination with segment therapy independently of the vegetative groove. By using point zero and an irritated point in the area of hip point (57) or sciatica zone (52), the line of treatment is established. Here, too this approach has turned out to be successful as additional points—although not well defined, but in need of treatment—can be found along this line (e.g., on the superior antihelical crus or the corresponding part of the cranial scapha).

Apart from the primary approach, the **supplementary** points play an important role in the treatment of coxalgia: first of all, analgesic and antiphlogistic points, such as the *shen men* point (55) and ACTH point (13), but also the prostaglandin point (on the dorsal part of the lobule), thalamus point (26 a), and muscle-relaxing Jerome point (29 b). In *acute processes*, the analgesia point should be considered in addition to thalamus point (26 a). It should be searched for on the ventral edge of the lobule and, in conditions of severe pain, needled in combination with the thalamus point (26 a).

In all symptoms of the locomotor system, the groups of muscles located close to the center of pain and affected by reflexes are a major component of the pain syndrome. Therefore, the muscle groups assigned to the symptom should be treated as well, not just through the Jerome point (29 b) and its counterpart on the back of the ear (retro-Jerome point), but also through the motor reflex zones on the back of the ear. With of coxalgia, the motor area of the lumbar and hip regions, as well as the thigh muscles, should be considered. For this purpose, the sulci of the superior and inferior antihelical crus on the back of the ear are searched for irritated points.

Practical Tip

With *chronically recurrent processes* and the associated emotional burdens they carry, both omega point II and the master omega point should be taken into consideration as supplementary points if they are irritated. Furthermore, a possible combination with body acupuncture can be considered, for which the local acupoints BL-29 and BL-30 are available. In cases of acute, singularly occurring symptoms, ear acupuncture is usually entirely sufficient to achieve a quick and lasting improvement.

9.8.6 Distortion and Contusion of Joints

With these forms of injury, it is essential to establish a proper diagnosis to exclude, above all, fractures or severe ligament injuries that require the appropriate conventional care. Here, acupuncture may only be used as an accompanying measure, e.g., for anesthesia or to reduce swelling. In the acute phase of joint distortions and contusions, it is always sensible not to economize on established accompanying measures, such as immobilization of the joint or application of cold compresses. In the initial phase, ear acupuncture is performed once or twice a day, followed by twice a week once the pain and swelling have subsided. Under the cover of the treatment—with the needles in place—body exercises may be started, although carefully and not beyond the limits of pain tolerance. In total, a series of approximately 10 sessions is usually sufficient.

The **primary** treatment is started by using the reflex zone (corresponding point) of the affected joint. For the knee joint, both knee points (49 a, 49 b) should be examined. The *shen men* point (55) and Jerome point (29 b) will also be found to be sensitive. When the joints of the upper extremity are affected, initially applying segment therapy has proved successful. Starting from the vegetative groove (zone of origin of sympathetic nuclei) and connecting it to point zero (82), a line of treatment is established in the area of scapha and helical brim for the detection of unnamed irritated points related to the affected joint. The zone of paravertebral chain of sympathetic ganglia (located in the antihelical wall) sometimes also contains sensitive points.

The vegetative groove can no longer be used for segment therapy because of limited diagnostic potential superior to the thoracolumbar transition. Nevertheless, even when the lower extremity is affected, a line of treatment may be established only through the corresponding joint points; along this line, injury-related yet undefined points can be found.

The ACTH point (13) is often sensitive on the second or third day after injury—and plays a role as **supplementary** point similar to the prostaglandin point.

Note. If the complaint is persistent, one should arrange for further radiological clarification, even if radiographs have initially been diagnostic, and after initial success by ear acupuncture. In particular, physicians who rarely deal with orthopedics or surgery should be reminded of this, which is of special importance with injuries of the wrist or carpus.

9.9 Neurological Disorders (Fig. 9.13)

Of the neurological syndromes, acute and chronically recurring pain conditions are among the best established indications for ear acupuncture. However, with other neurological syndromes of a similar chronic nature that are associated with paresis and paresthesia (such as the postapoplexy state), treatment by ear acupuncture is feasible, although only in combination with other therapeutic procedures and, if necessary, also with body acupuncture or scalp acupuncture. For these indications, spectacular healing results should not be expected, but rather alleviation or partial reversion at best, depending on the destroyed area and the accompanying functional disturbances. The promising case study by Faltz (1996) on multiple sclerosis should be mentioned in this context. This demonstrated that, even in a chronic syndrome with periodic attacks and an unfavorable prognosis, the combined use of ear and body acupuncture was able to bring about an impressive and relatively constant relief of symptoms.

Favorable results can usually be expected from treatment by ear acupuncture for the following neurological conditions involving pain, both the acute and chronically recurrent types.

9.9.1 Cephalalgia

Headache, with all its different variants, including migraine, is one of the most frequent of all symptoms. In most cases, only the chronically recurrent form of cephalalgia will be treated by ear acupuncture, either in the symptom-free period or in the acute phase. It is only when the patient is motivated by certain feelings—such as an intolerance of, or aversion to, drugs combined with a deep confidence in the body's power to heal itself—that the opportunity for ear acupuncture presents itself. Independently of the syndrome diagnosed by the pain therapist, neurological clarification should precede treatment, or at least be carried out in parallel. This is vitally important as a malignant process may be the underlying cause of cephalalgia; fortunately, however, this is seldom the case.

Another important step toward ear acupuncture is classification of the headache by means of the patient's history and clinical findings, not just in the Western sense (e.g., as cluster headache or Horton's syndrome), but also to grasp it as a syndrome: the challenge is to determine and differentiate the trigger mechanisms (e.g., bright light), accompanying symptoms (e.g., nausea), patterns of distribution (cervicooccipital), time course, duration, and similar criteria, in order to draw conclusions concerning the affected reflex zone to be treated according to its irritation. Very distinct sets of points can be determined in this way; these are essentially based on the selection of standard points listed below.

Using the inverted embryo as a mnemonic aid, it is easy to grasp why the most important points for treating headaches are found in the caudal part of the auricle. The following anatomical structures should be considered in the first place: antitragus, postantitragal fossa, and lobule.

During the *acute phase* of a headache, the following corresponding points along the sensory line are available as **primary** points: occiput point (29), sun point (35), and forehead point (33). In addition, the thalamus point (26 a) is very effective during this phase when combined with the analgesia point (at the ventral edge of the lobule). Furthermore, vegetative points I (51) and II (34) should also be considered.

From these "acute" points, different combinations are to be selected according to sensitivity and individual circumstances. It should be kept in mind that the limit is set at three to five needles per auricle. According to Chinese specifications, the *shen men* point (55) and the actual allergy point (78) (at the tip of the ear) are very effective in headache attacks, the latter point being stimulated during the acute phase by means of microphlebotomy.

Cephalalgia is expected to subside at the end of the session; a relatively stable and pain-free condition can be brought about in three or four sessions at intervals of 2 days.

This is followed by treatment in the *symptom-free phase* or interval. Here, mainly the

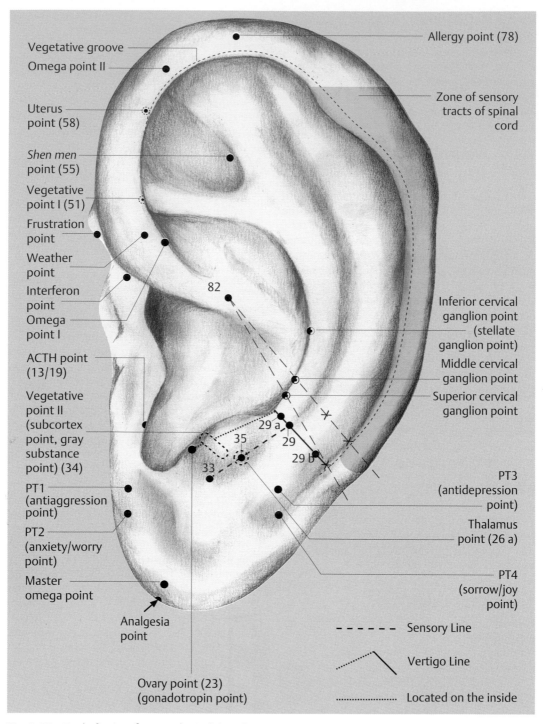

Vegetative groove

Omega point II

Uterus
point (58)

Shen men
point (55)

Vegetative
point I (51)

Frustration
point

Weather
point

Interferon
point

Omega
point I

ACTH point
(13/19)

Vegetative
point II
(subcortex
point, gray
substance
point) (34)

PT1
(antiaggression
point)

PT2
(anxiety/worry
point)

Master
omega point

Analgesia
point

Ovary point (23)
(gonadotropin point)

Allergy point (78)

Zone of sensory
tracts of spinal
cord

Inferior cervical
ganglion point
(stellate
ganglion point)

Middle cervical
ganglion point

Superior cervical
ganglion point

PT3
(antidepression
point)

Thalamus
point (26 a)

PT4
(sorrow/joy
point)

Sensory Line

Vertigo Line

Located on the inside

82

29 a

35   29

29 b

33

Fig. 9.13   Pool of points for neurological disorders.

supplementary points need to be selected, including those reflex zones which relate to the trigger mechanisms or accompanying circumstances of the individual case at hand. These reflex zones include the psychotropic points on the lobule, such as PT1 (antiaggression point), PT2 (anxiety/worry), PT4 (sorrow/joy point) and PT3 (antidepression point), and also the master omega point and omega point I. It should be kept in mind that often only a few or just one of these recommended points may be sensitive. In case of symptoms originating from the cervical spine region and caused by a bad posture, the segmental approach may be considered. Here, the vegetative groove at the cervical spine level, C1 to C7, is of great help when starting the search for additional sensitive points. Depending on the symptoms, the muscle-relaxing Jerome point (29 b) may be treated too.

In cases of *tension headache*, the search for points is extended to the thoracic spine level. While searching along the line of treatment, starting from the vegetative groove, one will often encounter the shoulder point (65) in the zone of paravertebral muscles and ligaments.

> **Practical Tip**
>
> In chronic headache (e.g., the common case of *permanent cephalalgia* in which temporarily occurring phases of aggravation predominate), vegetative point II (gray substance point, 34) is usually found also to be irritated; in this case, it is one of the most effective **supplementary** points.

With respect to trigger mechanisms (which play a major role especially in migraine; see below), the following points need to be considered: the weather point, uterus point (58), and ovary point (23).

According to the concept of Chinese medicine, headache is caused by a disturbance in the *qi* of the blood (*xui*) in three pairs of channels (small intestine/bladder, triple burner/gallbladder, and large intestine/stomach channels), by either external or internal disease factors. The corresponding areas on the auricle are treated depending on the channel pair involved, and the needling technique is carried out to sedate (*xie fa*) or tonify (*bu fa*), depending on whether the

headache has been assigned to repletion (*shi*) or to vacuity (*xu*).

Headaches assigned more to the vacuity (*xu*) type are caused, according to the classical expression, by relative dominance of *yang* with general weakness of *yin*, but on the other hand also by weakness in *qi*. Unlike headaches of the repletion (*shi*) type, they can be less well treated by ear acupuncture; combination with **body acupuncture** is recommended here. In case of *cervicooccipital headache*, for example, in which the pair of the small intestine/bladder channels (*tai yang*) is predominantly affected, the local body acupoints BL-2 and BL-10—and perhaps the extra point EX-HN 3 (*yin tang*) at the nasal root—should be included. Accordingly, when the headache radiates into the temple area, i.e., into the pair of the triple burner/gallbladder channels (*shao yang*), the local points of this channel pair, e.g., GB-14 and GB-20, are added.

▶ Particularly promising is the treatment of *classical migraine* with ear acupuncture. Its typical triad of symptoms demarcates this syndrome easily from other headaches. The symptoms include strict hemicrania (albeit alternating between sides), nausea (sometimes with vomiting), and extreme sensitivity to light. In extreme cases, ear acupuncture will have to attack two disorders simultaneously: on the one hand, a considerable addiction to painkillers, which can no longer be fed because of drug intolerance and, on the other hand, the syndrome of migraine itself. ◀

If patients arrive for their first treatment during an *acute attack* of migraine, the predominant symptoms are nausea and vomiting in addition to the headache itself. For the **primary** choice of points, information will initially derive from these symptoms as the practitioner will search for irritated points in the corresponding areas of the solar plexus zone and stomach zone. While doing this, an irritated zone will usually be found between point zero (82)—the start point of the solar plexus zone—and the bordering stomach zone (87), as well as right at the beginning of the stomach zone (87) itself. During the acute phase, vegetative points I (51) and II (34) belong to the points of first choice and should be included in the treatment accordingly. Predominant among the analgesic points in the region of the antitragus, lobule, and postantitragal fossa is the sun point (35) in combination with the thalamus point (26 a) and analgesia point.

The occiput point (29) and forehead point (33), as well as the *shen men* point (55), may be considered as **supplementary** points.

In each individual case, a different combination of points may be established, depending on individual circumstances and sensitivities. Especially in migraine, however, treatment must be started on the ipsilateral auricle with respect to the site of the complaints.

Once the symptoms have subsided or if the patient is seen during the symptom-free period, the thalamus point (26 a) and analgesia point are usually no longer found to be irritated, and this solar plexus zone and stomach zone are also found to be normal. The preferred points of treatment during this phase are the sun point (35), occiput point (29), and forehead point (33), as well as vegetative points I (51) and II (34) and occasionally the *shen men* point (55). On the other hand, a point at the cervical level of the zone of paravertebral chain of sympathetic ganglia may be found to be sensitive; and it is recommended that the practitioner search specifically for the inferior cervical ganglion point as well. Depending on their sensitivity, the master omega point and omega point II will also be available as treatment points.

One important aspect in selecting points for the *preventive treatment* of migraine, i.e., during attack-free intervals, is the consideration of possible trigger mechanisms. This will often bring the decisive breakthrough.

Note. Caution is advised in case of noticeable psychogenic causes. Here, it is far too readily assumed that lasting results can be achieved by means of the following psychotropic points: the frustration point, PT1 to PT4, and point R (psychotherapeutic point).

This is not, however, feasible. If there are lasting psychogenic problems, accompanying psychotherapy should be initiated. In fact, the willingness to undergo such therapy is definitely promoted by ear acupuncture treatment.

Practical Tip

Migraine attacks triggered by changes in the weather are primarily treated by including the weather point on the ascending helix.

In cases of migraine associated with menstruation, the ovary point (23) and uterus point (58) may be included in the treatment, although not only hormonal factors, but also psychogenic factors contribute to the syndrome. In this case, the previously listed psychotropic points will often be irritated as well.

If there are clues in the patient's history or clinical findings that specific foods or other allergens might trigger a migraine, experience shows that ear acupuncture can only compensate the acute attack or lower the frequency of attacks in the intervals if the exposure to allergens is undiminished. Treatment that focuses on the cause by incorporating a rotation diet or avoidance of allergens is essential. During the accompanying treatment by ear acupuncture, the following points should be considered: the allergy point (78), thymus point in the antihelical wall (zone of nervous control points of endocrine glands), and omega point I.

If trigger factors are present, leading to symptoms ranging from myospasms in the region of the thoracic-cervical muscles to cervical migraine, the attempt is made to identify an effective set of points primarily derived from the segmental approach as defined by **ear geometry**. Most important are the vegetative groove, for example, and the zone of paravertebral muscles and ligaments, *as well as* the retroauricular reflex zones of the involved muscle groups in the neck and shoulder. The underlying causes, such as a bad posture or continuing emotional stress, can be influenced only to a certain extent by ear acupuncture. In such cases, therefore, it is essential to initiate an appropriate concomitant therapy, compensation through regular physical exercise (e.g., sports activities), and training in mental and physical relaxation techniques.

The approach outlined by Chinese medicine essentially corresponds to the one recommended for cephalalgia. This may be supplemented by combination with **body acupuncture** if specific points related to trigger mechanisms are available, e.g., the acupoint KI-6 if migraine is associated with menstruation, or acupoint CV-17 in case of psychogenic factors.

9.9.2 Facial Neuralgia, Trigeminal Neuralgia

Neuralgia in the region of the face and head, as well as trigeminal neuralgia, is among those syndromes which are most difficult to treat. The treatment is very difficult with ear acupuncture as well, especially when the disorder has been chronic over many years. The prognosis depends very much on the cause. Trigeminal neuralgia due to trauma (i.e., caused by an accident) or postoperative trigeminal neuralgia has a better prognosis than the essential form. Nevertheless, a therapeutic attempt is justified even in the latter case, as considerable alleviation may be achieved here too.

Practical Tip

In cases of *persistent pain* with temporary aggravation, the initial treatment may be carried out daily, or at intervals of 2 to 3 days depending on the course, until a distinct alleviation is noticed. In case of *pain attacks*, treatment takes place twice a week during the symptom-free period and may be reduced to weekly intervals once the attacks fail to recur. Such a therapeutic attempt involves approximately 10 sessions; if these are successful, up to five more treatments should be added for stabilization, depending on the sensitivity of the affected reflex zones.

According to the image of the inverted embryo, the head and sensory organs are projected primarily in the area of lobule, antitragus, and end of the scapha. Consequently, this is the main area to search for sensitive reflex zones in cases of *trigeminal neuralgia*. Depending on the localization of the pain and the predominant involvement of one of the three branches of the trigeminal nerve (ophthalmic, maxillary, and mandibular), one can expect different sensitivities of the following points: the forehead point (33), cheek zone (11), upper jaw point (Chinese) (5), lower jaw point (Chinese) (6), and perhaps eye point (8) and trigeminal zone.

In the *acute phase*, the following analgesic points predominate: the thalamus point (26 a), sun point (35), forehead point (33), and analgesia point (at the ventral edge of the lobule).

Similarly to the situation of pain syndromes of the head (such as cephalalgia), an attack may be stopped by microphlebotomy of the allergy point (78) at the tip of the ear, as long as this point is sensitive.

The trigeminal zone at the dorsal edge of the lobule usually exhibits several sensitive points that should be needled using the sieving technique. With respect to the maximum number of needles per session (four or five needles per ear), sieving counts as one needle. If the number of reflex zones found to be sensitive exceeds the maximum number of needles permissible per auricle, the extra points should be documented for further treatment, possibly the next day.

For continued or intermediate treatment, suitable **supplementary** points should be searched for in the vegetative groove at the level of the cervical spine zone, primarily C1 to C3. Along the established line of treatment, special attention should be paid to the zone of paravertebral chain of sympathetic ganglia, in particular, to the superior and middle cervical ganglion points. On the other hand, the following points may play an important role: the weather point (as weather may be a trigger factor), ACTH point (13), and vegetative point II (34), as well as the occiput point (29) and Jerome point (29 b).

According to the concept of Chinese medicine, the syndrome of trigeminal neuralgia is primarily caused by the effect of wind and cold in the head area or by emotions such as rage, fury, and anger. Consequently, treatment should include the liver zone (97) and gallbladder zone (96). On the other hand, the following projection zones may also be examined, depending on the affected channel (or channel pair): the stomach zone (87), large intestine zone (91), and urinary bladder zone (92).

Taking into consideration the rather intricate course of the disease, one should immediately consider combination with **body acupuncture**. The selection of points depends on the pain center and phase of the disease, which may be acute or chronic. For example, for chronic pain symptoms in the region of the first trigeminal branch, the local acupoints BL-3, TB-23, ST-8 as well as GB-3 and GB-15 should be considered. If the second trigeminal branch is predominantly involved, acupoints along the stomach (ST), small intestine (SI), and large intestine (LI) channels, such as ST-3 and ST-6, LI-20, and SI-18, should primarily be chosen. If the disease process involves the third trigeminal branch, the local points TW-17 as well as ST-5 to ST-7 should be considered.

Body acupuncture is usually added after ear acupuncture treatment has been successful but has no long-lasting effect. This is mainly true for the chronic long-term forms of trigeminal neuralgia. Regular repeat treatments (i.e., series of five to six sessions) have proved necessary here, even after periods of 6 to 9 months.

9.9.3 Herpes Zoster Neuralgia

The cause of the shingles syndrome is usually a temporary weakness in the body's defense system or, if occurring repeatedly, a manifest immunodeficiency. The possibility of malignancy or HIV infection must also be considered here.

In the wake of the latently developing disease process, the herpes virus present in the body becomes active and attacks the corresponding spinal ganglia. The vesicular skin eruption associated with the inflammation of the nerve appears only after prodromal pain and uncharacteristic concomitant symptoms. Against this backdrop, it is often possible to apply ear acupuncture as an adjuvant measure as early as in the prodromal phase. Apart from a relatively swift relief from pain, ear acupuncture makes it possible to alleviate the acute course of the disease, or avoid it altogether, and to prevent chronicity of the postherpetic neuralgia.

Especially in view of the possible complications of herpes zoster in the facial area, the patient must be informed about the available types of conventional medical drug therapies. Furthermore, it is possible to combine both therapies. In this case, ear acupuncture is primarily used for pain relief.

In the *acute phase*, the **primary** therapeutic access will be achieved via of the affected segment. For this purpose, the vegetative groove is examined at the level of the corresponding section of the spinal column zone. In connection with point zero (82), one or possibly two lines of treatment are established that refer to the affected segment. Along these lines, special attention should be paid to sensitive points in the sensory portion of the zone of spinal cord (on the helical brim) and

in the zone of paravertebral chain of sympathetic ganglia (in the antihelical wall).

It goes without saying that, in this phase of the disease, the analgesic points play a major role in the selection of points: the *shen men* point (55) and thalamus point (26 a), as well as the analgesia point (on the ventral edge of the lobule).

If skin eruptions have already appeared, the urticaria zone (71) on the cranial scapha as well as the allergy point (78) are also used.

In addition, it has proved helpful to use **body acupuncture** and needle the area around the vesicular skin eruptions at a distance of 3 to 4 cm by using the superficial needle technique. This may be supplemented by including the appropriate distal points on the channel(s) corresponding to this area.

Once a successful response is observed after the first two or three treatments carried out at intervals of 1 to 2 days, the following points may be preferred: the ACTH point (13), interferon point with its immunostimulating effect, and thymus gland point.

Practical Tip

Especially in the *chronically recurrent* course of the disease, combination with body acupuncture may be considered; the body acupoints SP-6, SP-10, LI-11, and GV-14 may be used.

While acute herpes zoster neuralgia can be well controlled with ear acupuncture alone, chronic herpes zoster neuralgia is more difficult to treat. In this case, freedom from pain is achieved only with great effort, i.e., frequent treatments, even if ear acupuncture is combined with body acupuncture. However, a therapeutic attempt with ear acupuncture is still justified, because it at least alleviates the pain in many cases. In view of the chronicity of the illness, the above selection of points is expanded as necessary by including irritated psychotropic points, among which the master omega point is usually also found to be sensitive.

Treatment of *acute herpes zoster* initially takes place at intervals of 1 to 2 days (with approximately three or four sessions), then twice a week, and finally, when only minor symptoms remain, once a week. A total of 10 to 15 sessions are likely to be necessary, provided that the symptoms are not due to an underlying severe chronic disease.

Treatment of *chronic postherpetic neuralgia* starts with two sessions per week until relief from the pain is clearly noticed, and is then continued at weekly intervals. The series of initial treatment may require 10 to 20 sessions; with improvement, after 4 to 8 months, repeat treatments in series of five or six sessions each are indicated. The longer the chronic postherpetic neuralgia has already existed, the lengthier will be its treatment, i.e., more sessions and more frequent series of repeat treatments are to be expected.

Because the symptoms appear unilaterally, the ipsilateral auricle with regard to the site of symptoms is treated first. With *acute herpes zoster*, a relatively swift alleviation of pain within the first 12 hours following acupuncture treatment indicates favorable prospects for the therapy, whereas such tendencies appearing only after three or four treatments predict a more difficult course.

In cases of *postherpetic neuralgia*, the first signs of improvement are not expected until after five or six treatments; the pain will decrease to a tolerable level only after 10 to 12 treatments. At this point, treatment may be interrupted; however, the patient must be advised to return for repeat treatment as soon as possible if the condition gets worse.

According to the concept of Chinese medicine, the pair of lung and large intestine channels is involved. Consequently, the lung zone (101)—if found sensitive—should be stimulated with several needles (the sieving technique). Furthermore, the stomach and liver channels are considered to be affected as well; hence, the corresponding areas of the stomach zone (87) and liver zone (97) should also be needled. How the latter Chinese point selection has come about remains open; in cases of herpes zoster, irritated points are indeed often found in both the liver zone (97) and stomach zone (87) when using the segmental lines of treatment.

9.10 Skin Diseases (Fig. 9.14)

It is important to differentiate between primary and secondary afflictions when treating diseases of the skin. The secondary ones usually represent concomitant symptoms of underlying internal illnesses. Frequently, they are also associated with psychogenic factors. In terms of holistic medicine, this differentiation must be taken into consideration when the choice of points for the following conditions is mainly based on symptoms.

9.10.1 Skin Allergy

Skin allergies are known to have various manifestations. In generalized forms (e.g., urticaria, generalized eczema), systemic immune mechanisms react inadequately throughout the skin or in the skin and mucosa; in localized forms (e.g., contact dermatitis), isolated pathological skin reactions occur.

When selecting the points for ear acupuncture, this differentiation is relevant in so far as very few projection zones on the auricle are expected to be sensitive in localized allergic skin reactions.

Note. The life-threatening form of *acute urticaria* is an indication for ear acupuncture only in exceptional cases. Preventive treatment is started during the symptom-free period and has favorable prospects comparable to those in pollinosis

The **primary** therapeutic access is the urticaria zone (71), which usually exhibits several sensitive points. These should be needled using the sieving technique. Furthermore, the allergy point (78) may be needled—also in the sense of microphlebotomy—from the inside or outside depending on its sensitivity. Next, the zone of nervous control points of endocrine glands in the antihelical wall is examined for sensitivity of the thymus gland point and adrenal gland point. Within the endocrine zone (22), the ACTH point (13) is usually found to be sensitive.

Primarily, the omega point I as well as vegetative points I (51) and II (34) are available as **supplementary** points.

According to Chinese medicine, the skin is assigned to the lung and large intestine channels. Considering the involvement of this channel pair, the lung zone (101) and large intestine zone (91) should be included in the treatment.

In cases of a localized disease process (e.g., *allergic eczema*), the general choice of points described above is expanded by the representation zone corresponding to the affected part of the body. For example, with eczema of the hand,

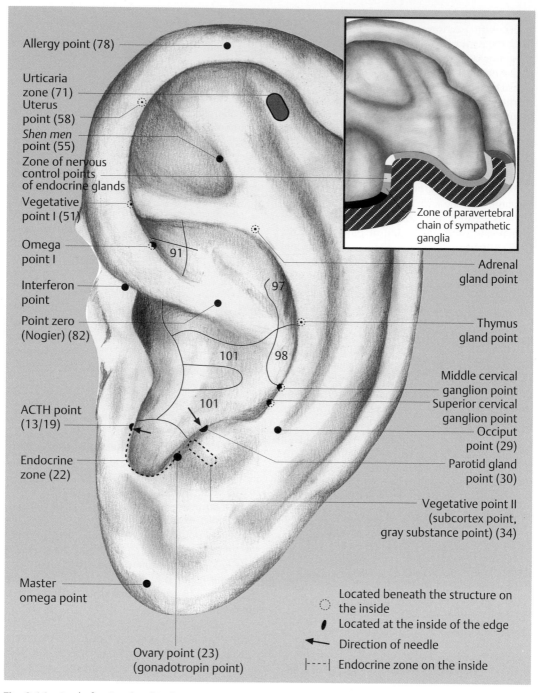

Allergy point (78)

Urticaria
zone (71)
Uterus
point (58)
Shen men
point (55)
Zone of nervous
control points
of endocrine glands
Vegetative
point I (51)
Omega
point I
Interferon
point
Point zero
(Nogier) (82)

ACTH point
(13/19)
Endocrine
zone (22)

Master
omega point

Ovary point (23)
(gonadotropin point)

Zone of paravertebral
chain of sympathetic
ganglia

Adrenal
gland point

Thymus
gland point

Middle cervical
ganglion point
Superior cervical
ganglion point
Occiput
point (29)
Parotid gland
point (30)

Vegetative point II
(subcortex point,
gray substance point) (34)

Located beneath the structure on
the inside
Located at the inside of the edge
Direction of needle
Endocrine zone on the inside

91
97
101
98
101

Fig. 9.14 Pool of points for skin diseases.

the representation zone of the hand/carpus will present one or more sensitive points. In contrast, both the thymus gland point and adrenal gland point, as well as the urticaria point (71), usually prove insensitive in localized processes.

Particularly in systemic, chronically recurrent skin allergies, it makes sense to combine ear acupuncture with **body acupuncture**. The following immunomodulatory body acupoints are available: LI-11, ST-36, SP-6, and GV-14.

Practical Tip

According to the functional correspondence of the skin and intestine in body acupuncture, it makes sense to stabilize the patient's probably disturbed intestinal flora (e.g., by means of symbiotic management) in parallel with the ongoing acupuncture treatment.

9.10.2 Generalized Pruritus

This condition usually occurs in connection with certain internal diseases, such as hematological anomalies, diseases of the liver (jaundice), and diabetes mellitus. The underlying basic disorder is taken into consideration when selecting supplementary points.

In most cases, however, the physician is confronted with the condition of *essential pruritus*, and the patient has already experienced some futile therapeutic attempts during several medical consultations.

In such cases, the **primary** therapeutic access will be found in the ACTH point (adrenal gland point) (13) and *shen men* point (55), as well as parotid gland point (30) on the tip of the antitragus.

In uncertain cases, it is also worth examining the urticaria zone (71) for sensitivity. The vegetative point II (34) on the inside of the antitragus should also be kept in mind; if irritated, the calming and harmonizing effect of this point on the body's autonomic system is utilized.

For the selection of **supplementary** points, it is helpful to pay attention to characteristic indications of the disease in the patient's history and to find representation zones that may be considered in the individual case and can be expected to be sensitive. Thus, any change for the worse when under emotional stress is a reason for examining the psychotropic points for sensitivity.

If the change is connected to the use of certain stimulants or spices, it may be helpful to include omega point I or the allergy point (78) in the treatment.

According to the concept of Chinese medicine, the lung zone (101) plays a major role here, as it does in all skin diseases.

With *secondary pruritus*, supplementary points may be found in certain reference zones related to the disease, depending on the underlying basic disorder. For example, in cases of liver disease (jaundice), the liver zone (97) and pancreas/gallbladder zone (96) may exhibit sensitive points.

Different factors are thought to be responsible for the appearance of *systemic pruritus of old age*. On the one hand, the skin is usually extremely dry and, during the natural process of aging, has lost its capacity to compensate for excessive oil-removing washing procedures. On the other hand, a hormonal deficiency due to old age may be involved. In addition to the usual skin care measures, ear acupuncture may be useful in this situation. The following supplementary points may prove sensitive: the ovary/gonadotropin point (23) and uterus point (58), and also points in the endocrine zone (22).

If pruritus appears in connection with *diseases of the hemopoietic system*, it is possible (according to Chinese considerations) to include further supplementary points in the treatment: point zero (82), the liver zone (97), and the spleen zone (98).

In difficult conditions, combination with **body acupuncture** is recommended. According to the Chinese school, weakness in the defense *qi* is assumed. Consequently, it makes sense to use the following body acupoints: SP-6 and SP-10, LI-11, and GV-14.

Approximately five or six treatments are required before a distinct alleviation of symptoms is perceived. An additional five to 10 sessions are recommended thereafter to achieve complete freedom from symptoms, or at least stabilization to produce a tolerable condition. Initially, treatment may take place twice a week and later, when improvement is noticed, one session per week will suffice. In case of chronicity of the symptoms, long-term therapy or repeat treatments will be required.

9.10.3 **Neurodermatitis**

Neurodermatitis is a general medical puzzle and therefore not treated here as a proven indication for ear acupuncture. Rather, it is discussed because the naturopath is relatively often confronted with these desperate patients, and some of them may actually be helped by ear acupuncture. The results are also modest in combination with body acupuncture, although encouraging results may be achieved depending on the individual circumstances. As with other intractable syndromes (e.g., bronchial asthma, optic atrophy), the patient is additionally burdened with the side effects of conventional medication, particularly those of corticosteroids in both systemic and topical applications. Hence, the aim of the ear acupuncturist is to reduce medication dosages to below the threshold of side effects or, in case of especially good results, to do entirely without it. In contrast to optic atrophy, optimal monitoring of the results by both physician and patient is possible in neurodermatitis.

The **primary** therapeutic approach takes place independently of the ongoing conventional medication, which should not initially be changed. Furthermore, the patient must be informed that a reduction of medication below the threshold dosage could result in freedom from annoying side effects, but that a hasty reduction in medication rather worsens the prospects. Unfortunately, exaggerated expectations on the part of the patient are the rule and must be put into perspective by the physician, especially in cases of neurodermatitis.

Invariably, a treatment series of approximately 10 sessions will be required. In my own experience, one should treat patients twice a week so that the response to ear acupuncture can be accurately assessed. Once results emerge, approximately 10 more sessions are required to achieve lasting success. Repeat treatments of 5 to 10 sessions each may or may not be necessary within 3 to 6 months. After the first signs of improvement, which are usually visible after six to 10 treatments, the current medication may be gradually reduced and then maintained at a low dosage level for the time being. After stabilization following the second series of approximately 10 sessions, a first attempt to discontinue medication may be undertaken.

The **primary** therapeutic set of points consists of the ACTH point (13) and other irritated points of the endocrine zone (22), as well as the adrenal gland point (in the antihelical wall at the T-12 level). In addition, the *shen men* point (55) and allergy point (78) may be found to be sensitive.

The psychotropic points must definitely be considered when choosing the primary points. It is known from experience that the master omega point, PT1, and PT2 usually prove to be sensitive; the other omega points and psychotropic points may, of course, also be found to be sensitive. A specific selection of these points is not possible against the backdrop of the individual patient's emotional state; the decisive criterion is sensitivity of the points.

Vegetative points I (51) and II (34), as well as calming and harmonizing points, such as the occiput point (29), and the points corresponding to the primarily affected body parts, serve as **supplementary** points.

According to considerations of Chinese medicine, which assign the organ that is the skin to the pair of lung/large intestine channels, the lung zone (101) and large intestine zone (91) should be examined for sensitive points. Likewise, to strengthen the defense *qi* in the superficial skin layer, the following body acupoints may be included: LU-9, LU-7, LI-4, LI-11, and also SP-6 and SP-10, and GV-14.

Neurodermatitis frequently requires combined treatments right from the start, in order to overcome the unknown multifactorial causes of this syndrome. It may also make sense to use, step by step and in parallel with ear acupuncture, other established naturopathic healing methods, such as homeopathy, special diets, or probiotic therapy. The aim is to eliminate in this way—but without succumbing to polypragmasy—further factors contributing to the disease.

9.11 **Treatment of Addictions (Fig. 9.15)**

Unlike diseases of the locomotor system, addiction is not one of the best indications for ear acupuncture, even though it is a relatively good one. Ear acupuncture must be viewed in comparison to many other therapies that are as good or as bad when it comes to effectiveness. Unless the optimal therapy is known, ear acupuncture may

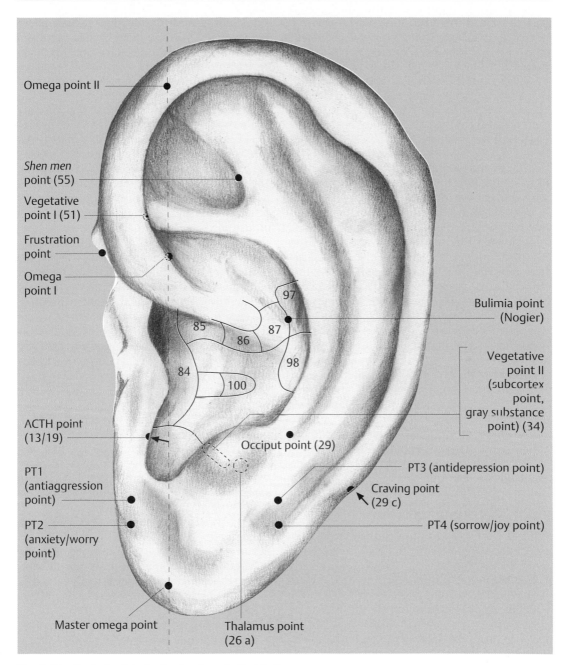

Fig. 9.15 Pool of points for the treatment of addictions.

be equal to other methods of treatment of addiction, although within certain limits.

So far, all scientific studies on addiction treatment by means of ear or body acupuncture give rise to criticism, no matter whether the results are positive or negative. In studies carried out at institutions or universities as projects for dissertations, the therapists have been inexperienced, briefly trained graduate students or research associates who were trying to treat this difficult syndrome by following a preset combination of points. On the other hand, when carried out by established practitioners, i.e., by physicians with many years of experience in the particularities of acupuncture, the studies have lacked the required design of a scholarly study because the numerous preconditions could hardly be fulfilled in the setting of an established practice. Nevertheless, for the sake of objectivity, the discussion of individual types of addictions should refer to studies of current interest.

In principle, every addiction therapy requires that patients are motivated to grapple with their addiction on their own initiative. This is true for all forms of addiction, whether it is nicotine addiction, bulimia, or alcoholism. As this motivation is decisive in the success or failure of ear acupuncture treatment, its role must be recognized or inspired by an experienced and competent physician. If this essential criterion is handled too permissively because of financial interests, failure is certain and can have serious consequences in case of severe addictions, such as alcoholism. Furthermore, failures are considerably damaging to a physician's good reputation, e.g., in cases of nicotine addiction.

The physician must make it quite clear to the patient which requirements need to be fulfilled by the patient and to what extent help may be expected from ear acupuncture.

9.11.1 Nicotine Addiction

When a patient approaches the physician with the desire for nicotine withdrawal, two points must be clarified:
1. How motivated is the patient?
   How many attempts have already been made to quit smoking and what were the motives in each case?
2. What can the patient expect from ear acupuncture?

Ear acupuncture alleviates the withdrawal symptoms and can entirely prevent irritability, nervousness, anxiety, and concentration problems during the first 4 to 5 days. The craving for cigarettes is considerably reduced, even converted into dislike. The psychological effect of ear acupuncture, which certainly also plays a role, takes

a back seat against this genuine somatic effect. The craving remains reduced beyond the first 4 to 5 days—although no longer with the initial impact, according to patient reports—but reappears with undiminished intensity after renewed exposure. If patients are likely to relapse during this phase, they should be promised the opportunity of a second treatment at short notice. Even after weeks and months, such phases carrying the risk of relapse may occur, with a strange increase being observed after 3 weeks and after 3 months. The potential second treatment is rarely used by patients, although its availability provides a reassuring sense of security. In principle, the effect of just one ear acupuncture treatment is sufficient. In difficult cases, further treatments may be carried out, if needed, at weekly intervals. In connection with withdrawal from nicotine, many publications recommend permanent needles. We ourselves do not use permanent needling, not even in this case, for reasons previously described in more detail (see Chapter 6.5 and p. 85).

If the physician realizes during the first visit that the patient has never seriously tried to quit smoking on their own, it is a good idea to motivate the patient to take this step, and to offer help by ear acupuncture should failure occur.

The actual ear needling for addiction therapy should, if possible, take place during a subsequent visit, having agreed during the first visit that the patient will abstain from smoking for the last 24 hours prior to treatment and will also prepares everything in their environment to avoid renewed exposure.

The 24-hour waiting period has two advantages:
1. The patient is actively integrated into the withdrawal process and already gets to know the withdrawal symptoms, including the contrast and relief that follows ear acupuncture treatment.
2. Furthermore, the search for sensitive points, particularly that for the craving point (29 c), is made easier and safer.

There are many different recommendations or "recipes" regarding the choice of points that are thought to be especially effective. Unfortunately, such standard procedures tempt the therapist into neglecting the patient's personal situation. Individually combined treatment regimens certainly agree with each other to a great extent, but they leave enough room for locating individual points that might be decisive for the particular patient.

Thus, the craving point (29 c) may play a predominant role in one smoker, whereas it may be more important for another smoker for the psychotropic points and vegetative points to be included in the treatment regimen, while the craving point (29 c) takes a back seat.

The following points have proved successful as **primary** points: first, the well-known points, such as the craving point (29 c), PT1, vegetative point I (51) and/or vegetative point II (34), *shen men* point (55), and ACTH point (13); the latter point is also called "stress control point" and is located in the endocrine zone (22). Furthermore, sensitive points are found at various locations within the lung zone (101). These points play a major role, particularly in long-term smokers with manifest chronic bronchitis. The bronchopulmonary plexus point (101) may be found to be sensitive, as may other, less well-defined points in the caudal area of the lung zone. Similarly, the mouth zone (84) may play an important role when selecting the primary points, e.g., in the typical smoker who smokes for pleasure and who in all probability shows primarily a sensitive craving point (29 c). If smoking is primarily induced by problems, the frustration point should be considered as the main psychotropic point and should be needled in combination with the previously listed PT1 as well as ACTH point (13).

The following points may play a role as **supplementary** points: the occiput point (29) and the psychotropic points PT2 and PT3, When selecting the individual set of points, the following projection zones should be kept in mind: the oppression point (83) in the solar plexus zone ("anxiety point"), master omega point, and omega point II. In long-term chain smokers who have repeatedly relapsed or in patients who need to quit smoking for health reasons (e.g., because of peripheral circulatory disturbances), withdrawal often turns out to be difficult and hard to treat. Two, three, or even more sessions may be required in such cases, and different sets of points may become apparent, depending on changes in symptoms during the course of treatment and on the associated sensitivities. In this situation, **body acupuncture** may be included by using, for example, the following body acupoints: GV-20, CV-17, ST-36, LU-9, or HT-7.

There are conflicting reports concerning success rates. One study in the literature reports an optimistic, but certainly too high, success rate of 80%; another report describes the poor results obtained in a 6-month follow-up study (at the Clinic for Anesthesia in Vienna, Austria) in which only one out of 33 patients actually quit smoking. In this study, however, acupuncture was carried out like a recipe in a cookbook, using the frequently proclaimed addiction triangles: frustration point/antiaggression point (PT1)/craving point (29 c), or one of the sensitive points in the lung zone (101), respectively.

▶ These two extreme examples clearly demonstrate that, on the one hand, it is very difficult to establish an objective study design because it is absolutely necessary to use individual sets of points. On the other hand, reservations against exaggerated reports of success seem in order. ◀

9.11.2 Bulimia, Obesity

Bulimia is much more difficult to treat than nicotine abuse, including when using ear acupuncture. Overweight and obesity may have many different causes and certainly do not simply result from overeating. The increase in weight, which is frequently observed after successful nicotine withdrawal, should be viewed as a shift in addiction with the underlying psychosocial problems remaining unchanged. To this end, in cases of obesity or bulimia, ear and body acupuncture provide effective help as a bridge or guidance toward dealing with the underlying personal problems, even more so than in the treatment of nicotine withdrawal. The patient must realize that, with the temporary help of ear acupuncture, weight loss is possible by changing eating habits and embarking on a well-balanced psychosocial lifestyle. The introduction of further therapeutic measures, including in cases of obesity or bulimia the patient's active cooperation, are required for reinforcement.

Furthermore, it is important to keep patients from focusing on short-term weight loss. Instead, they should concentrate primarily on a normalization of eating habits. This is especially true in light of the experience that rapid weight loss cannot last; weight is controlled centrally in the diencephalon via a form of feedback regulation, in which one's actual weight is almost identical under normal circumstances to the centrally stored ideal weight. Consequently, the effect of rapid weight loss is that another weight gain is going to take place for sure because the centrally stored ideal weight has not yet changed. Herein lies the problem for most overweight patients in terms of sustaining the reduced weight, as adjustment of the ideal weight to the changed actual weight takes place only after a delay, i.e., within about 2 months.

As with nicotine addiction, certain aspects must, therefore, be checked and clarified prior to treatment:

1. The possible causes of obesity should be determined both clinically and from the patient's history, and unsuccessful earlier attempts to reduce weight should be discussed.
2. It is important to check the patient's state of health, to consider existing underlying diseases if applicable, and to assess the indication for targeted weight loss.
3. The patient's motivation should be explored. In this connection, one should discuss the changes that patients must achieve on their own, in particular any changes in eating habits, lifestyle, etc.
4. The patient's expectations usually must be corrected.

Ear acupuncture does not induce weight loss, but it does reduce appetite. The patient feels full rather more quickly and, as a result, will reduce the usual amount of food eaten. This effect lasts for approximately 5 to 7 days, at which time another treatment is required. After two to four sessions, the intervals may be extended to 2 to 3 weeks, depending on the patient's need in terms of maintaining appetite control. Under the cover of ear acupuncture, the patient is supposed to normalize their eating habits and come to terms with the underlying psychosocial problems. Contrary to widespread belief, one cannot get rid of these problems just by needling the psychotropic (PT) points.

A series of 10 to 15 sessions will be sufficient to initiate physiological weight loss. After cessation of treatment for 3 to 6 months, repeat treatments may be carried out with a series of five sessions each.

If no effect is observed after the second session, at the latest, it is not wise to continue with the treatment.

In part, the **primary** choice of points emphasizes those already described for nicotine addiction: the craving point (29 c), vegetative points I (51) and II (34), PT1, and a point in the liver zone (97) that is regularly found to be sensitive. The latter point, which is located close to the antihelix and not defined in more detail, is also called the "bulimia point." Nearby, on the helical crus and within the stomach zone (87), another sensitive point may often be found. Aside from PT1, the frustration point plays a major role. In view of the considerable psychosomatic component, especially in cases of overweight with a matching medical history, the remaining psychotropic points should be examined as **supplementary** points, in particular PT3 and PT4.

Beyond this, the *shen men* point (55) and occiput point (29) have proved successful. Furthermore, the three omega points must be listed: omega point I can usually be detected, followed by omega point II and then by the master omega point. The mouth zone (84), esophagus zone (85), and cardia zone (86) may be found to be sensitive as well.

Depending on their sensitivity and the patient's history, only a maximum of four or five individual points from those listed above are selected and needled. The remaining points found during the first examination and considered in need of treatment are documented and, after rechecking their sensitivity, used in subsequent sessions as further sets of points. This applies, for example, when the points used initially—such as the craving point (29 c), psychotropic points, and *shen men* point (55)—are no longer found to be sensitive during the further course of treatment. This happens fairly often.

Experience has shown that using the following points as a basic combination provides success: craving point (29 c) and PT1, a point in the stomach zone (87) close to the solar plexus zone, as well as the "bulimia point." Depending on sensitivity and medical history, one of the psychotropic points, such as PT3, or one of the omega or vegetative points is recommended.

It is interesting to note that patients relatively often report unintentional beneficial side effects of ear acupuncture. For example, cephalalgia, insomnia, chronically recurrent gastritis, or high blood pressure often improve or are eliminated completely. The latter effect must not be overlooked, as medication may need to be reduced accordingly.

Nutritional instructions in connection with the treatment for bulimia and obesity have proved unsuccessful, whereas it is a good idea to introduce the general basics of a balanced and suitable diet and advise the patient to engage in regular physical exercise.

9.11.3 Alcohol and Drug Addictions

Treatment of alcoholism and drug addiction requires a comprehensive therapeutic approach. Ear acupuncture is used here as one of several supportive measure. The therapy of both types of addiction requires practical experience as well as comprehensive psychiatric and psychotherapeutic knowledge. Hence, treatment should be carried out in a hospital endowed with such provisions, at least during the detoxification phase.

Note. We strongly advise against any attempt at undertaking the detoxification of an outpatient by ear acupuncture alone.

Even when the patient seems to meet the highest prerequisites and vehemently pushes for outpatient "detoxification," a physician lacking an expert background in this area must not be tempted into making this risky step simply by relying on the alleviating effect of acupuncture on the withdrawal symptoms. Such an arrangement may result in serious complications, including the life-threatening delirium tremens.

At this point, it is referred to the work of Kossovski and Marx, which is based on many years of practical experience in treating alcoholic individuals with the aid of ear acupuncture in a hospital setting.

Especially in the United States (NADA founded in 1985 [Smith 1984]), but also in Germany (German NADA, founded in 1993), ear acupuncture has been used more and more in recent years. In addiction centers both in hospitals and increasingly also in outpatient departments, the use of acupuncture has been very successful as a supportive measure for drug addicts.

The necessary follow-up as well as continuous care are guaranteed by **daily ear acupuncture** during the *first 30 days* after withdrawal. According to NADA's therapeutic concept, treatment takes place in group sessions during all phases of the therapy.

The *second phase*, in which emotional and psychological complaints predominate, begins after

approximately 30 days and often lasts for more than 6 months. During this period, ear acupuncture is carried out two or three times per week.

In the subsequent *third phase* of withdrawal, which deals mainly with social reintegration, ear acupuncture takes a back seat and is performed just once or twice a week for relaxation.

During the course of these three phases, ear acupuncture is only part of a complex therapeutic concept consisting of daily urine and breath monitoring as well as the principle of noninterference on the part of caregivers and therapists (i.e., the social worker, the physician in charge, the drug team, and the psychotherapist). This approach creates a kind of substitute for the actual social net, because the various institutions collaborate closely with one another. The huge success of the NADA model lies, above all, in the synergistic nature of the therapeutic concept described above. A publication by Raben (2004) in the *Deutsche Zeitschrift für Akupunktur* offers a good overview. Additional work concerning the topic of addictions can be found predominantly in international publications such as Avants et al (2000), Bullock et al (2002), and Margolin et al (2002).

The following recommendation for the choice of points should be understood as a basis for supportive ear acupuncture in combination with multidisciplinary treatment in a hospital or outpatient department; a more comprehensive treatise would go beyond the introductory character of this book.

When choosing the points for withdrawal treatment, it is recommended that the detoxification phase and weaning phase are differentiated.

Detoxification Phase

The following points predominate in the *detoxification phase:* the thalamus point (26 a), vegetative points I (51) and II (34), and the *shen men* point (55).

Consideration should also be given to the liver zone (97), kidney zone (95), and lung zone (101), as well as the occiput point (29). Furthermore, the practitioner should search for sensitive points in the solar plexus zone and stomach zone (87), such as the oppression point (83). In addition, the craving point (29 c) and vegetative point II (34) are usually found to be sensitive.

Up to five needles per auricle are inserted during each of the daily treatments. Depending on the sensitivities of the individual points, different combinations of points may be treated from day to day.

Weaning Phase

Once the detoxification phase has been completed (after approximately 1 week), the following psychotropic points may predominantly be included in the treatments involved in the *weaning phase*, depending on their sensitivity: PT1 and the frustration point, PT2, PT3, and PT4. Furthermore, of special significance are the master omega point and omega point II, both of which are often neglected. Points found to be sensitive during the detoxification phase—i.e., vegetative point II (34), the thalamus point (26 a), and the craving point (29 c)—usually lose their sensitivity during the weaning phase and therefore become therapeutically less important.

Irritated points are occasionally also found in the liver zone (97) and spleen zone (98), as well as in the endocrine zone (22), and are used as **supplementary** points.

Within the framework of long-term therapy, repeated treatments are carried out at long intervals as dictated by need, e.g., in case of "drug dreams." Here too, vegetative points I (51) and II (34), the heart zone (100), the psychotropic zones, and sometimes also the omega points are most likely to be found sensitive.

A standardized set of points is recommended by NADA for the treatment of any kind of addiction—drugs, alcohol, pharmaceuticals, or nicotine. When applied daily, it has proved successful in tens of thousands of patients within the framework of NADA's therapeutic concept.

This "setting" consists of the following points: the *shen men* point (55), vegetative point I (51) (this is called sympathetic point in the United States of America), kidney zone (95), liver zone (97), and lung zone (101) (**Fig. 9.16**).

Drug addicts exhibit symptoms of *yin* vacuity and, as a result, symptoms of *yang* repletion. The general symptoms of *yin* vacuity are anxiety, irritability, chronic dryness of the mouth,

and burning of the palms and soles. Similar additional characteristic symptoms are found in kidney *yin* vacuity and liver *yin* vacuity, see also Maciocia (1977).

From this, an indication to involve the kidney zone (95) and liver zone (97) can be deduced. The *shen men* point (55), with its analgesic effect, is thought to affect heart *yin* vacuity with its symptoms of emotional overexcitability, palpitations, etc. in terms of a soft termination of the rising fire of repletion (*yang* repletion of the heart).

The setting of the five points lies at the heart of the established NADA protocol. Components of the protocol are group therapy, low-threshold access, non-verbal communication during group treatment, and a special, respectful approach to the patient/client. Experience has shown that the other elements of the NADA protocol, especially group therapy, are on a par with ear acupuncture of the five points. This applies especially to individuals with addiction. NADA cannot alleviate all the discomfort of withdrawal, nor does it completely suppress the craving. In this situation, trust in other group members who have persevered for a longer period of time is immensely important. These psychological aspects of the NADA protocol should not be underestimated. It should be mentioned that the NADA protocol is being increasingly applied in general psychiatric practice and recently also in the therapy treatment of posttraumatic stress disorders.

Ear acupuncture according to the "NADA protocol" is mainly performed by specially trained, nonmedical staff. However, the physician should not turn down the opportunity to benefit from using a points concept tailored to suit individual patients displaying varying individual symptoms.

The choice of points given here can be used for treating alcoholism as well as drug addiction. From these points, individual combination of points, or even general ones, may be established.

Note. It should be emphasized yet again that treatment by ear acupuncture can only serve as a support during withdrawal treatment.

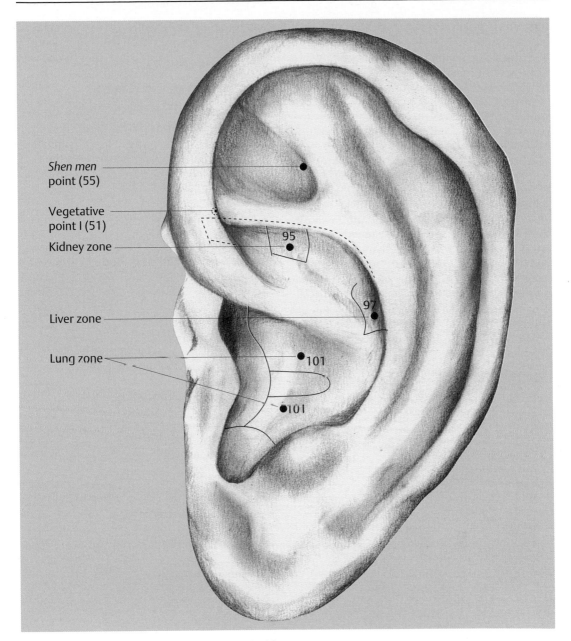

Fig. 9.16 "NADA setting" for the treatment of addictions.

10 Examples of Therapy for Use in Practice

The following condensed examples of therapy represent the common range, as well as the particularities, of syndromes frequently in need of treatment in general practice that are usually successfully treated by means of ear or body acupuncture. They also serve as compact practical instructions for a therapeutic approach, as well as a source of quick reference.

Apart from certain painful diseases of the locomotor system where good results may be achieved with a fixed set of points, the decisive factor is usually the selection of points tailored to the individual patient. Consequently, the following practical examples of therapy should be understood as aids rather than "point recipes."

We would like to emphasize once again that disorders may need to be evaluated by a specialist and that patients must be informed about the options provided by conventional medicine.

10.1 Diseases of the Eye

10.1.1 Hordeolum (Stye)/ Conjunctivitis

Pool of Feasible Points (Fig. 10.1)
- Eye point (8).
- Allergy point (78) (microphlebotomy).
- *Shen men* point (55).
- Apex of tragus point (12).
- ACTH point.
- Thymus gland point.
- Interferon point.

Pool of Feasible Points in Body Acupuncture
ST-1, ST-2, ST-41, BL-1, BL-2, TB-3, GB-1, GB-14, GB-20, LR-2, LR-3, LI-4, LI-11, KI-6, GB-20, LU-5.

Acute: Ipsilateral Ear
First Session
- Eye point (8).
- Allergy point (78) (microphlebotomy).
- *Shen men* point (55).
- Apex of tragus point (12).

Second Session
- ACTH point.
- Thymus gland point.
- Interferon point.

Third Session
- The same as the first session.

Preventive Treatment in the Symptom-free Period
- Thymus gland point.
- Interferon point.
- Allergy point (78).

Combination with Body Acupuncture
BL-1, BL-2, BL-6, LI-4, LI-11, TB-23, GB-1, GB-14, GB-20, GB-37, LR-2, LR-3, LU-5, ST-1, ST-2, ST-41, KI-6.

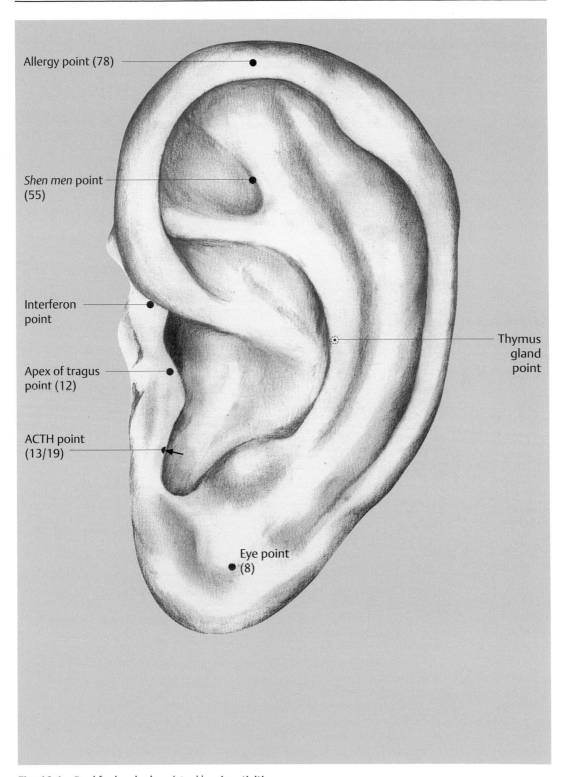

Allergy point (78)

Shen men point
(55)

Interferon
point

Apex of tragus
point (12)

ACTH point
(13/19)

Thymus
gland
point

Eye point
(8)

Fig. 10.1 Pool for hordeolum (stye)/conjunctivitis.

10.1.2 Macular Degeneration (Dry)/Optic Atrophy

Points are chosen from the same pool for both disorders. The selection of points differs according to their degree of irritation.

Pool of Feasible Points (Fig. 10.2)
- Eye points 24 a and 24 b.
- Segmental treatment line: vegetative groove—cervical spine.
- Superior and/or middle cervical ganglion point.
- *Shen men* point (55).
- ACTH point.
- Vegetative point II (34) (sieving technique).
- Sensory line (29, 35, 33).
- Psychotropic points (e.g., PT1–PT4).
- Master omega point.
- Liver zone (97) (according to Chinese indications).

Macular Degeneration

Preventive Treatment in the Symptom-free Period
Primary Selection of Points
- Eye points 24 a and 24 b.
- Segmental treatment line: vegetative groove—cervical spine.
- Superior and/or middle cervical ganglion point.

Supplementary Points
- *Shen men* point (55).
- ACTH point.
- Vegetative point II (34) (sieving technique).
- Sensory line (29, 35, 33).
- Psychotropic points (e.g., PT1–PT4).
- Master omega point.
- Liver zone (97) (according to Chinese indications).

The initial series of treatments spans 15 sessions. Treatment takes place daily or every other day. Once the condition has stabilized, treatment changes to a preventive approach. Treatment is initially once a week; if there is no progression of the disorder, maintenance treatment of one session every 2 to 4 weeks depending on the condition may take place under the supervision of an eye specialist.

Optic Atrophy

First Session
- Eye points 24 a and 24 b.
- Segmental treatment line: vegetative groove—cervical spine.
- Vegetative point II (34) (sieving technique).
- PT2.

Second Session
- Superior and/or middle cervical ganglion point.
- *Shen men* point (55).
- Sensory line (29, 35, 33).

Third Session
- The same as the first session, if necessary including the master omega point.

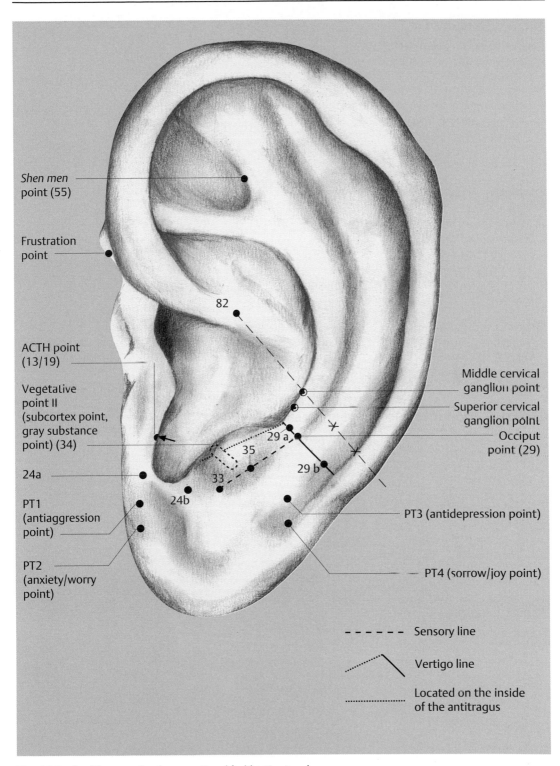

Shen men
point (55)

Frustration
point

82

ACTH point
(13/19)

Vegetative
point II
(subcortex point,
gray substance
point) (34)

24a

PT1
(antiaggression
point)

PT2
(anxiety/worry
point)

Middle cervical
ganglion point

Superior cervical
ganglion point

Occiput
point (29)

29 a

35

29 b

33

24b

PT3 (antidepression point)

PT4 (sorrow/joy point)

- - - - - - Sensory line

Vertigo line

Located on the inside
of the antitragus

Fig. 10.2 Pool for macular degeneration (dry)/optic atrophy.

10.1.3 Glaucoma

Pool of Feasible Points (Fig. 10.3)
- Eye points 24 a and 24 b.
- Forehead point (33).
- Sensory line (29, 35, 33).
- Superior and/or middle cervical ganglion point.
- Vegetative point II (34) (sieving technique), vegetative point I.
- Psychotropic points (e.g., PT-1–PT4).
- ACTH point.

Preventive Treatment in the Symptom-free Period

Primary Point Selection
- Sensory line (29, 35, 33).
- Eye points 24 a and 24 b.
- Forehead point (33).
- Superior and/or middle cervical ganglion point.

Supplementary Points
- Vegetative point II (34) (sieving technique), vegetative point I.
- Psychotropic points (e.g., PT1–PT4).
- ACTH point.

Combination with Body Acupuncture
BL-6, GB-37.

Example

First Session
- Eye points 24 a and 24 b.
- Sensory line (29, 35, 33).
- Vegetative point II (34) (sieving technique).
- ACTH point.

Second Session
- Superior and/or middle cervical ganglion point.
- Psychotropic points (e.g., PT1–PT4), depending on sensitivity.
- Vegetative point II (34) (sieving technique).
- Forehead point (33).

Third Session
- Eye points 24 and 24 b.
- Superior and/or middle cervical ganglion point.
- ACTH point.
- Vegetative point I.

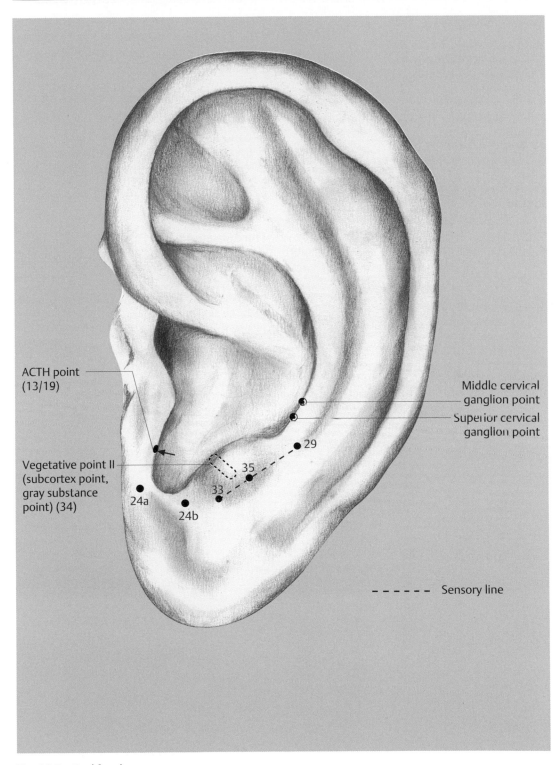

ACTH point
(13/19)

Vegetative point II
(subcortex point,
gray substance
point) (34)

24a

24b

33

35

29

Middle cervical
ganglion point

Superior cervical
ganglion point

– – – – – – Sensory line

Fig. 10.3 Pool for glaucoma.

10.1.4 **Myopia**

Pool of Feasible Points (Fig. 10.4)
- Eye points 24 a and 24 b.
- Superior and/or middle cervical ganglion point.
- Liver zone (97).
- Kidney zone (95).
- Vegetative point II (34) (sieving technique), vegetative point I.
- Sensory line (29, 35, 33).
- Psychotropic points (e.g., PT1–PT4).

Preventive Treatment in the Symptom-free Period
Primary Point Selection
- Eye points 24 a and 24 b.
- Superior and/or middle cervical ganglion point.
- Liver zone (97).
- Kidney zone (95).

Supplementary Points
- Vegetative point II (34) (sieving technique), vegetative point I.
- Sensory line (29, 35, 33).
- Psychotropic points (e.g., PT1–PT4).

Combination with Body Acupuncture
ST-1, GB-1, GB-20, GB-37.

Example
First Session
- Superior and/or middle cervical ganglion point.
- Kidney zone (95).
- Liver zone (97).
- Psychotropic points (e.g., PT1–PT4), depending on sensitivity.

Second Session
- Eye points 24 a and 24 b.
- Vegetative point II (34) (sieving technique).
- Sensory line (29, 35, 33).
- Psychotropic points (e.g., PT1–PT4), depending on sensitivity.

Third Session
- Superior and/or middle cervical ganglion point.
- Eye points 24 a and 24 b.
- Vegetative point I.
- Psychotropic points (e.g., PT1–PT4), depending on sensitivity.

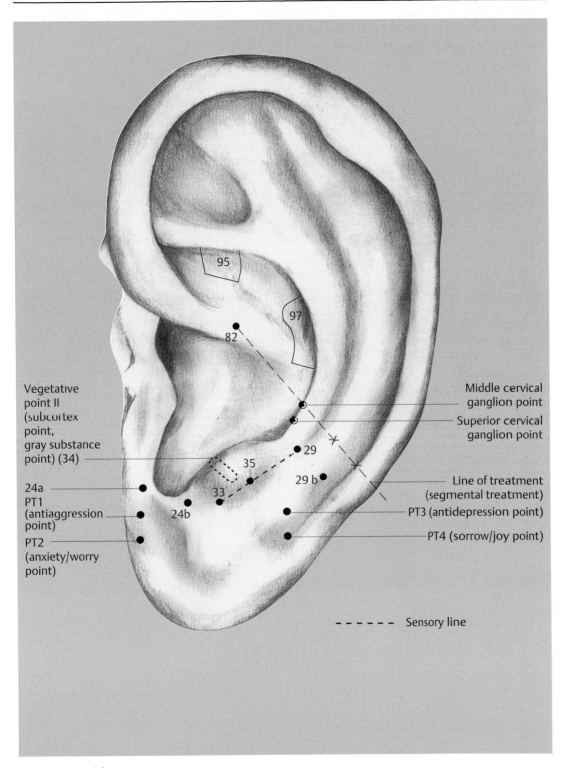

Fig. 10.4 Pool for myopia.

10.2 ENT (Ear, Nose, and Throat) Diseases

10.2.1 Globus Sensation

Pool of Feasible Points (Fig. 10.5)
- Segmental treatment line: cervical spine—vegetative groove.
- Larynx/pharynx point (15).
- Esophagus zone (85), cardia zone (86).
- Solar plexus point.
- Vegetative point I and II.
- Liver zone (97).
- Psychotropic points (e.g., PT1–PT4).

Primary Point Selection
- Segmental treatment line: cervical spine—vegetative groove.
- Larynx/pharynx point (15).
- Esophagus zone (85), cardia zone (86).
- Solar plexus point.

Supplementary Points
- Vegetative point I and II.
- Liver zone (97).
- Psychotropic points (e.g., PT1–PT4).

Combination with Body Acupuncture
CV-17, PC- 6, LR-2.

Example

First Session
- Larynx/pharynx zone (15).
- Esophagus zone (85), cardia zone (86).
- Solar plexus point.
- Vegetative point I.

Second Session
- Segmental treatment line: cervical spine—vegetative groove.
- Vegetative point II.
- Liver zone (97).
- Psychotropic points (e.g., PT1–PT4), depending on sensitivity.

Third Session
- Solar plexus point.
- Vegetative point II.
- Larynx/pharynx zone (15).
- Psychotropic points (e.g., PT1–PT4), depending on sensitivity.

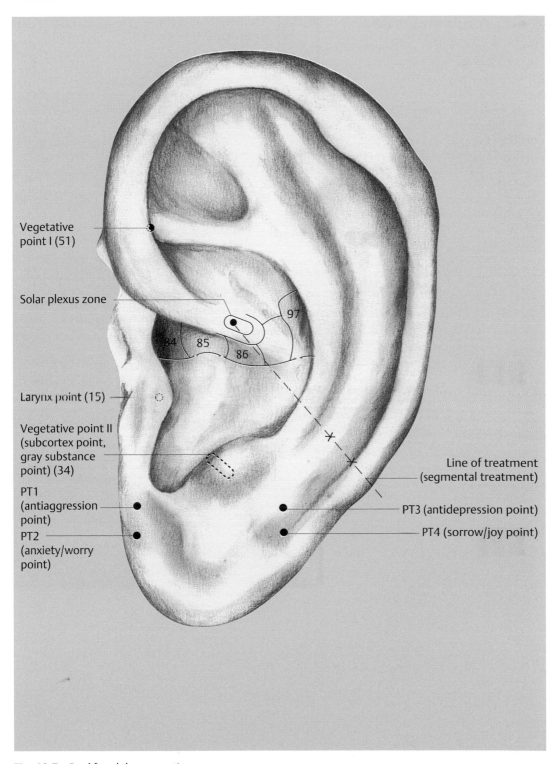

Fig. 10.5 Pool for globus sensation.

10.2.2 **Vestibular Vertigo**

Note. It is important to differentiate between systematic types of vertigo and nonsystematic types, for which ear acupuncture is of little help.

Pool of Feasible Points (Fig. 10.6)
- Von Steinburg's line of vertigo, including the nausea point (29a), occiput point (29), Jerome point (29 b), and additional points on the medial aspect of the antitragus, depending on sensitivity.
- Segment therapy—cervical spine section, including the superior cervical ganglion point, medial cervical ganglion point, and points along the vegetative groove.
- Inner ear point (9).
- If necessary, vegetative points I (51) and II (34).

Initially, treatment takes place every 2 to 3 days with changing point sets.

First Session
- Von Steinburg's line of vertigo.
- Inner ear point (9).
- Vegetative point I (51) or vegetative point II (34).

Second Session
- Segment therapy with ganglion points and the vegetative groove.

Third Session
- The same as the first session.

After approximately four sessions, treatment may take place once a week without changing point sets.

Treatment may be successful immediately after the first session, but may not appear until the fifth or sixth session. A total of approximately 10 sessions is required.

Combination with Body Acupuncture
GB-24, GB-40, GB-34, GV-20, LR3, LR-14, GV-20, SP-6.

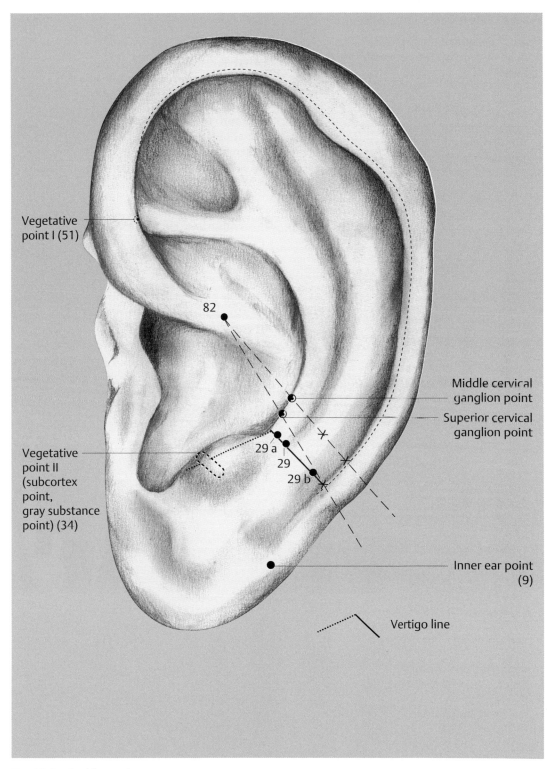

Vegetative
point I (51)

82

Middle cervical
ganglion point

Superior cervical
ganglion point

29 a

29

29 b

Vegetative
point II
(subcortex
point,
gray substance
point) (34)

Inner ear point
(9)

Vertigo line

Fig. 10.6 Pool for vertigo.

10.2.3 Meniere's Disease

Pool of Feasible Points (Fig. 10.7)
- Segmental treatment line of the vegetative groove.
- Superior and/or middle cervical ganglion point.
- Sensory line (29, 35, 33).
- Kinetosis point (nausea point) (29 a).
- Von Steinburg's line of vertigo.
- Vegetative points I and II.
- Inferior cervical ganglion point (stellate ganglion).
- PT1 to PT4.
- Jerome point (29 b).
- Weather point (= vegetative point).
- Liver zone (97).

Acute
Primary Point Selection
- Segmental treatment line of vegetative groove.
- Superior and/or middle cervical ganglion point.
- Sensory line (29, 35, 33).
- Kinetosis point (nausea point) (29 a).
- Von Steinburg's line of vertigo.

Supplementary Points
- Vegetative points I and II.
- Inferior cervical ganglion point (stellate ganglion).
- PT1 to PT4.
- Jerome point (29 b).
- Weather point (= vegetative point).

Preventive Treatment in the Symptom-free Period
Primary Point Selection
- Sensory line (29, 35, 33).
- Kinetosis point (nausea point) (29 a).
- Weather point (vegetative point).
- Von Steinburg's line of vertigo.

Supplementary Points
- Vegetative points I and II.
- PT1 to PT3.
- Jerome point (29 b).
- Liver zone (97).

Example
First Session
- Kinetosis point (29 a).
- Von Steinberg's line of vertigo.
- Weather point (= vegetative point)
- PT1 to PT4.

Second Session
- Sensory line (29, 35, 33).
- Jerome point (29 b).
- Liver zone (97).
- PT1 to PT4.

Third Session
- Sensory line (29, 35, 33).
- Vegetative point II.
- Weather point (= vegetative point).
- (PT1–PT4).

Fourth Session
The same as the first session.

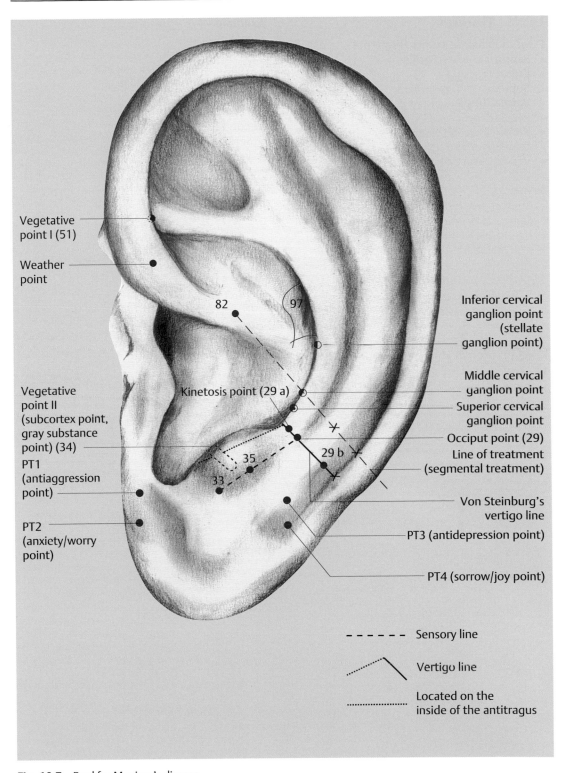

Fig. 10.7 Pool for Meniere's disease.

10.2.4 **Tinnitus**

Pool of Feasible Points (Fig. 10.8)
- Sensory line (29, 35, 33).
- Segment therapy C2 to C7 with ganglion points.
- Vegetative points I and II.
- PT1 to PT4.
- Kidney zone (95).
- Liver zone (97).
- Von Steinburg's line of vertigo.

Primary Point Selection
- Sensory line (29, 35, 33).
- Ganglion points of segments C2 to C7.
- Vegetative point I and II.
- Von Steinburg's line of vertigo.

Supplementary Points
- PT1 to PT4.
- Kidney zone (95).
- Liver zone (97).

Combination with Body Acupuncture
CV-17, GV-20, LR-3, GB-2, GB-8, GB-43, HT-7, PC-6, KI-3, KI-7, SI 19.

Example
First Session
- Ganglion points of segments C2 to C7.
- Vegetative point II (sieving technique).
- Kidney zone (95).
- PT1 to PT4.

Second Session
- Sensory line (29, 35, 33).
- Vegetative point I.
- Liver zone (97).
- Von Steinburg's line of vertigo.
- PT1 to PT4.

Third Session
- The same as the first session. If necessary, replace the kidney point (95) with von Steinberg's line of vertigo.

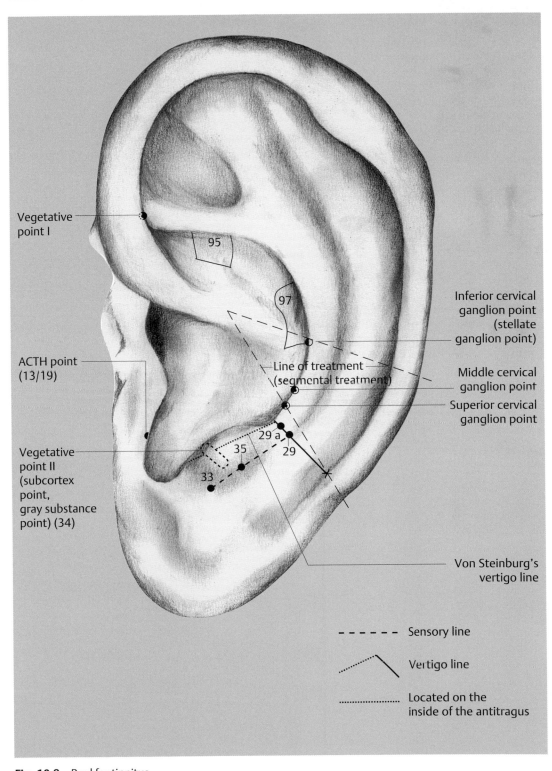

Vegetative point I

95

97

Inferior cervical ganglion point (stellate ganglion point)

ACTH point (13/19)

Line of treatment (segmental treatment)

Middle cervical ganglion point

Superior cervical ganglion point

Vegetative point II (subcortex point, gray substance point) (34)

29 a

35

29

33

Von Steinburg's vertigo line

— — — — — Sensory line

Vertigo line

Located on the inside of the antitragus

Fig. 10.8 Pool for tinnitus.

10.2.5 Sudden Hearing Loss

Pool of Feasible Points (Fig. 10.9)
- Superior and/or middle cervical ganglion.
- Vegetative point II (34), vegetative point I.
- Sensory line (29, 35, 33).
- Psychotropic points (e.g., PT1–PT4)..
- Jerome point (29 b).
- Von Steinburg's line of vertigo.

Primary Point Selection
- Superior and/or middle cervical ganglion point.
- Vegetative point II (34), vegetative point I.
- Sensory line (29, 35, 33).
- Von Steinburg's line of vertigo.

Supplementary Points
- Psychotropic points (e.g., PT1–PT4).
- Jerome point (29 b).

Combination with Body Acupuncture
TB-9, TB-16, TB-17, SI-3, CV-17, LR-3, GV-20, ST-36.

Example

First Session
- Sensory line (29, 35, 33).
- Psychotropic points (e.g., PT1–PT4), depending on sensitivity.
- Jerome point (29 b).
- Vegetative point II (34).

Second Session
- Superior and/or middle cervical ganglion point.
- Vegetative point I.
- Von Steinburg's line of vertigo.
- Psychotropic points (e.g., PT1–PT4), depending on sensitivity.

Third Session
- Von Steinburg's line of vertigo.
- Superior and/or middle cervical ganglion point.
- Jerome point (29 b).
- Vegetative point I.

Fourth Session
- The same as the first session.

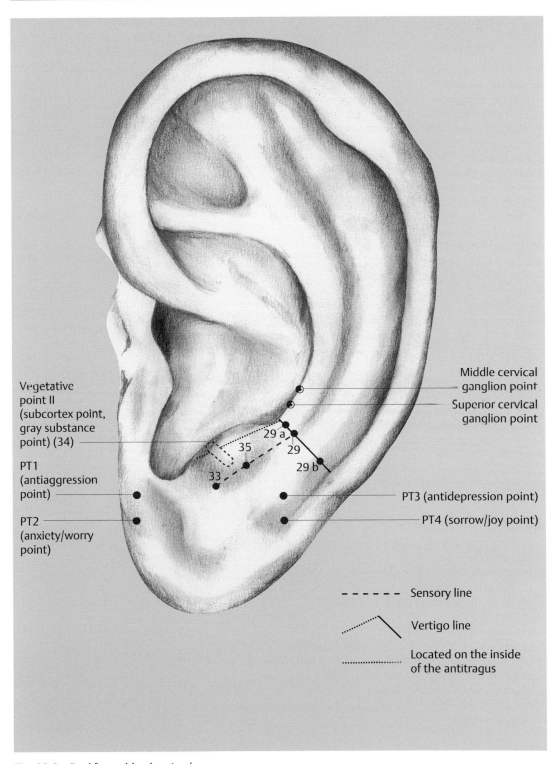

Vegetative point II (subcortex point, gray substance point) (34)

PT1 (antiaggression point)

PT2 (anxiety/worry point)

Middle cervical ganglion point

Superior cervical ganglion point

29 a
35
29
33
29 b

PT3 (antidepression point)

PT4 (sorrow/joy point)

– – – – – Sensory line

·········· Vertigo line

··········· Located on the inside of the antitragus

Fig. 10.9 Pool for sudden hearing loss.

10.3 Respiratory Diseases

10.3.1 Pollinosis

Treatment during the Attack (Fig. 10.10)
- Allergy point (78) followed by microphlebotomy.
- Thymus gland point.
- Superior and/or middle cervical ganglion point.
- ACTH point or *shen men* point (55).
- Eye point (8).
- Inner nose point (16).
- Interferon point.
- Vegetative point I (51) or vegetative point II (34).
- Master omega or omega point I.
- Occiput point (29).
- Lung zone (101).
- Kidney zone (95).
- PT1.

Treatment is carried out every 2 to 3 days. Once the individual's condition improves, prophylactic treatment follows with one or two sessions per week.

Preventive Treatment in the Symptom-free Period (Fig. 10.10)
The treatment series involves 10 to 15 sessions, starting with four to six sessions twice a week and then once a week after about 8 to 12 weeks, depending on results.

The first treatment should be initiated approximately 5 to 6 weeks prior to the start of the pollen season.

Primary Point Selection
- Allergy point (78) without microphlebotomy.
- Thymus gland point.
- Interferon point.
- Inner nose point (16).
- ACTH point (in cases of "hay fever").

Supplementary Points
Depending on the patient's history and load factors:
- Vegetative point I (51) or vegetative point II (34).
- Master omega or omega point I.
- Occiput point (29).
- Lung zone (101).
- Kidney zone (95).
- PT1.

Combination with Body Acupuncture
- Local points: LI-20, BL-1, BL-2, LI-20, TB 23, GB-1; EX-HN3 (*yin tang*), EX-HN5 (*tai yang*).
- Distal points: SP-6, SP-10, LI-3, LI-4, LI-11, GB-20, GB-37.

Example: Prevention
First Session
- Inner nose point (16).
- Eye point (8).
- Superior and/or middle cervical ganglion point.
- Allergy point (78).

Second Session
- Interferon point.
- Thymus gland point.
- Vegetative point I (51).
- PT1.

Third Session
- Allergy point (78).
- Interferon point.
- Thymus gland point.
- Lung zone (101).
- Occiput point (29).

Fourth Session
- The same as the second session.

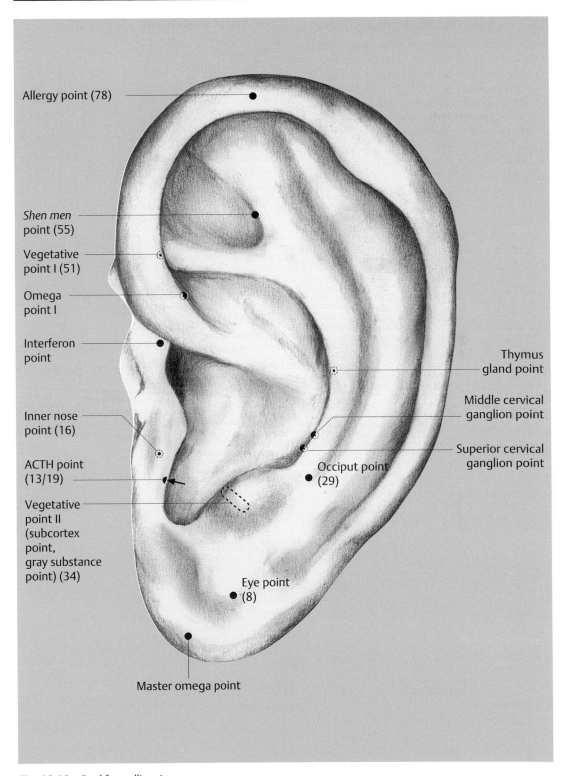

Allergy point (78)

Shen men
point (55)

Vegetative
point I (51)

Omega
point I

Interferon
point

Inner nose
point (16)

ACTH point
(13/19)

Vegetative
point II
(subcortex
point,
gray substance
point) (34)

Thymus
gland point

Middle cervical
ganglion point

Superior cervical
ganglion point

Occiput point
(29)

Eye point
(8)

Master omega point

Fig. 10.10 Pool for pollinosis.

10.3.2 **Allergic Bronchial Asthma**

Treatment during the Attack (Fig. 10.11)

- Allergy point (78) in combination with microphlebotomy.
- Thymus gland point.
- Stellate ganglion point (= inferior cervical ganglion point); if necessary segment therapy.
- Bronchopulmonary plexus point.
- Occiput point (29).
- ACTH point (13) and/or *shen men* point (55).
- Asthma point (31).
- Interferon point.
- Kidney zone (95).
- Master omega point, omega point I, and omega point II.
- Antiaggression point, anxiety point.
- Vegetative point I (51) or vegetative point II (34).
- Lung zone (191).
- Psychotropic points: PT1 to PT4.

Combination with Body Acupuncture

Distal points: LU-5, GV-20, GV-5, GV-7, GV-9, SP-6, SP-10, LI-4, LI-11.

Preventive Treatment in the Symptom-free Period (Fig. 10.11)

Primary Point Selection

- Allergy point (78) without microphlebotomy.
- Thymus gland point.
- Sensitive points in the lung zone (101) by using the sieving technique, including the bronchopulmonary plexus point.
- Interferon point.
- Kidney zone (95).
- ACTH point.

Supplementary Points

- Mast omega point, omega point I, and omega point II.
- Vegetative point I (51) or vegetative point II (34).
- Psychotropic points: PT1 to PT4.

Combination with Body Acupuncture

Local points: LU-1, CV-17, BL-12, BL-13, BL-17, TB-15, ST-12 to ST-15, KI-27, GV-14, GV-20.

Example: Prevention

First Session

- Lung point (101), sieving technique.
- Bronchopulmonary plexus point.
- Allergy point (78).
- ACTH point.
- Interferon point.

Second Session

- Lung zone (101).
- Thymus gland point.
- Interferon point.
- Kidney zone (95).
- Psychotropic points: PT1 to PT4, depending on sensitivity.
- Vegetative point I (51).

Third Session

- Lung point (101), sieving technique.
- Bronchopulmonary plexus point.
- Allergy point (78).
- Psychotropic points: PT1 to PT4, depending on sensitivity.
- Vegetative point II (34).
- Master omega point.

Fourth Session

- The same as the second session + omega point II.

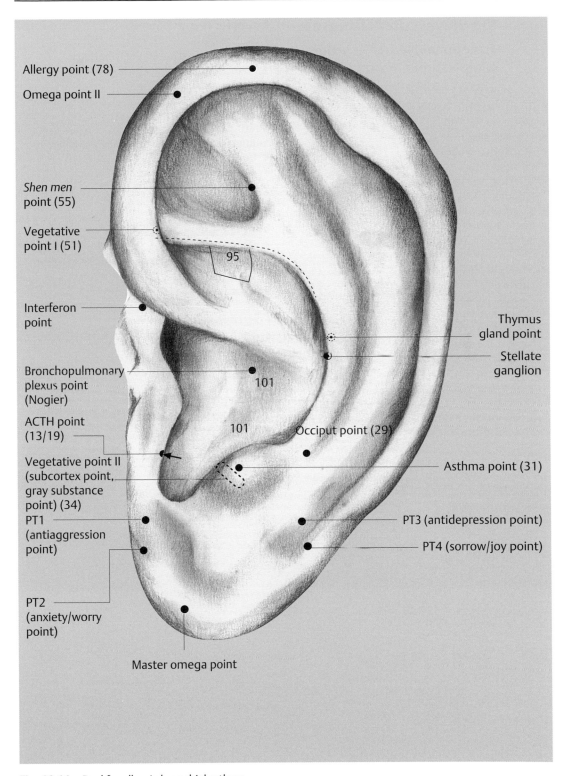

Allergy point (78)

Omega point II

Shen men point (55)

Vegetative point I (51)

95

Interferon point

Bronchopulmonary plexus point (Nogier)

ACTH point (13/19)

Vegetative point II (subcortex point, gray substance point) (34)

PT1 (antiaggression point)

PT2 (anxiety/worry point)

101

101

Master omega point

Thymus gland point

Stellate ganglion

Occiput point (29)

Asthma point (31)

PT3 (antidepression point)

PT4 (sorrow/joy point)

Fig. 10.11 Pool for allergic bronchial asthma.

10.4 Cardiovascular Diseases

10.4.1 Functional Heart Disorders (Palpitations, Paroxysmal Tachycardia)

Pool of Feasible Points (Fig. 10.12)
- Heart point (100).
- Cardiac plexus point.
- Vegetative point I (51).
- PT1 to PT4.
- Inferior cervical ganglion point (stellate ganglion).
- Vegetative point II (34).
- Occiput point (29).
- Small intestine point (89).

Primary Point Selection
- Heart point (100).
- Cardiac plexus point.
- Vegetative point I (51).
- PT1 to PT4.

Supplementary Points
- Inferior cervical ganglion (stellate ganglion).
- Vegetative point II (34).
- Occiput point (29).
- Small intestine point (89).
- Psychotropic points (e.g., PT1–PT4).

Treatment takes place every 2 to 3 days. Depending on the stabilization of the condition, this is extended to weekly intervals, 5 to 10 treatments suffice.

Example
First Session
- Cardiac plexus point.
- Vegetative point I.
- Heart point (100).
- PT1 to PT4.

Second Session
- Inferior cervical ganglion (stellate ganglion).
- Vegetative point II (34).
- Occiput point (29).
- Small intestine point (89).

Third Session
- Cardiac plexus point.
- Heart point (100).
- Inferior cervical ganglion (stellate ganglion).
- Vegetative point I (51) and vegetative point II (34).

Fourth Session
- The same as the third session, depending on sensitivity.

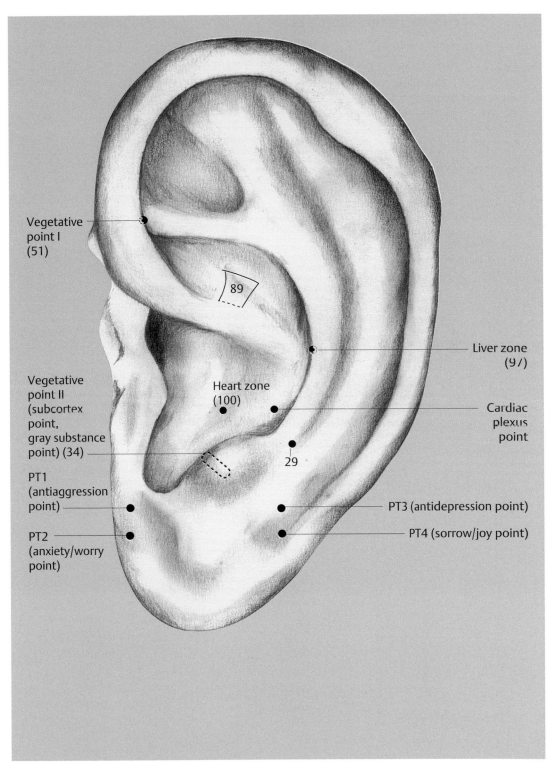

Vegetative
point I
(51)

89

Liver zone
(97)

Vegetative
point II
(subcortex
point,
gray substance
point) (34)

Heart zone
(100)

Cardiac
plexus
point

PT1
(antiaggression
point)

29

PT3 (antidepression point)

PT2
(anxiety/worry
point)

PT4 (sorrow/joy point)

Fig. 10.12   Pool for functional heart disorders.

10.5 Gastrointestinal Diseases

10.5.1 Hiccups

Pool of Feasible Points (Fig. 10.13)
- Point zero (82, diaphragm point).
- Vagus nerve branch point (112).
- Solar plexus points (several points).
- Vegetative point I (51).
- Vegetative point II (34).

Primary Point Selection
- Point zero (82, diaphragm point).
- Vagus nerve branch point (112).
- Solar plexus points (several points).

Supplementary Points
- Vegetative point I (51).
- Vegetative point II (34).
- PT1 to PT4.

In persisting cases of singultus, two or three treatments produce a positive result. In order to achieve stabilization and lasting effects in chronic conditions, 5 to 10 treatments at weekly intervals are known to be required. The procedure in chronically recurrent types is similar: long-term treatment must be expected and a customized selection of points is required depending on the findings and the patient's history.

Example

First Session
- Solar plexus points.
- Point zero.
- Psychotropic points (e.g., PT1–PT4), depending on sensitivity.
- Vegetative point II (34).

Second Session
- Vagus nerve branch point (112).
- Point zero.
- Vegetative point I (51).
- Psychotropic points (e.g., PT1–PT4), depending on sensitivity.

Third Session
- Solar plexus points.
- Vagus nerve branch point (112).
- Vegetative point II (34).
- Psychotropic points (e.g., PT1–PT4), depending on sensitivity.

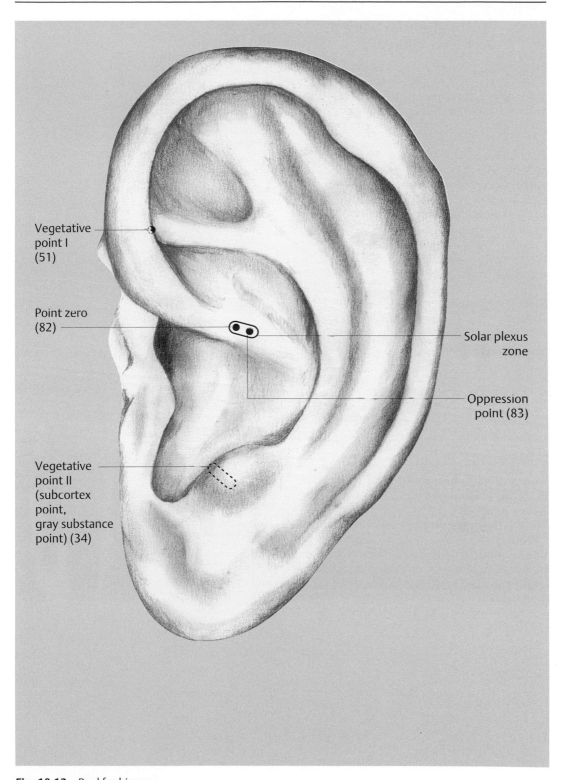

Vegetative
point I
(51)

Point zero
(82)

Solar plexus
zone

Oppression
point (83)

Vegetative
point II
(subcortex
point,
gray substance
point) (34)

Fig. 10.13 Pool for hiccups.

10.5.2 Gastroenteritis, Nausea, Vomiting, Diarrhea

Supporting treatment is possible as follows, after largely emptying the gastrointestinal system, replacing fluids, and being under consideration for the necessary conventional medical measures.

Pool of Feasible Points (Fig. 10.14)
- Point zero (82)—solar plexus points.
- Retro-point zero.
- Stomach point (87).
- Duodenum point (88).
- Ileum—jejunum point (89).
- Colon—sigmoid point (90, 91).
- Vegetative points I and II.
- Jerome point (29 b).

Primary Point Selection
- Point zero (82)—solar plexus points.
- Retro-point zero.
- Stomach point (87).
- Duodenum point (88).
- Ileum—jejunum point (89).
- Colon—sigmoid point (90, 91).

If several points within one area are sensitive, the sieving technique must be applied.

Supplementary Points
- Vegetative points I and II.
- Jerome point (29 b).

Depending on the stage of the acute phase, the treatment intervals should be shorter. If possible, treatment should take place twice a day; stabilization is known to set in after one or two treatments, and treatment can be continued as necessary.

Example
First Session
- Solar plexus points.
- Point zero.
- Stomach point (87).
- Vegetative point II (34).

Second Session
- Retro-point zero.
- Duodenum zone (88).
- Ileum—jejunum zone (89).
- Colon—sigmoid zone (90, 91).

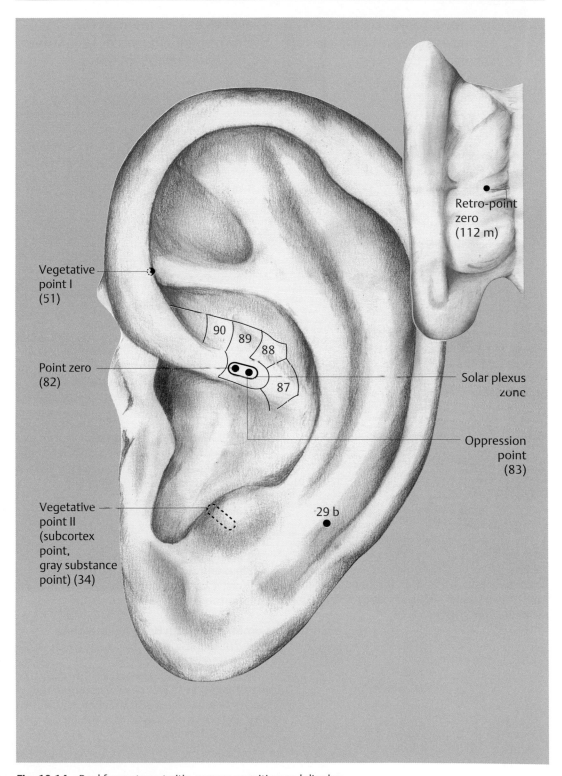

Fig. 10.14 Pool for gastroenteritis, nausea, vomiting and diarrhea.

10.5.3 Inflammatory Intestinal Diseases (Crohn's Disease, Ulcerative Colitis)

Pool of Feasible Points (Fig. 10.15)

- Ileum—jejunum zone (89).
- Colon. sigmoid zone (90, 91).
- Point zero (82)—solar plexus zone.
- Retro-point zero.
- *Shen men* point (55).
- Urogenital plexus zone.
- Psychotropic points (e.g., PT1–PT4, master omega point).
- Vegetative points I and II.
- Jerome point (29 b).
- Interferon point.
- Allergy point.
- ACTH point.
- Thymus gland point.

Primary Point Selection

- Ileum—jejunum zone (89).
- Colon—sigmoid zone (90, 91).
- Point zero (82)—solar plexus zone.
- Retro-point zero.
- *Shen men* point (55).
- Urogenital plexus zone.

Supplementary Points

- Psychotropic points (e.g., PT1–PT4, master omega point).
- Vegetative points I and II, Jerome point (29 b).
- Interferon point.
- Allergy point.
- ACTH point.
- Thymus gland point.

Treatment can be carried out without restrictions in combination with medication and measures from conventional medicine, as well as during symptom-free periods.

Preventive Treatment in the Symptom-free Period of Ulcerative Colitis and Crohn's Disease

Example

First Session

- Colon—sigmoid zone (90, 91) or ileum—jejunum zone (89) (each with the sieving technique).
- Vegetative point II (34) (1–2 points).
- PT1 and PT3.
- Interferon point.
- Allergy point.

Second Session

- PT1 and PT2.
- Vegetative point I.
- Rectum zone (81) (not in Crohn's disease).
- Master omega point.
- Thymus gland point.

Third Session

- Colon (90) or ileum—jejunum (89).
- Vegetative point II (34) (one or two points).
- PT1 and PT4.
- Interferon point.
- Allergy point.

Fourth Session

- Possibly the same as the first session, modified according to the available, i.e. sensitive, points. All combinations are possible, and the order is not imperative.

The initial treatment series involves 15 sessions. Treatment initially takes place twice a week. If there is no recurrence of the condition, one session can be undertaken every 2 to 4 weeks, depending on results. Therapy is more successful and longer lasting if combined with colon rehabilitation and repeated annually.

Combination with Body Acupuncture

BL-20, BL-21, BL-23, KI-3, CV-4, CV-12, GV-4, ST-36, SP-6.

In these disorders, ear and body acupuncture should be part of a complex treatment including dietary therapy (colon rehabilitation, elimination diet) and psychotherapy. This is the only way to achieve good results.

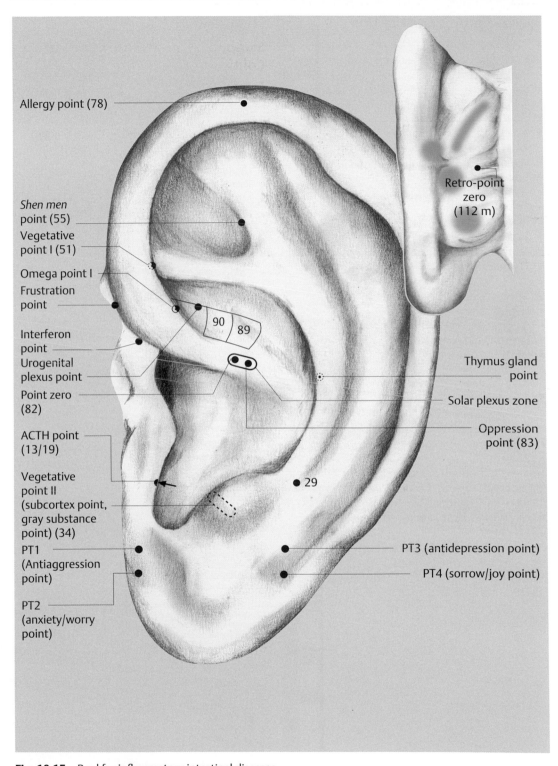

Fig. 10.15 Pool for inflammatory intestinal diseases.

Allergy point (78)

Retro-point zero (112 m)

Shen men point (55)

Vegetative point I (51)

Omega point I

Frustration point

Interferon point

Urogenital plexus point

Point zero (82)

ACTH point (13/19)

Vegetative point II (subcortex point, gray substance point) (34)

PT1 (Antiaggression point)

PT2 (anxiety/worry point)

90 89

29

Thymus gland point

Solar plexus zone

Oppression point (83)

PT3 (antidepression point)

PT4 (sorrow/joy point)

10.5.4 Chronic Obstipation

> **Practical Tip**
>
> If there are clues in the patient's history that it is present, a diagnosis of habitually delayed transit should be ruled out; neither ear nor body acupuncture is sufficiently effective in such cases.

Pool of Feasible Points (Fig. 10.16)
- Hypogastric plexus point.
- Colon zone (91).
- Hemorrhoid zone (81).
- Point zero (82).
- Retro-point zero.
- Vegetative point I (51).
- Motor intestine zone on the back of the ear.
- Psychotropic points (PT1–PT4).

Primary Selection of Points
- Hypogastric plexus point.
- Colon zone (91).
- Hemorrhoid zone (81).
- Point zero (82).
- Retro-point zero .

Supplementary Points
- Vegetative point I (51).
- Motor intestine zone on the back of the ear.
- Psychotropic points (PT1–PT4).

Treatment is initially carried out every 2 days using alternating sets of points; once an improvement is noticed, this changes to once a week. A series of 10 to 15 sessions is required.

Combination with Body Acupuncture
The *shu/mu* technique using BL-25 to ST-25. Furthermore, LI-4, LI-11, CV-6, TB-12, ST-36, GB-25, GB-26, GB-31.

Example
First Session
- Colon zone (91).
- Point zero (82).
- Vegetative point I (51).
- Psychotropic points (e.g., PT1–PT4), depending on sensitivity.

Second Session
- Hemorrhoid zone (81).
- Hypogastric plexus point.
- Retro-point zero.
- Motor intestine zone on the back of the ear.
- Psychotropic points (e.g., PT1–PT4), depending on sensitivity.

Third Session
- Colon zone (91).
- Hypogastric plexus point.
- Vegetative point I (51).
- Psychotropic points (e.g., PT1–PT4), depending on sensitivity.

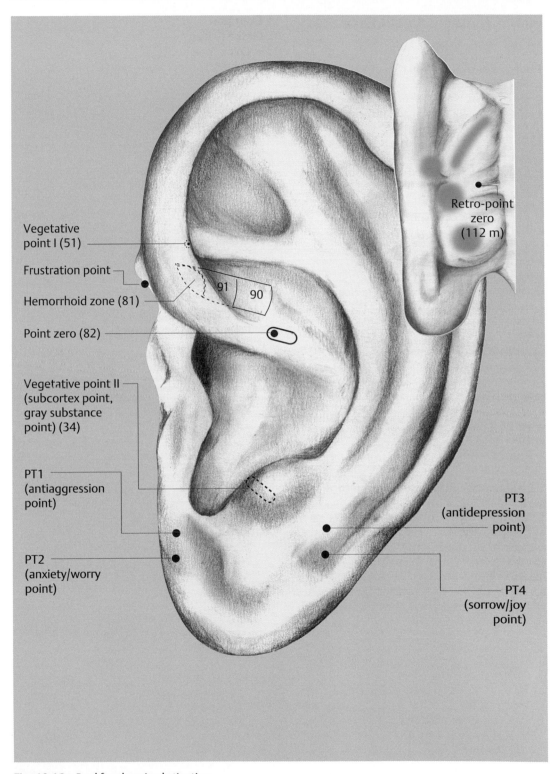

Vegetative
point I (51)

Frustration point

Hemorrhoid zone (81)

Point zero (82)

Vegetative point II
(subcortex point,
gray substance
point) (34)

PT1
(antiaggression
point)

PT2
(anxiety/worry
point)

91

90

Retro-point
zero
(112 m)

PT3
(antidepression
point)

PT4
(sorrow/joy
point)

Fig. 10.16 Pool for chronic obstipation.

10.6 Gynecological Diseases

10.6.1 Infertility

Pool of Feasible Points (Fig. 10.17)
- Uterus point (58).
- Ovary/testis point (according to Nogier).
- Ovary (gonadotropin) point (23).
- Urogenital plexus point.
- Psychotropic points (e.g., PT1–PT4, master omega point).
- Vegetative points I and II.
- Jerome point (29 b).
- ACTH point.
- Liver zone (97).
- Kidney zone (95).

Primary Point Selection
- Uterus point (58).
- Ovary/testis point (according to Nogier).
- Ovary (gonadotropin) point (23).
- Urogenital plexus point.

Supplementary Points
- Psychotropic points (e.g., PT1–PT4, master omega point).
- Vegetative points I and II.
- Jerome point (29 b).
- ACTH point.
- Liver zone (97).
- Kidney zone (95).

Combination with Body Acupuncture
KI-3, BL-23, and, if necessary, ST-26.

Initially, a series of 10 treatments is carried out, if possible once a day or every other day. Depending on sensitivity, two or three areas per ear are selected and treated in an alternating manner with other sensitive points. The combination of points is determined by their detectability and varies depending on the individual.

Example
First Session
- Uterus point (58).
- Ovary (gonadotropin) point (23), urogenital plexus point.
- Jerome point (29 b).
- Psychotropic points (e.g., PT1–PT4), depending on sensitivity.

Second Session
- Ovary/testis point (according to Nogier).
- Uterus point (according to Nogier).
- ACTH point.
- Liver zone (97).
- Kidney zone (95).
- Psychotropic points (e.g., PT1–PT4), depending on sensitivity.

Third Session
- The same as the first session; if required, exchange Jerome point (29 b) for vegetative point I (51) or vegetative point II (34).

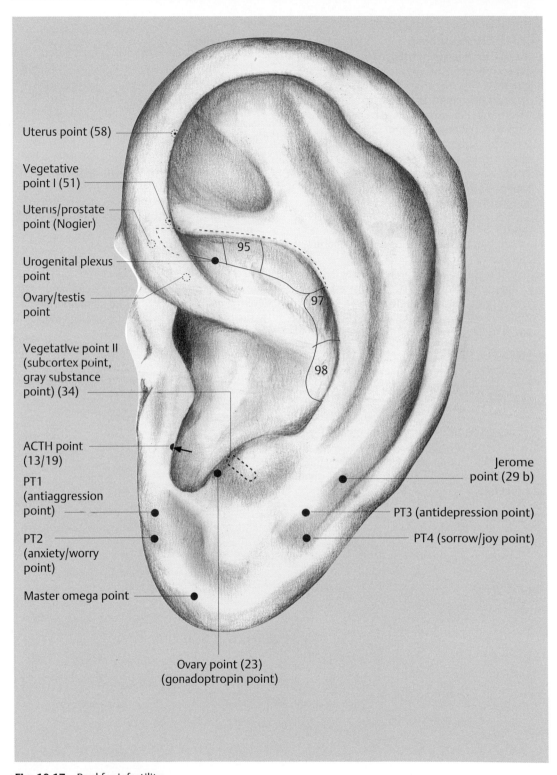

Uterus point (58)

Vegetative
point I (51)

Uterus/prostate
point (Nogier)

Urogenital plexus
point

Ovary/testis
point

Vegetative point II
(subcortex point,
gray substance
point) (34)

ACTH point
(13/19)

PT1
(antiaggression
point)

PT2
(anxiety/worry
point)

Master omega point

95

97

98

Jerome
point (29 b)

PT3 (antidepression point)

PT4 (sorrow/joy point)

Ovary point (23)
(gonadoptropin point)

Fig. 10.17 Pool for infertility.

10.6.2 Loss of Libido/Erectile Dysfunction

Pool of Feasible Points (Fig. 10.18)
- Libido points penis/clitoris point (according to Nogier).
- Ovary/testis point (according to Nogier).
- Urogenital plexus point.
- Ovary (gonadotropin) point (23).
- Zone of paravertebral chain of ganglia (level L5/S1), checking for sensitive points.
- Psychotropic points: e.g., PT1 to PT4, master omega point, frustration point.
- Vegetative points I and II.

Primary Selection of Points
- Libido points penis/clitoris point (according to Nogier).
- Ovary/testis point (according to Nogier).
- Urogenital plexus point.
- Ovary (gonadotropin) point (23).
- Zone of paravertebral chain of ganglia (level L5/S1), checking for sensitive points.

Supplementary Points
- Psychotropic points: e.g., PT1 to PT4, master omega point, frustration point.
- Vegetative points I and II.

Treatment begins with two sessions per week and can be reduced to one session per week after improvement sets in after five or six sessions. A total of approximately 10 to 15 sessions should be expected.

Example
First Session
- Libido points penis/clitoris point (according to Nogier).
- Psychotropic points: (e.g., PT1–PT4), depending on sensitivity.
- Vegetative point I (51).

Second Session
- Ovary/testis point (according to Nogier).
- Zone of paravertebral chain of ganglia (level L5/S1), checking for sensitive points.
- Vegetative points II (34).
- Psychotropic points: (e.g., PT1–PT4), depending on sensitivity.
- Ovary (gonadotropin) point (23).

Third Session
The same as the first session, depending on sensitivity; possibly exchange the libido point of the penis/clitoris point (according to Nogier) for the ovary (gonadotropin) point (23).

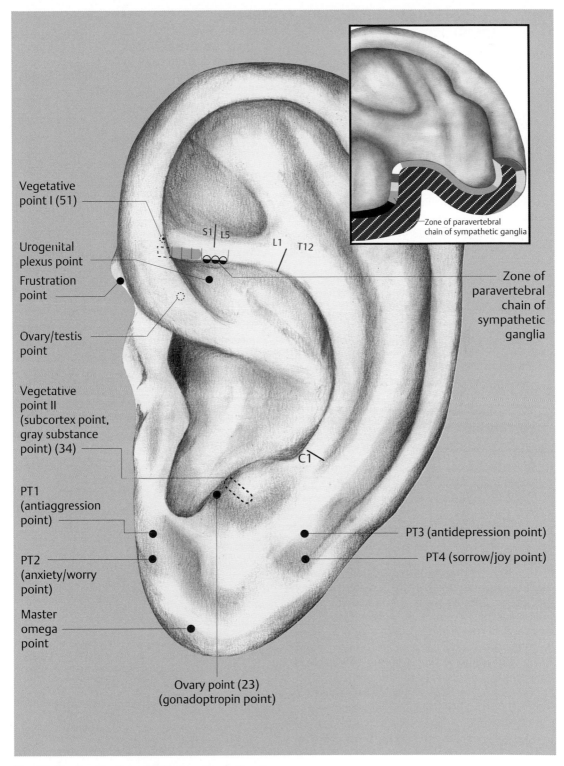

Vegetative point I (51)

Urogenital plexus point

Frustration point

Ovary/testis point

Vegetative point II (subcortex point, gray substance point) (34)

PT1 (antiaggression point)

PT2 (anxiety/worry point)

Master omega point

S1 | L5

L1   T12

Zone of paravertebral chain of sympathetic ganglia

Zone of paravertebral chain of sympathetic ganglia

C1

PT3 (antidepression point)

PT4 (sorrow/joy point)

Ovary point (23) (gonadoptropin point)

Fig. 10.18   Pool for loss of libido/erectile dysfunction.

10.6.3 Premenstrual Syndrome (PMS)

Pool of Feasible Points (Fig. 10.19)

- Zone of paravertebral chain of ganglia (level L5/S1), checking for sensitive points.
- Urinary bladder zone (92).
- Urogenital plexus point.
- Ovary point (23).
- Uterus point (58).
- Uterus (according to Nogier).
- Mamma ("zone of nervous control points of endocrine glands").
- Mammary gland point (44).
- Psychotropic points: PT1 to PT4, frustration point, master omega point.
- Vegetative points I and II.

Primary Point Selection

- Zone of paravertebral chain of ganglia (level L5/S1), checking for sensitive points.
- Urinary bladder zone (92).
- Urogenital plexus point.
- Ovary point (23).
- Uterus point (58).
- Uterus (according to Nogier).
- Mamma ("zone of nervous control points of endocrine glands").
- Mammary gland point (44).

Supplementary Points

- Psychotropic points: PT1 to PT4, frustration point, master omega point.
- Vegetative points I and II.

Combination with Body Acupuncture

GB-34, GB-4, GB-10, SI-5, TB-6, CV-17, LR-3, LR-13, LR-14.

The first treatment of two sessions per week begins approximately 1 week before the expected discomfort starts and continues during menstruation. A total of approximately five sessions per treatment occurs over the course of two cycles. This generally results in considerable improvement of or freedom from symptoms.

Depending on the course of the condition, therapy may continue for another two cycles.

Example

First Session

- Urogenital plexus point.
- Mammary gland point (44).
- Zone of paravertebral chain of ganglia (level L5/S1), checking for sensitive points.
- Vegetative point I (51).
- Psychotropic points: PT1 to PT4, depending on sensitivity.
- Uterus point (58).

Second Session

- Mamma ("zone of nervous control points of endocrine glands").
- Ovary point (23).
- Uterus (according to Nogier).
- Vegetative point II.
- Psychotropic points: PT1 to PT4, depending on sensitivity.

Third Session

- The same as the first session. If necessary, repeated treatment of the ovary point (23) and mamma ("zone of nervous control points of endocrine glands").

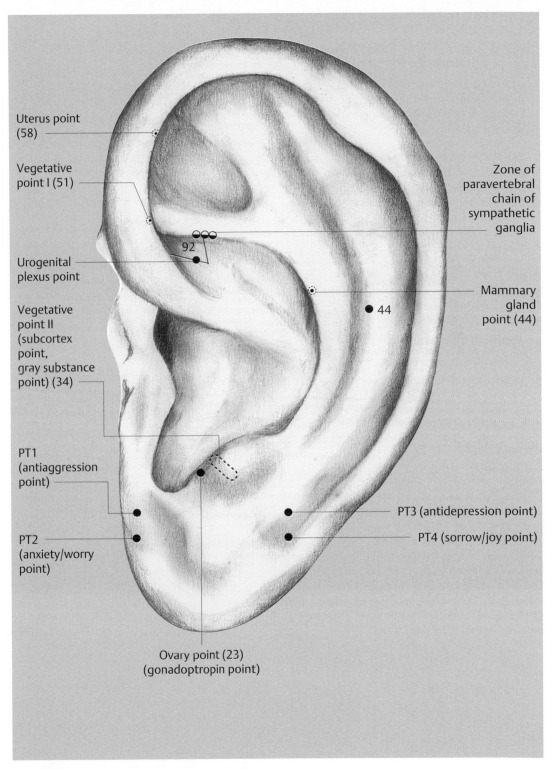

Uterus point (58)

Vegetative point I (51)

Urogenital plexus point

Vegetative point II (subcortex point, gray substance point) (34)

PT1 (antiaggression point)

PT2 (anxiety/worry point)

92

Zone of paravertebral chain of sympathetic ganglia

Mammary gland point (44)

44

PT3 (antidepression point)

PT4 (sorrow/joy point)

Ovary point (23) (gonadoptropin point)

Fig. 10.19 Pool for premenstrual syndrome (PMS).

10.7　Urological Diseases

10.7.1　Prostatitis (Abacterial, Chronically Recurrent)

Pool of Feasible Points (Fig. 10.20)
- Prostate/uterus point (according to Nogier).
- Prostate zone (93).
- Urinary bladder zone (92).
- Urogenital plexus point.
- Zone of paravertebral chain of ganglia (level L5/S1), checking for sensitive points.
- *Shen men* point (55).
- Immunomodulatory points: allergy point, interferon point, thymus gland point.
- Psychotropic points: e.g., PT1 to PT4, frustration point.

Primary Point Selection
- Prostate/uterus point (according to Nogier).
- Prostate zone (93).
- Urinary bladder zone (92).
- Urogenital plexus point.
- Zone of paravertebral chain of ganglia (level L5/S1), checking for sensitive points.
- Shen men point (55).

Supplementary Points
- Immunomodulatory points: allergy point, interferon point, thymus gland point.
- Psychotropic points: e.g., PT1 to PT4, frustration point.

Initially, treatment is carried out every other day. When the condition improves, treatment is reduced to two sessions per week. Improvement is expected after a series of 8 to 10 treatments. In general, lasting freedom from symptoms can only be expected in combination with colon rehabilitation and several repeated treatment series. Again, the patient must be informed about options from conventional therapy, and supervision by a specialist is warranted.

Example
First Session
- Urogenital plexus point.
- Prostate zone (93).
- *Shen men* point (55).
- Interferon point.

Second Session
- Prostate/uterus point (according to Nogier).
- Zone of paravertebral chain of ganglia (level L5/S1), checking for sensitive points.
- Allergy point.
- Psychotropic points: PT1 to PT4, depending on sensitivity.

Third Session
- The same as the second session, if necessary including the thymus gland point.

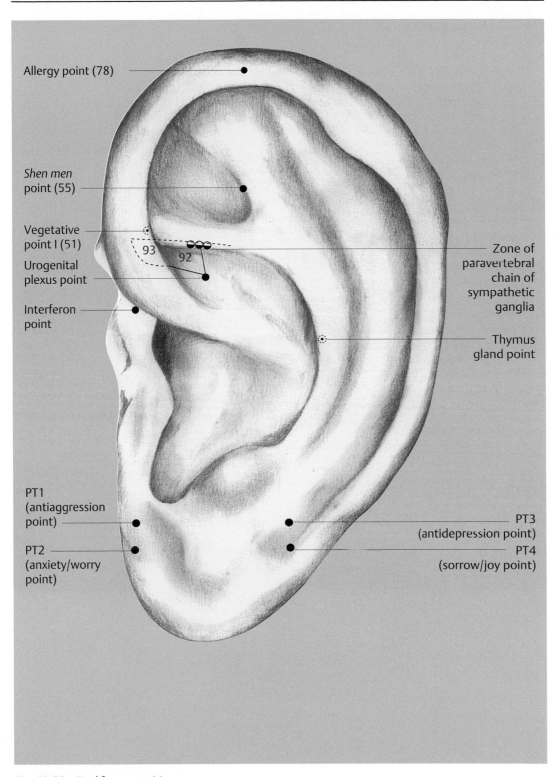

Allergy point (78)

Shen men point (55)

Vegetative point I (51)

Urogenital plexus point

Interferon point

93

92

Zone of paravertebral chain of sympathetic ganglia

Thymus gland point

PT1 (antiaggression point)

PT2 (anxiety/worry point)

PT3 (antidepression point)

PT4 (sorrow/joy point)

Fig. 10.20 Pool for prostatitis.

10.7.2 Urinary Incontinence
Pool of Feasible Points (Fig.10.21)
- Urinary bladder zone (92).
- Urogenital plexus point.
- Zone of paravertebral chain of ganglia (level L5/S1), checking for sensitive points.
- Point zero (82, diaphragm point).
- Psychotropic points: e.g., PT1 to PT4, master omega point, frustration point.
- Vegetative points I and II.
- Kidney zone (95).

Primary Point Selection
- Urinary bladder zone (92).
- Urogenital plexus point.
- Zone of paravertebral chain of ganglia (level L5/S1), checking for sensitive points.
- Point zero (82, diaphragm point).

Supplementary Points
- Psychotropic points: e.g., PT1 to PT4, master omega point, frustration point.
- Vegetative points I and II.
- Kidney zone (95).

Example
First Session
- Urogenital plexus point.
- Point zero (82).
- Vegetative point I (51).

Second Session
- Zone of paravertebral chain of ganglia (level L5/S1), checking for sensitive points.
- Urinary bladder zone (92).
- Vegetative point II (34).
- Psychotropic points: e.g., PT1 to PT4, depending on sensitivity.

Third Session
- Urogenital plexus point.
- Vegetative point I (51).
- Urinary bladder zone (92).
- Psychotropic points: e.g., PT1 to PT4, depending on sensitivity.

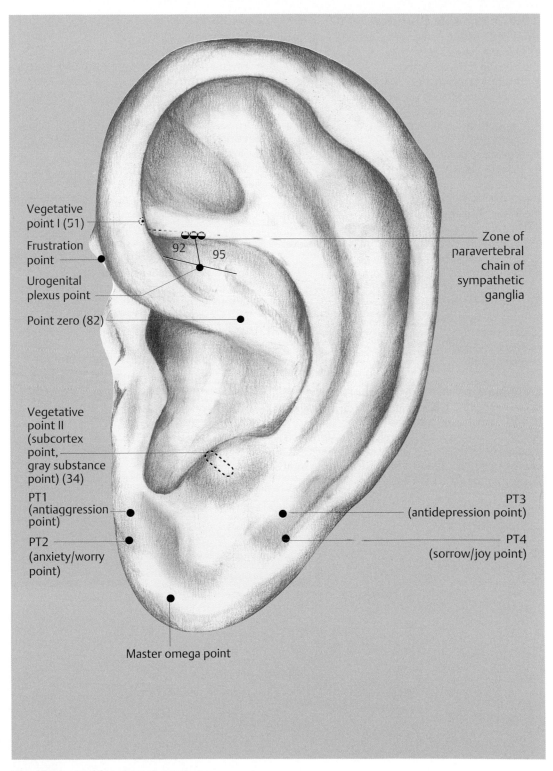

Vegetative point I (51)

Frustration point

Urogenital plexus point

Point zero (82)

92   95

Zone of paravertebral chain of sympathetic ganglia

Vegetative point II (subcortex point, gray substance point) (34)

PT1 (antiaggression point)

PT2 (anxiety/worry point)

PT3 (antidepression point)

PT4 (sorrow/joy point)

Master omega point

Fig. 10.21 Pool for urinary incontinence.

10.7.3 Irritable Bladder
Pool of Feasible Points (Fig. 10.22)
- Urinary bladder zone (92).
- Urogenital plexus point.
- Zone of paravertebral chain of ganglia (level L5/S1), checking for sensitive points.
- Point zero (82, diaphragm point).
- Psychotropic points: e.g., PT1 to PT4, frustration point.
- Vegetative points I and II.
- Kidney zone (95).

Primary Point Selection
- Urinary bladder zone (92).
- Urogenital plexus point.
- Zone of paravertebral chain of ganglia (level L5/S1), checking for sensitive points.
- Point zero (82, diaphragm point).

Supplementary Points
- Psychotropic points: e.g., PT1 to PT4, frustration point.
- Vegetative points I and II.
- Kidney zone (95).

Combination with Body Acupuncture
KI-7, BL-20, BL-23, BL-28, BL-40, CV-3, SP-6, SP-9.

Initial treatment is carried out daily or twice a day. When the condition improves, treatment is reduced to two sessions per week. Usually, treatment can be successfully completed with a total of approximately 10 sessions.

Example
First Session
- Urinary bladder zone (92).
- Psychotropic points: e.g., PT1 to PT4, depending on sensitivity.
- Kidney zone (95).
- Vegetative point I (51).

Second Session
- Urogenital plexus point.
- Point zero (82).
- Vegetative point II (34).
- Psychotropic points: e.g., PT1 to PT4, depending on sensitivity.

Third Session
- Zone of paravertebral chain of ganglia (level L5/S1), checking for sensitive points.
- Kidney zone (95).
- Vegetative point I (51).
- Psychotropic points: e.g., PT1 to PT4, depending on sensitivity.
- Urinary bladder zone (92).

Fourth Session
- The same as the third session.

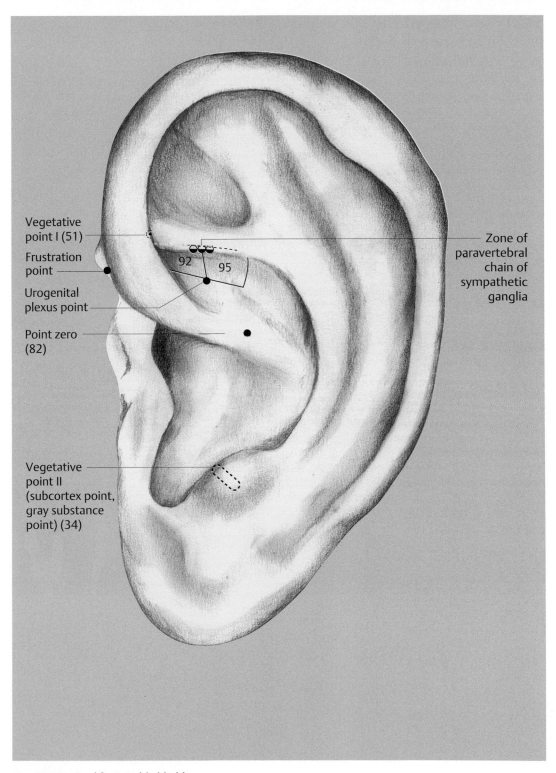

Vegetative
point I (51)

Frustration
point

Urogenital
plexus point

Point zero
(82)

Vegetative
point II
(subcortex point,
gray substance
point) (34)

Zone of
paravertebral
chain of
sympathetic
ganglia

92

95

Fig. 10.22 Pool for irritable bladder.

10.8 Diseases of the Locomotor System

10.8.1 Achillodynia

Pool of Feasible Points (Fig. 10.23)
- Calcaneus point (47).
- Ankle point.
- Knee point (49 b).
- *Shen men* point (55).
- Jerome (29 b).
- Sensitive points between ankle point and calcaneus point.
- Retro-Jerome point .
- Retro-knee point (French).

Primary Point Selection
- Calcaneus point (47).
- Ankle point.
- Sensitive points between the ankle point and calcaneus point.

Supplementary Points
- *Shen men* point (55).
- Jerome (29 b).

Combination with Body Acupuncture

KI-3, KI-5, BL-57, BL-58, BL-60, BL-61, locally at the insertion of the Achilles tendon.

In acute conditions, treatment is carried out three times a week depending on the course of the pain, and if necessary daily with alternating sets of points. After the complaint has eased, another three sessions are carried out at weekly intervals, until freedom from symptoms is achieved.

Example

First Session
- Ankle point.
- Knee point (49 b).
- Sensitive points between ankle point and calcaneus point.
- *Shen men* point (55).

Second Session
- Calcaneus point (47).
- Sensitive points between the ankle point and calcaneus point.
- Jerome point (29 b).
- Retro-knee point (French).

Third Session
- Sensitive points between the ankle point and calcaneus point.
- Ankle point.
- *Shen men* point (55).
- Retro-Jerome point.

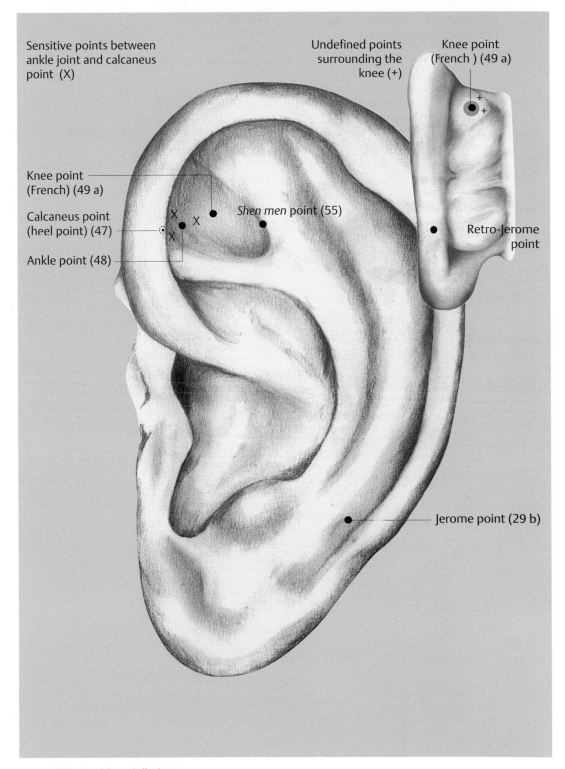

Sensitive points between
ankle joint and calcaneus
point (X)

Undefined points
surrounding the
knee (+)

Knee point
(French) (49 a)

Knee point
(French) (49 a)

Calcaneus point
(heel point) (47)

Ankle point (48)

Shen men point (55)

Retro-Jerome
point

Jerome point (29 b)

Fig. 10.23 Pool for achillodynia.

10.8.2 Epicondylitis, Epicondylopathy (Tennis Elbow)

For point selection, differentiation between lateral and medial epicondylitis is irrelevant.

Pool of Feasible Points (Fig. 10.24)
- Elbow point (66) (ipsilateral).
- Points in proximity to 66.
- Retro-elbow point (elbow joint zone).
- *Shen men* point (55).
- Jerome point (29 b).

Primary Point Selection
- Elbow point (66) (ipsilateral).
- Points in proximity to 66.
- Retro-elbow point.

Supplementary Points
- *Shen men* point (55).
- Jerome point (29 b).

Combination with Body Acupuncture
Point selection is according to the affected pathways.

Depending on the course of the pain, treatment may be carried out daily with alternating sets of points. Once the complaint has subsided, another three sessions are carried out at weekly intervals.

Example
First Session
- Elbow point (66).
- *Shen men* point (55).

Second Session
- *Shen men* point (55).
- Jerome point (29 b).
- Two or three sensitive points in proximity to 66.

Third Session
- Elbow point (66).
- *Shen men* point (55).

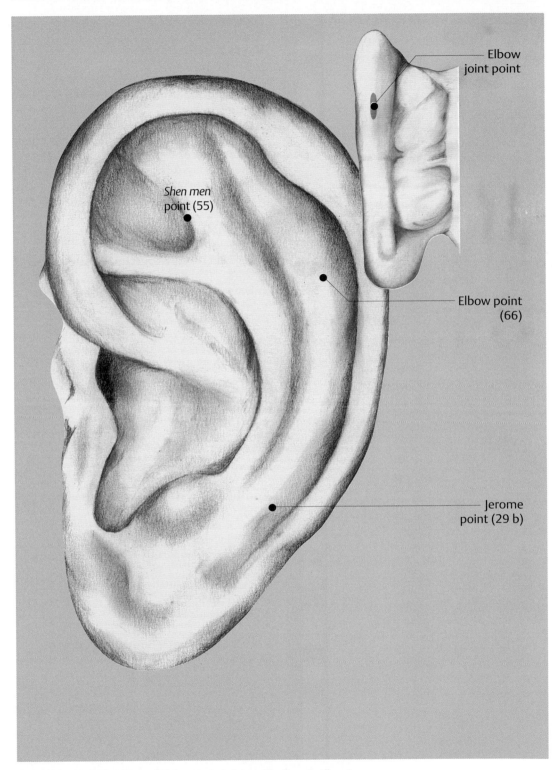

Fig. 10.24 Pool for epicondylitis or epicondylopathy (tennis elbow).

10.8.3 **Shoulder–Arm Syndrome**

Pool of Feasible Points (Fig. 10.25)
- Segment therapy: vegetative groove at level C7 to T8.
- Shoulder joint point (64).
- Shoulder point (65).
- Retro-shoulder joint point.
- Retro-shoulder point.
- Jerome point (29 b).
- *Shen men* point (55).
- Occiput point (29).
- Thalamus point (26a).
- Analgesia point.
- ACTH point.

Acute

Primary Point Selection
- Segment therapy: vegetative groove at level C7 to T8.
- Shoulder joint point (64).
- Shoulder point (65).
- Retro-shoulder joint point.
- Retro-shoulder point.

Supplementary Points
- Jerome point (29 b).
- *Shen men* point (55).
- Occiput point (29).
- Thalamus point (26 a).
- Analgesia point.
- ACTH point.

Combination with Body Acupuncture
Here, differentiation is required between:
- Lateral shoulder pain: LI-15 or TB-14; ST-36, ST-38, as well as GB-34.
- Dorsal shoulder pain: SI-9, SI-11, SI-12, BL-60, SI-3, and ST-38.

In the acute phase, treatment takes place either every day or every other day. Approximately five sessions are required. Once the complaint has improved, sessions can be reduced to two and later one per week. Depending on the severity of the condition, a total of approximately 10 sessions are required.

Combination with Oral Acupuncture (Gleditsch)
The third molar–retromolar space of the upper jaw, at the maxillary tuberosity.

Preventive Treatment in the Symptom-free Period
In chronic conditions, treatment is started with two sessions per week, which can be reduced to one session per week depending on the course of the condition. Point combinations differ from patient to patient. Generally, two series of 10 sessions each with a treatment break of 1 to 2 weeks are required.

Example: Dorsal Shoulder Pain

First Session
- Segment therapy: vegetative groove at level C7 to T8.
- Shoulder joint point.
- *Shen men* point (55).
- Retro-shoulder point.

Combination with Body Acupuncture
SI-9, SI-12, BL-60, SI-3.

Second Session
- Segment therapy: vegetative groove at level C7 to T8.
- Shoulder point (65).
- Jerome point (29 b).
- Retro-shoulder joint point.

Combination with Body Acupuncture
SI-11, BL-60, ST-38.

Third Session
- Segment therapy: vegetative groove at level C7 to T8.
- Shoulder joint point (64).
- ACTH point.
- Retro-shoulder point.

Combination with Body Acupuncture
SI-3, ST-38.

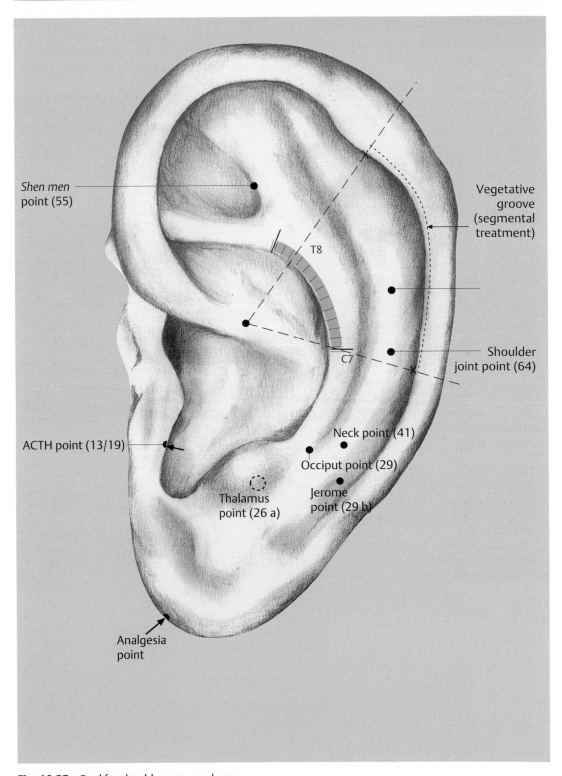

Shen men point (55)

Vegetative groove (segmental treatment)

T8

C7

Shoulder joint point (64)

ACTH point (13/19)

Neck point (41)

Occiput point (29)

Thalamus point (26 a)

Jerome point (29 b)

Analgesia point

Fig. 10.25 Pool for shoulder–arm syndrome.

10.8.4 Cervicobrachial Syndrome

Pool of Feasible Points (Fig. 10.26)
- Thalamus point (26 a).
- *Shen men* point (55).
- Retro-thalamus point.
- Jerome point (29 b).
- Segment therapy: cervical segment, including points in the zone of paravertebral chain of sympathetic ganglia (e.g., middle cervical ganglion point and also undefined points).
- Neck point (scapha).
- Vegetative groove (helical groove).
- Zone of sensory tracts of spinal cord on the helical brim.
- Neck zone (back of ear).
- Segment therapy: thoracic segment, including points in the zone of paravertebral chain of sympathetic ganglia (e.g., stellate ganglion).
- Shoulder point (scapha).
- Vegetative groove.
- Zone of sensory tracts of spinal cord on the helical brim.
- Shoulder zone (back of ear).

Four treatments are usually required at intervals of 3 to 6 days, depending on the intensity of the pain. If the treatment intervals are shorter, i.e., 3 days or less, alternation of different sets of points is recommended.

First Session
- Thalamus point (26 a).
- Segment therapy—cervical segment (ganglion points and points of sensory tracts of spinal cord).
- Segment therapy—thoracic segment (vegetative groove and shoulder points).
- Shoulder zone (back of ear).

Second Session
- Retro-thalamus point.
- Segment therapy—cervical segment (points in the area of the neck zone, points of the vegetative groove).
- Segment therapy—thoracic segment (stellate ganglion point and points of the sensory tract of the spinal cord).
- Neck zone (back of ear).
- Jerome point (29 b).
- Occiput point (29).

Third Session
- The same as the first session.

No more than five or six needles per ear should be used.

When maintaining treatment intervals of at least 3 to 4 days, a regular repetition of treatment can be carried out using all sets of points according to their sensitivity.

Combination with Body Acupuncture
- Depends on the affected pathway; e.g., in cases of acute symptoms along the triple burner, use BL-5, GB-34, and GB-41, whereas in chronic conditions, the following body points are more appropriate: BL-10, GB-10, GV-13, GV-14, SI-11, SI-12, SI-14, BL-15.

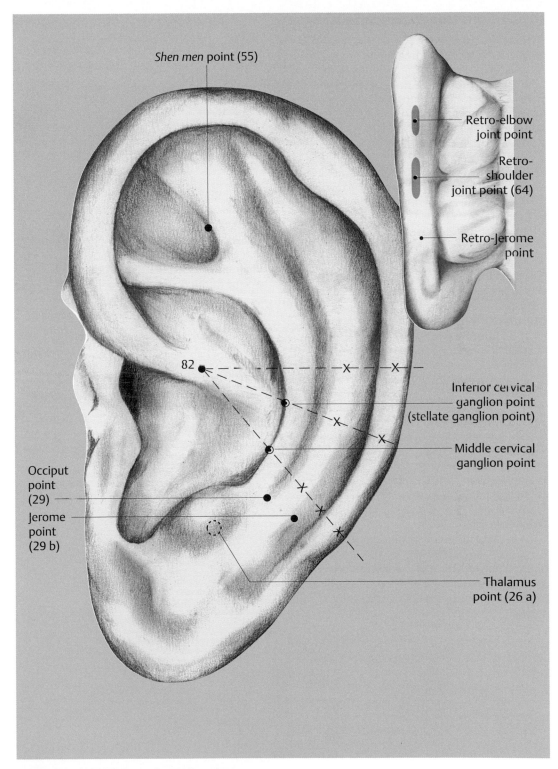

Fig. 10.26 Pool for cervicobrachial syndrome.

10.8.5 Lumbago–Sciatica Syndrome

Acute (Fig. 10.27)

- Sciatica zone (52), primarily on the ipsilateral side. Depending on the number of sensitive points, approximately three or four points are needled using the sieving technique.
- Thalamus point (26 a).
- Analgesia point.
- Retro-thalamus point.
- *Shen men* point (55).
- Segment therapy, e.g., points in the sciatica zone (52), in combination with the thigh point or knee points (49 a, 49 b).
- Occiput point (29).
- Jerome point (29 b).
- Zone of lumbar-gluteal motor tract (back of ear).

Initial treatment takes place as needed, either daily or every other day with alternating sets of points.

Example

First Session

- Sciatica zone (52) (sieving technique) .
- Thalamus point (26 a).
- Vegetative point I .
- Jerome point (29 b).

Second Session

- Segment therapy (psychotropic points).
- Retro-thalamus point.
- *Shen men* point (55).
- Zone lumbar-gluteal motor tract (back of ear).
- Occiput point (29).

Third Session

- The same as the first session.

Approximately five or six sessions are required. Once the symptoms have improved significantly, treatment is continued during the symptom-free period.

Preventive Treatment in the Symptom-free Period

In case of chronically recurrent symptoms, points are selected according to the patient's history and findings:

- Jerome point (29 b).
- ACTH point (13).
- *Shen men* point (55).
- Segment therapy: various lines of treatment are established by using sensitive points in the L1 to L5 section.
- Psychotropic points, depending on sensitivity:
- Frustration point.
- PT1 to PT4.
- If required, point R (Bourdiol).
- Vegetative point I (51), vegetative point II (34).

When using individual sets of points, it should be kept in mind that the upper limit is five or six needles per ear, and that needles used in the sieving technique are counted as one needle. Approximately 10 sessions are required initially, and these are carried out at weekly intervals.

Combination with Body Acupuncture

This is carried out in accordance with the pathways affected, e.g., in cases of a lateral radiation of pain: GB-30, GB-31, GB-34, GB-39, BL-62.

- In cases of pain along the midline or pain radiating from there: BL-10, BL-58, BL-62, BL-40, GV-26, GV-3, GV-4.

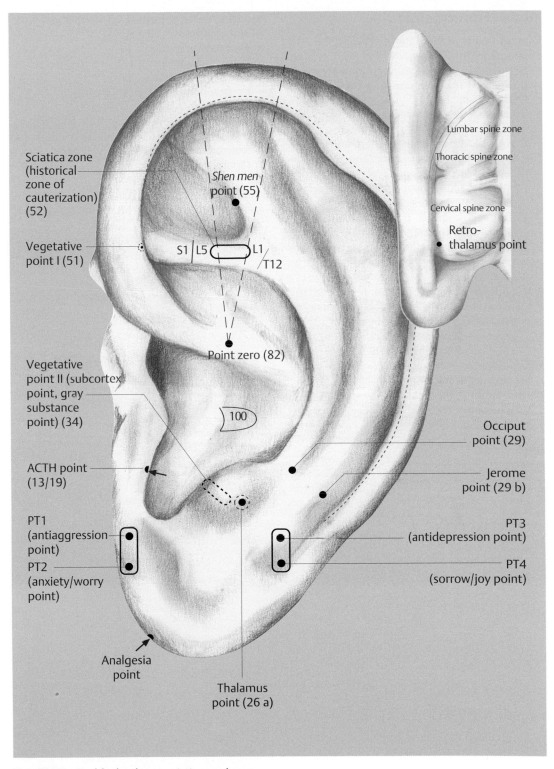

Fig. 10.27 Pool for lumbago–sciatica syndrome.

10.8.6 **Fibromyalgia**

Pool of Feasible Points (Fig. 10.28)

Primary points

- Segment therapy: using alternating treatment lines along sensitive points in the various affected areas:
  - Cervical segment, including points of the paravertebral chain of sympathetic ganglia, e.g., middle cervical ganglion, and also undefined points of the neck zone (muscle and ligament zone—scapha), vegetative groove (under helical brim), and sensory tracts of the spinal cord (helical brim).
  - Thoracic segment, including points of the paravertebral chain of sympathetic ganglia (e.g., stellate ganglion), shoulder zone (scapha), vegetative groove, and spinal cord (helical brim).
  - Lumbar segment, including the sciatica zone (inferior crus), undefined points of the paravertebral chain of sympathetic ganglia, vegetative groove, muscle and ligament zone, as well as spinal cord.
- Shoulder zone (cervical spine—back of ear).
- Neck zone (thoracic spine—back of ear).
- Retro-joint points.
- Jerome point (29 b).

Supplementary Points

- Thalamus point (26 a).
- *Shen men* point (55).
- Retro-thalamus point.
- Jerome point (29 b).
- Occiput point (29).
- ACTH point.
- Vegetative points I and II.
- Psychotropic points, depending on sensitivity: frustration point, PT1 to PT4, if required, point R (Bourdiol), master omega, and omega point II.

In chronic conditions, usually 15 to 20 sessions are required, depending on the intensity of the pain. Initially, treatment is carried out every 2 to 3 days. With shorter treatment intervals, e.g., 1 to 2 days, alternating sets of points are generally recommended for each session.

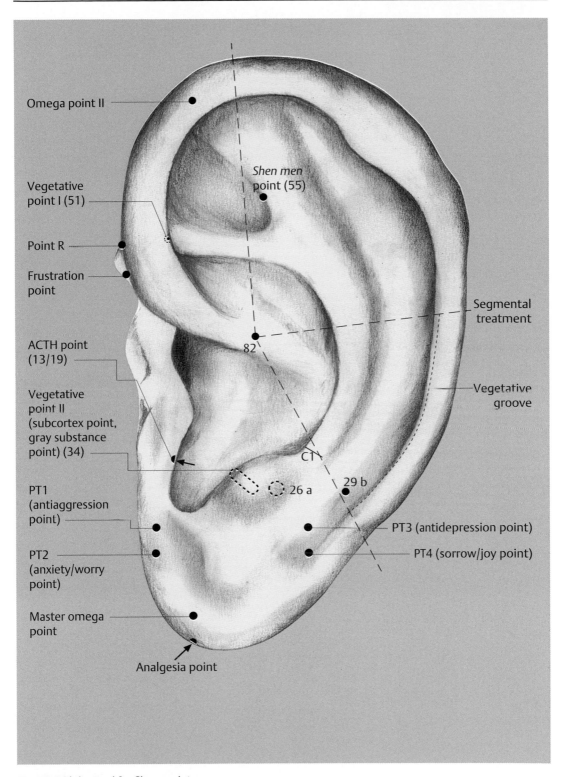

Fig. 10.28(a) Pool for fibromyalgia.

Example

First Session

- Segment therapy—cervical segment (vegetative groove, ganglion points, and points in the muscle and ligament zone).
- Jerome point (29 b).
- Master omega point.
- Thalamus point (26 a).

Second Session

- Segment therapy: lumbar segment—sciatica zone (inferior crus), undefined points of paravertebral chain of sympathetic ganglia, vegetative groove, as well as muscle and ligament zone.
- Neck zone (cervical spine—back of ear).
- Occiput point (29).
- Retro-thalamus point.

Third Session

- Segment therapy thoracic segment (vegetative groove, points in the shoulder zone, stellate ganglion point, and points of the sensory tracts of spinal cord).
- Retro-joint point: pelvis and hip.
- PT3.
- *Shen men* point (55).

Fourth Session

- The same as the first session.

Combination with Body Acupuncture

For example, BL-23, GB-34, HT-6, LR-3, GV-20, KI-3, PC-6.

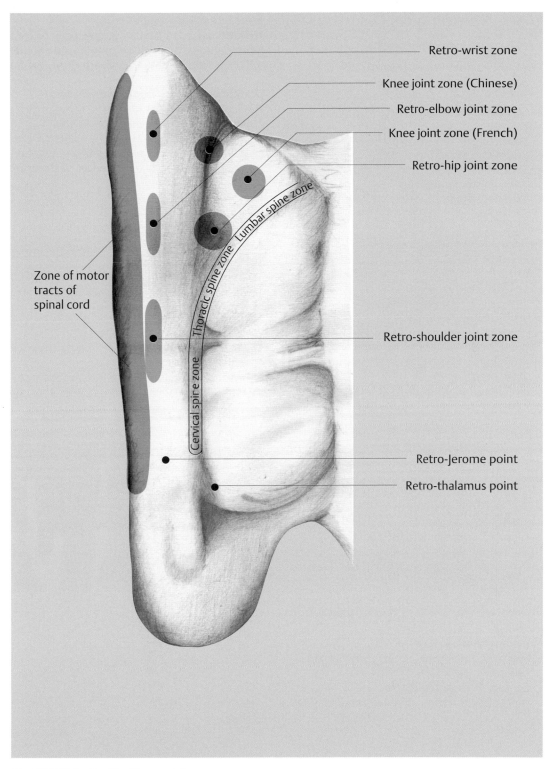

Retro-wrist zone

Knee joint zone (Chinese)

Retro-elbow joint zone

Knee joint zone (French)

Retro-hip joint zone

Lumbar spine zone

Thoracic spine zone

Zone of motor tracts of spinal cord

Cervical spire zone

Retro-shoulder joint zone

Retro-Jerome point

Retro-thalamus point

Fig. 10.28(b)   Pool for fibromyalgia.

10.9 Neurological Disorders

10.9.1 Tension Headache

Pool of Feasible Points (Fig. 10.29)

- Segment therapy: vegetative groove at level C1 to T5.
- Sensory line (29, 35, 33).
- Psychotropic points: PT1 to PT4, frustration point, master omega point.
- Jerome point (29 b).
- *Shen men* point (55).
- Thalamus point (26 a).
- Analgesia point.

Acute

Primary Point Selection

- Segment therapy: vegetative groove at level C1 to T5.
- Sensory line (29, 35, 33).

Supplementary Points

- Psychotropic points: PT1 to PT4, frustration point, master omega point.
- Jerome point (29 b).
- *Shen men* point (55).
- Thalamus point (26 a).
- Analgesia point.

Combination with Body Acupuncture

For example, BL-10, BL-60, SI 3, TB 5, GB-20, LI-4.

Depending on the degree of pain, treatment takes place, if necessary, daily, with alternating sets of points. After the discomfort has subsided, preventive treatment is given during the symptom-free period.

Initially, treatment is carried out twice a week, changing to only once a week once the pain has improved or subsided. A total of 5 to 10 sessions must be expected.

Preventive Treatment in the Symptom-free Period

Primary Point Selection

- Segment therapy: vegetative groove at level C1 to T5.
- Sensory line according to Nogier: forehead point (33), sun point (35), occiput point (29).

Supplementary Points

- Vegetative point I and/or Jerome point (29 b).
- Psychotropic points: PT1 to PT4, frustration point, omega points.

Combination with Body Acupuncture

HT-3, HT-7, GV-20, CV-17.

Depending on the intensity of the pain, 6 to 10 sessions at intervals of 3 to 6 days are required. with shorter treatment intervals, e.g., 3 days or less, varying sets of points must be selected for each session.

Example

First Session

- Segmental treatment line C2/C3.
- Jerome point (29 b).
- Occiput point (29).
- Psychotropic points: PT1 to PT4, depending on sensitivity.

Second Session

- Sensory line (29, 35, 33).
- Jerome point (29 b).
- Vegetative point I.
- Psychotropic points: PT1 to PT4, depending on sensitivity.

Third Session

- Segmental treatment line C2/C3.
- Sensory line (29, 35, 33).
- Psychotropic points: PT1 to PT4, depending on sensitivity.

Fourth Session

- The same as the first or second session.

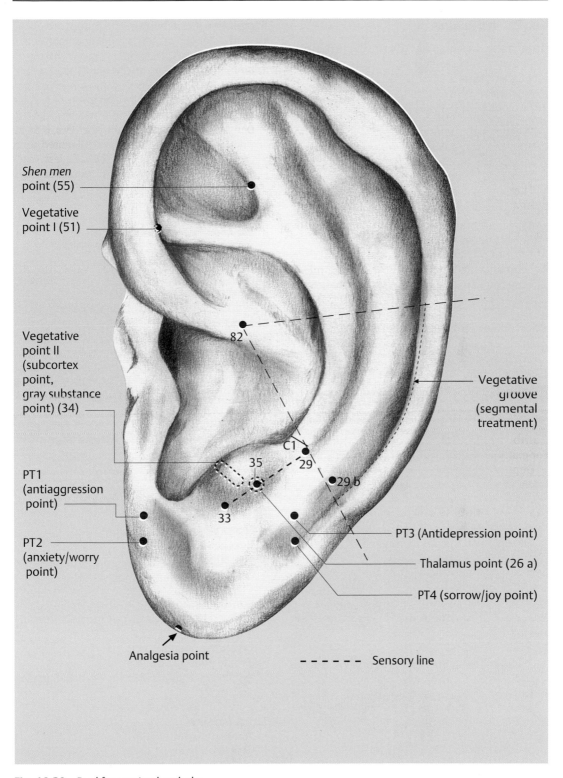

Shen men point (55)

Vegetative point I (51)

Vegetative point II (subcortex point, gray substance point) (34)

PT1 (antiaggression point)

PT2 (anxiety/worry point)

Analgesia point

82

C1

35

29

29 b

33

Vegetative groove (segmental treatment)

PT3 (Antidepression point)

Thalamus point (26 a)

PT4 (sorrow/joy point)

- - - - - - Sensory line

Fig. 10.29 Pool for tension headache.

10.9.2. **Migraine**

Treatment During the Attack (Fig. 10.30)

Primary Point Selection

- Thalamus point (26 a).
- Analgesia point.
- Sun point (35).
- Occiput point (29).
- Forehead point (33).
- *Shen men* point (55).
- Sensitive points in the solar plexus zone, such as the oppression point (83), or in the stomach zone.

or

- Thalamus point (26 a) or retro-thalamus point.
- Sun point (35).
- Occiput point (29).
- Segment therapy: e.g., superior and middle cervical ganglion points, vegetative groove, etc.

Depending on the intensity of the pain, the treatment is carried out at intervals of 2 days using alternating sets of points. After the symptoms have subsided, this is followed by preventive treatment in the symptom-free period.

Combination with Body Acupuncture

Distal points: BL-58, BL-60, SI-3, TB-5, GB-37, GB-39, GB-43, KI-3, PC-7, LI-4, ST-44, SP-6, HT-7.

Preventive Treatment in the Symptom-free Period

Primary Point Selection

Treatment is initially carried out twice a week. When attacks become less frequent or are absent, treatment should then be given only once a week. In total, 5 to 10 sessions will be required.

- Sensory line according to Nogier: forehead point (33), sun point (35), and occiput point (29).
- Sensitive points in the solar plexus zone.

Supplementary Points

Depending on the trigger mechanism:

- Weather point (body acupuncture: TB-15, GB-20).
- Ovary point/gonadotropin point (23) (body acupuncture: SP-6, KI-3).
- Vegetative point I and/or II.
- Uterus point (58) (body acupuncture: SP-6, KI-3).
- Segment therapy: vegetative groove in the cervical segment.
- Jerome point (29 b).
- Psychotropic points: PT1 to PT4, frustration point, omega points (body acupuncture: HT-3, HT-7, GV-20, CV-17).

Combination with Body Acupuncture

Local points: BL-2, BL-10, GB-3, GB-20, EX-HN5 (*tai yang*), LI-20, ST-8, GV-20, TB 15, SP-6, KI-3.

Example: Weather-dependent Migraine

First Session

- Sensory line (29, 35, 33).
- Weather point.
- Vegetative point II (34).
- Frustration point.

Second Session

- Segment therapy: vegetative groove at level C1 to T5.
- Vegetative point I (51).
- Jerome point (29 b).
- Psychotropic points: PT1 to PT4, depending on sensitivity.

Third Session

- Weather point.
- Vegetative point II (34).
- Jerome point (29 b).
- Master omega point.

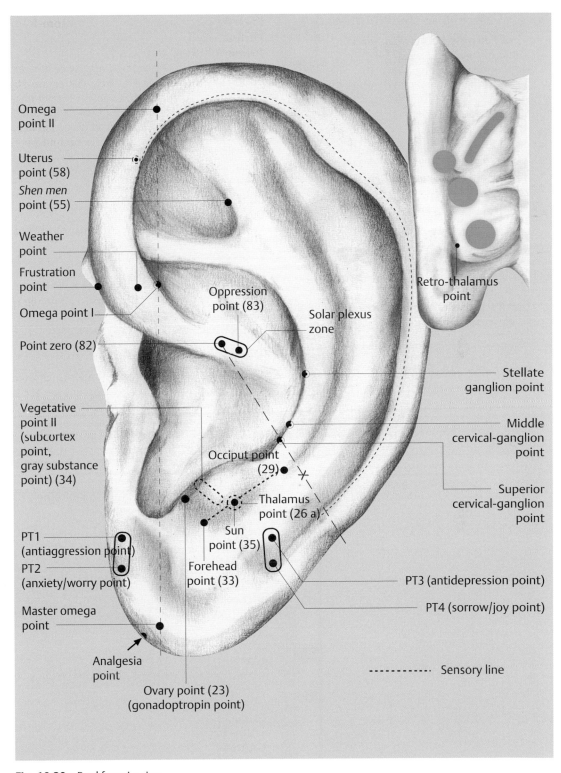

Fig. 10.30 Pool for migraine.

10.9.3 Herpes Zoster Neuralgia

Pool of Feasible Points (Fig. 10.31)

- Thalamus point (26 a).
- Retro-thalamus point.
- Segment therapy: vegetative groove, zone of sensory tracts of spinal cord in the affected segment.
- *Shen men* point (55).
- Analgesia point.
- ACTH point (13).
- Ear geometry.
- Sun point (35).
- Occiput (29).

Treatment is initially carried out every 2 days with alternating sets of points, depending on the course of the disease.

Combination with Body Acupuncture

LR-3, PC-6, BL-60, CV-14, CV-15, CV-5.

Locally: around the blister area, segmentally, e.g., GB-34, GB-40, LR-5, in cases of thoracic herpes zoster.

Example

First Session

- Thalamus point (26 a).
- Ear geometry.
- ACTH point.

Second Session

- Retro-thalamus point.
- *Shen men* point (55).
- Analgesia point.
- Ear geometry with other sensitive points, if warranted.
- Sun point (35).
- Occiput point (29).

Third Session

- The same as the first session.

Once an improvement is noticed, treatment frequency should be changed to two sessions a week and, finally, one a week.

If reactive emotional stress is suspected, PT1 and/or the master omega point may be treated, depending on their sensitivity.

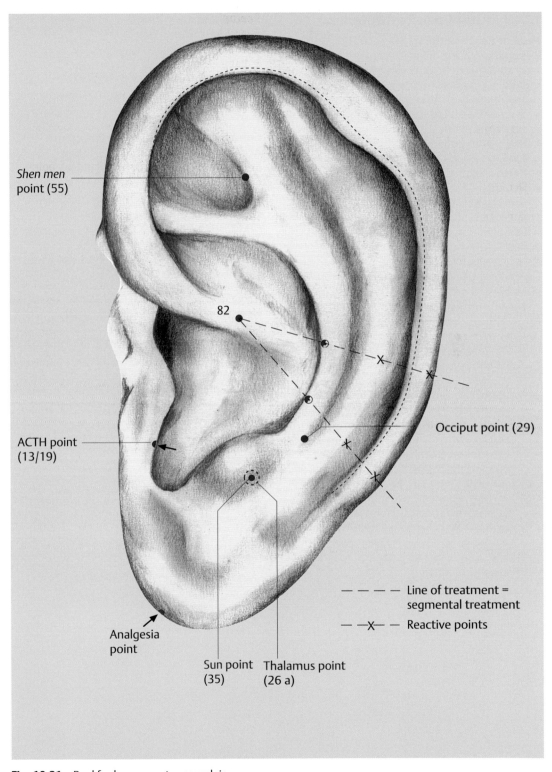

Fig. 10.31 Pool for herpes zoster neuralgia.

Shen men point (55)

82

ACTH point (13/19)

Occiput point (29)

Analgesia point

Sun point (35)

Thalamus point (26 a)

– – – – – Line of treatment = segmental treatment

– X – – Reactive points

10.9.4 Apoplexy, Postapoplexy

Pool of Feasible Points (Fig. 10.32)

Depending on the affected body parts (extremities) and/or functions, corresponding areas (segmentally or direct) are selected and sensitive supplementary points located.

- Segment therapy, cervical, thoracic, lumbar segments.
- Retro-joint points.
- Thalamus point (26 a).
- Retro-thalamus point.
- Jerome point (29 b).
- Sensory line according to Nogier (29, 35, 33).
- Vegetative point II (sieving technique).
- Von Steinburg's line of vertigo.

Primary Point Selection

- Segment therapy: using alternating treatment lines along sensitive points in the corresponding affected segments:
  - Cervical segment, including points of the paravertebral chain of sympathetic ganglia, e.g., middle cervical ganglion and also undefined points in the neck zone (muscle and ligament zone—scapha), vegetative groove (under the helical brim), as well as sensory tracts of the spinal cord (helical brim).
  - Thoracic segment, including points of the paravertebral chain of sympathetic ganglia (e.g., stellate ganglion), shoulder zone (scapha), vegetative groove, and spinal cord (helical brim).
  - Lumbar segment, including the sciatica zone (inferior crus), undefined points of the paravertebral chain of sympathetic ganglia, vegetative groove, muscle and ligament zone, as well as spinal cord.
- Retro-joint points.

Supplementary Points

- Thalamus point (26 a).
- Retro-thalamus point.
- Jerome point (29 b).
- Sensory line according to Nogier (29, 35, 33).
- Vegetative point II (sieving technique).
- Von Steinburg's line of vertigo.

Combination with Scalp Acupuncture According to Yamamoto

Basic points A, C and D, Y point: kidney.

Combination with Body Acupuncture

- Upper extremity: LI-4, LI-11, LI-15, TB-5.
- Lower extremity: GB-34, GB-14, ST-31, ST-36, ST-41.
- Facial palsy: GB-2, GB-14, SI-18, TB-17, TB-3, LI-20, GV-26, ST-1, ST-3, ST-4, ST-6, ST-7.
- Speech disorder: GV-23, CV-15.

For this disorder, up to 15 to 20 sessions may be required. Initially, treatment is carried out at intervals of 2 to 3 days, depending on the course of the condition. Symptoms tend to improve even within the first six sessions of treatment. With shorter treatment intervals, e.g., 1 to 2 days, alternating sets of points are recommended for each session.

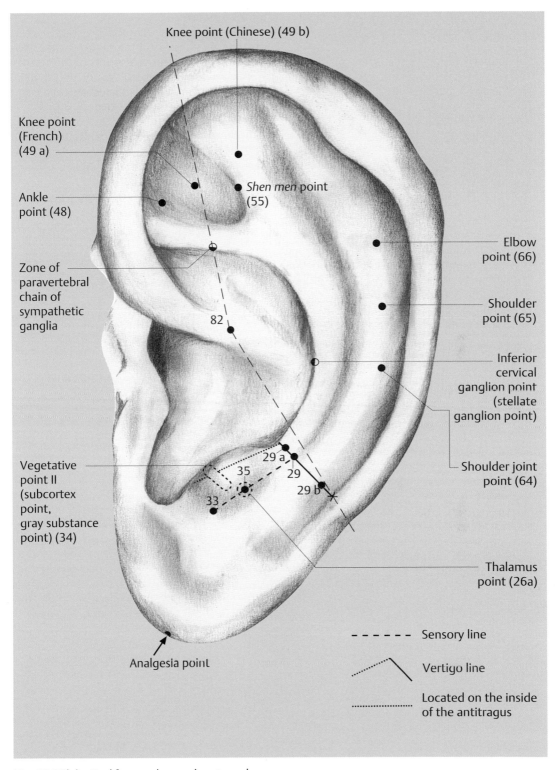

Knee point (Chinese) (49 b)

Knee point
(French)
(49 a)

Ankle
point (48)

Zone of
paravertebral
chain of
sympathetic
ganglia

Shen men point
(55)

82

Vegetative
point II
(subcortex
point,
gray substance
point) (34)

35

29 a

29

29 b

33

Analgesia point

Elbow
point (66)

Shoulder
point (65)

Inferior
cervical
ganglion point
(stellate
ganglion point)

Shoulder joint
point (64)

Thalamus
point (26a)

– – – – – Sensory line

Vertigo line

Located on the inside
of the antitragus

Fig. 10.32(a) Pool for apoplexy and postapoplexy.

Example: Partial Hemiparesis of the Right Upper and Lower Extremity

First Session
- Segment therapy: cervical segment (vegetative groove, ganglion points, and points in the muscle and ligaments zone).
- Jerome point (29 b).
- Thalamus point (26 a).
- Retro-joint points: hand, elbow or shoulder joint.
- Scalp acupuncture according to Yamamoto: basic point A.
- Body acupuncture: LI-4, LI-15, GB-34, ST-41, CV-15.

Second Session
- Segment therapy: lumbar segment (sciatica zone [inferior crus], undefined points of paravertebral chain of sympathetic ganglia, vegetative groove, as well as muscle and ligaments zone).
- Retro-joint point: knee or hip joint.
- Vegetative point II (sieving technique).
- Retro-thalamus.
- Scalp acupuncture according to Yamamoto: basic point C.
- Body acupuncture: LI-11, GB-39, ST-36, GV-23.

Third Session
- Segment therapy: thoracic segment (vegetative groove, points of the shoulder zone, stellate ganglion point, and points of the sensory tracts of the spinal cord).
- Retro-joint points: pelvis and hip.
- Sensory line according Nogier (29, 35, 33).
- Von Steinburg's line of vertigo.
- Scalp acupuncture according to Yamamoto: basic point D.
- Body acupuncture: LI-4, LI-15, TB-5, GB-34, ST-41, CV-15.

Fourth Session
- The same as the first or second session.

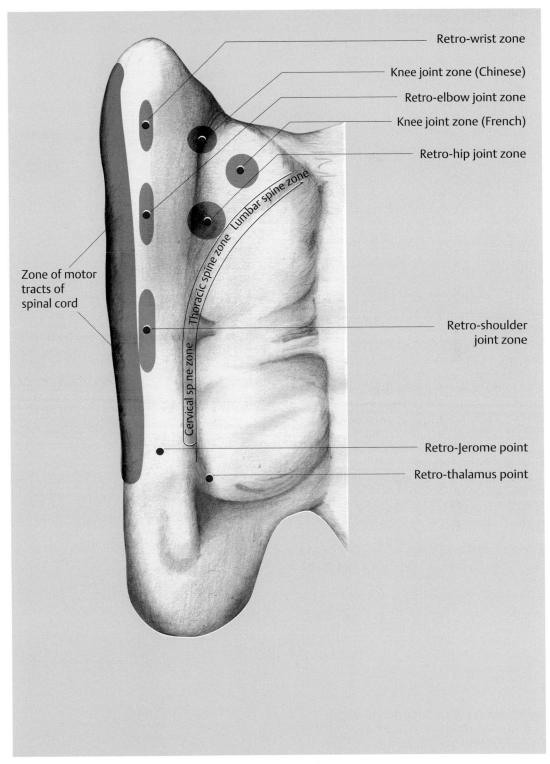

Retro-wrist zone

Knee joint zone (Chinese)

Retro-elbow joint zone

Knee joint zone (French)

Retro-hip joint zone

Zone of motor tracts of spinal cord

Thoracic spine zone

Lumbar spine zone

Cervical spine zone

Retro-shoulder joint zone

Retro-Jerome point

Retro-thalamus point

Fig. 10.32(b)   Pool for apoplexy and postapoplexy.

10.10 **Skin Diseases**

10.10.1 **Urticaria**

Pool of Feasible Points (Fig. 10.33)
- Urticaria zone (sieving technique).
- Allergy point (78), followed by micro-phlebotomy.
- Thymus gland point.
- Interferon point.
- ACTH point.
- *Shen men* point (55).
- Lung zone (101).
- Colon zone (91).
- Vegetative point I (51) or vegetative point II (34).
- Master omega or omega point I.
- Occiput point (29).
- Kidney zone (95).
- PT-1.

Preventive Treatment in the Symptom-free Period
The treatment series consists of 10 to 15 sessions. The first four to six sessions are carried out twice per week, after which treatment takes place once a week. Prior to treatment, basic care should be initiated with colon rehabilitation (symbiosis control), because acupuncture by itself will not produce a lasting therapeutic effect.

Primary Point Selection
- Allergy point (78, without microphlebotomy).
- Thymus gland point.
- Interferon point.
- ACTH point.

Supplementary Points
Depending on patient's history and exposure factors:
- Vegetative point I (51) or vegetative point II (34).
- Master omega or omega point I.
- Occiput point (29).
- Lung zone (101).
- Kidney zone (95).
- PT1.

Combination with Body Acupuncture
LI-4, LI-10, LI-11, PC-3, PC-6, PC-7, BL-13, BL-40, LU-7, SP-6, SP-10, ST-36, GV-14.

Example
First Session
- ACTH point.
- Allergy point (78).
- Interferon point.
- Vegetative point II (34).
- Omega 1 point.

In combination with Body Acupuncture
LI-4, LI-11, SP-6, ST-36.

Second Session
- Thymus gland point.
- Interferon point.
- Lung zone (101).
- Kidney zone (95).
- PT1.

In combination with Body Acupuncture
LI-10, PC-6, BL-40, LU-7, GV-14.

Third Session
- Allergy point.
- Vegetative point I (51).
- Thymus gland point.
- ACTH point.
- Master omega point.

In combination with Body Acupuncture
SP-6, ST-36, LI-4, LI-11.

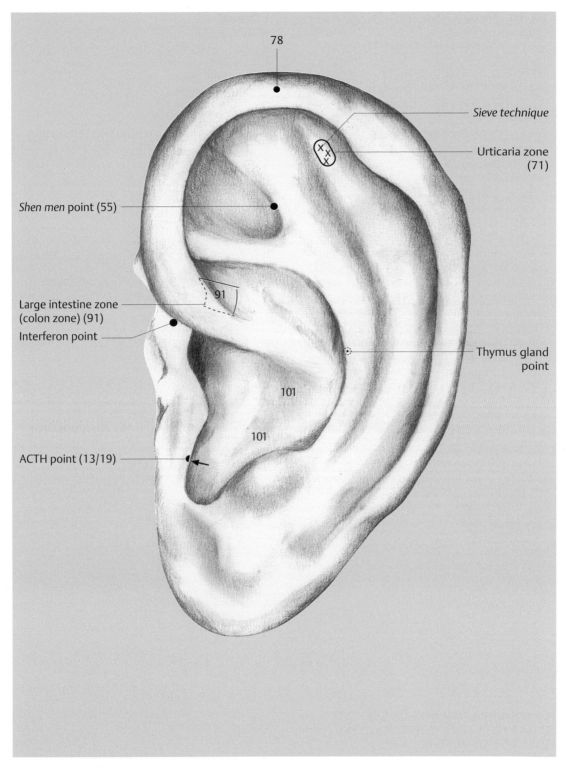

78

Sieve technique

Urticaria zone
(71)

Shen men point (55)

Large intestine zone
(colon zone) (91)

Interferon point

91

101

101

Thymus gland
point

ACTH point (13/19)

Fig. 10.33 Pool for urticaria.

10.11 Psychological Disorders

10.11.1 Sleep Disturbances

Note. Drug abuse, physical causes, and serious mental problems should be ruled out before treatment begins. Parallel treatment is possible, if warranted.

Pool of Feasible Points (Figure 10.34)
- Jerome point (29 b).
- Retro-Jerome point.
- Vegetative point I (51).
- Vegetative point II (34).
- Psychotropic points: PT1 to PT4.
- Heart zone (100).

If no serious concurrent diseases are present (e.g., pharmacomania, chronic pain conditions), approximately 5 to 10 sessions are required. Treatment is initially carried out twice a week. When improvement is noticed after four to five sessions, treatment changes to once a week.

It is recommended to use alternating sets of points and to needle in the evening, if possible.

Combination with Body Acupuncture
Depending on the constitution; general sleep-promoting points: SP-6, Ex-HN3 (*yin tan*), GV-20, KI-6, CV-17, PC-6, PC-7, HT-7, KI-3.

Example
First Session
- Jerome point (29 b).
- Occiput point (29).
- Vegetative point I (51).
- If warranted, PT1.

Second Session
- Retro-Jerome point.
- Vegetative point II (34).
- Heart zone (100).
- If warranted, PT2 or frustration point.

Third Session
- The same as the first session.

It is crucial that each of these points is found to be sensitive.

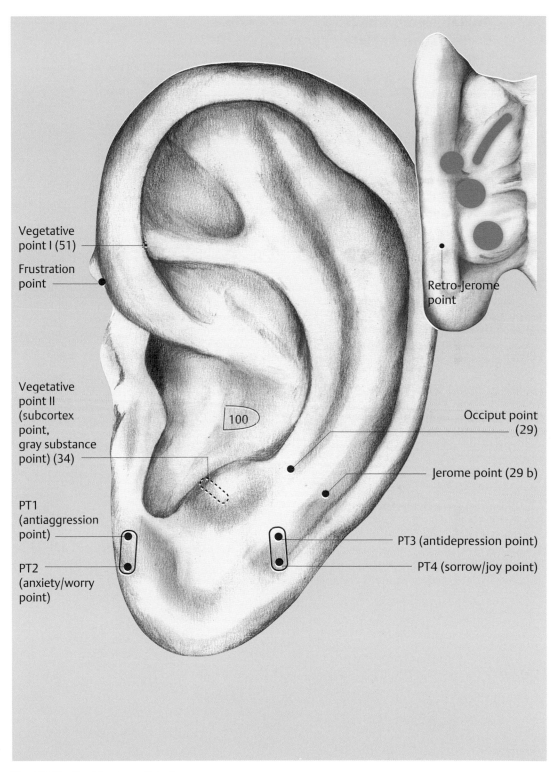

Vegetative
point I (51)

Frustration
point

Vegetative
point II
(subcortex
point,
gray substance
point) (34)

PT1
(antiaggression
point)

PT2
(anxiety/worry
point)

Retro-Jerome
point

100

Occiput point
(29)

Jerome point (29 b)

PT3 (antidepression point)

PT4 (sorrow/joy point)

Fig. 10.34 Pool for sleep disturbances.

10.11.2 Anxiety Syndrome (e.g., Examination Anxiety, Fear of Flying)

Pool of Feasible Points (Fig. 10.35)
- Jerome point (29 b).
- Retro-Jerome point.
- Occiput (29).
- Vegetative point I (51).
- Vegetative point II (34).
- Psychotropic points (PT1–PT4), frustration point.
- Heart zone (100).
- Point zero (82).
- Kidney zone (95).
- *Shen men* point (55).
- Master omega point.

Primary Point Selection
- Kidney zone (95).
- Point zero (82).
- Vegetative point II (34).
- Heart zone (100).
- *Shen men* point (55).

Supplementary Points
- Jerome point (29 b).
- Retro-Jerome point.
- Occiput (29).
- Vegetative point I (51).
- Psychotropic points (PT1–PT4), frustration point, master omega point.

Combination with Body Acupuncture
GV-20, CV-17, CV-15, HT-7, ST-36, KI-3, BL-23.

Approximately six sessions are required. Treatment is carried out twice a week, beginning around 2 to 3 weeks before the examination. Sets of points are selected individually and may be as follows:

Example
First Session
- Point zero (82).
- Vegetative point II (34) (sieving technique).
- PT2.
- Heart zone (100).
- *Shen men* point (55).
- Body acupuncture: GV-20, KI-3.

Second Session
- Kidney zone (95).
- Jerome point (29 b).
- PT1 and PT3.
- Master omega point.
- Body acupuncture: HT-7, ST-36, CV-14.

Third Session
- *Shen men* point (55).
- PT2 and PT4.
- Vegetative point II (34).
- Heart zone (100).
- Body acupuncture: BL-23, KI-3, CV-15.

Last Session—1 Day before the Examination
- Point zero (82).
- Vegetative point II (34) (sieving technique).
- Heart (100).
- *Shen men* point (55).
- Body acupuncture: GV-20, CV-15, KI-3.

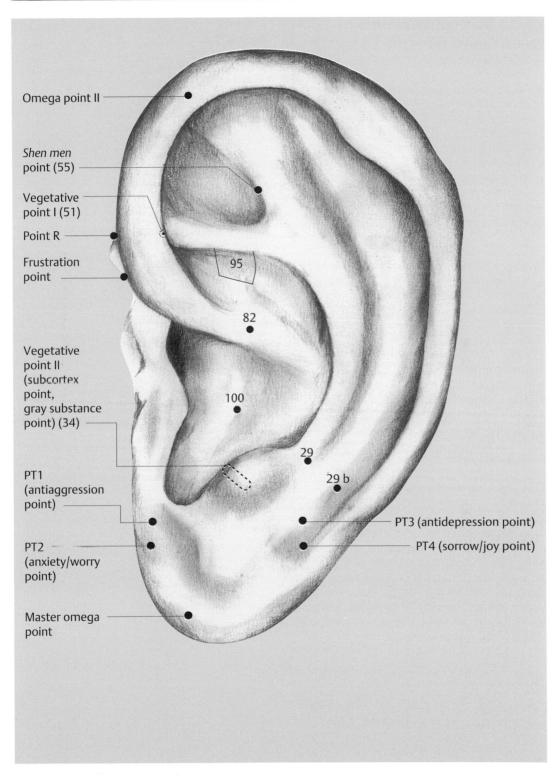

Omega point II

Shen men point (55)

Vegetative point I (51)

Point R

Frustration point

95

82

Vegetative point II (subcortex point, gray substance point) (34)

100

29

29 b

PT1 (antiaggression point)

PT3 (antidepression point)

PT2 (anxiety/worry point)

PT4 (sorrow/joy point)

Master omega point

Fig. 10.35 Pool for anxiety syndrome.

10.11.3 **Burnout Syndrome**

Pool of Feasible Points (Fig. 10.36)
- Psychotropic points (PT1–PT4), frustration point.
- Master omega point, omega point II.
- Point R (Bourdiol).
- Heart zone (100).
- Point zero (82).
- Kidney zone (95).
- *Shen men* point (55).
- Retro-Jerome point.
- Occiput (29).
- Vegetative point I (51).
- Vegetative point II (34).
- Jerome point (29 b).

Primary Point Selection
- Psychotropic points (PT1–PT4), frustration point.
- Master omega point, omega point II.
- Point R (Bourdiol).
- Kidney zone (95).

Supplementary Points
- Jerome point (29 b).
- Retro-Jerome point.
- Occiput point (29).
- Vegetative point I (51).
- Heart zone (100).
- Point zero (82).

Combination with Body Acupuncture
KI-3, HT-7, SP-6, LU-7, BL-23, BL-20, GV-20, PC-5, PC-6.

In severe conditions, psychotherapy should be the primary focus. Depending on the course, more than 20 adjuvant sessions may be necessary. Initially, treatment is three times a week (Monday, Wednesday, Friday). Once the condition stabilizes, weekly or biweekly treatment intervals are desirable. The selection of points differs from session to session.

Example

First Session
- PT1 and PT3.
- Master omega point.
- Omega point II.
- Vegetative point II (34).
- Body acupuncture: SP-6, HT-7.

Second Session
- PT2.
- Kidney zone (95).
- Jerome point (29 b).
- Occiput point (29).
- Vegetative point I (51).
- Body acupuncture: BL-23, KI-3.

Third Session
- Master omega point.
- Omega point II.
- Vegetative point II (34).
- PT3 and PT4.
- Vegetative point II (34).
- Body acupuncture: LU-7, BL-20, GV-20.

Fourth Session
- If required, the same as the first session.

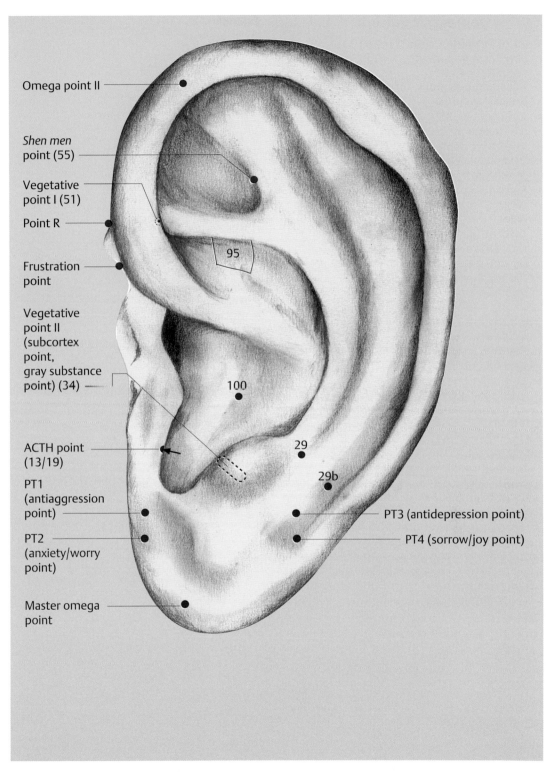

Omega point II

Shen men
point (55)

Vegetative
point I (51)

Point R

Frustration
point

Vegetative
point II
(subcortex
point,
gray substance
point) (34)

ACTH point
(13/19)

PT1
(antiaggression
point)

PT2
(anxiety/worry
point)

Master omega
point

95

100

29

29b

PT3 (antidepression point)

PT4 (sorrow/joy point)

Fig. 10.36 Pool for burnout syndrome

10.11.4 **Depressive Episode**

Pool of Feasible Points (Fig. 10.37)
- Psychotropic points (PT1–PT4).
- Point R (Bourdiol).
- Master omega point.
- Frustration point.
- Kidney zone (95).
- Occiput point (29).
- Vegetative point I (51).
- Vegetative point II (34).
- Jerome point (29 b).
- Retro-Jerome point.

Primary Point Selection
- Psychotropic points (PT1–PT4).
- Frustration point.
- Master omega point.
- Kidney zone (95).
- *Shen men* point (55).

Supplementary Points
- Jerome point (29 b).
- Retro-Jerome point.
- Occiput point (29).
- Vegetative point I (51).
- Vegetative point II (34).

Combination with Body Acupuncture
For example in liver *qi* stagnation: BL-18, LR-3, CV-12, GB-34, ST-36.

For this condition, psychotherapeutic treatment is the focus of the therapeutic efforts, and acupuncture has become an established adjuvant treatment. A total of 15 to 20 sessions of acupuncture treatment will be required as follows: Initially, the patient is needled twice a week. Once the condition has stabilized, treatment is carried out at weekly intervals. The sets of points will be selected according to the course of the condition and alternate from session to session.

Example
First Session
- PT1 and PT3.
- Master omega point.
- Point R.
- Frustration point.
- Vegetative point II (34).
- Body acupuncture: GB-34, CV-17.

Second Session
- PT2.
- Kidney zone (95).
- Jerome point (29 b).
- Occiput point (29).
- Vegetative point I (51).
- Body acupuncture: LR-3, BL-18.

Third Session
- Master omega point.
- Point R.
- PT3 and PT4.
- Vegetative point II (34).
- Body acupuncture: ST-36, CV-12.

Fourth Session
- If required, the same as the first session.

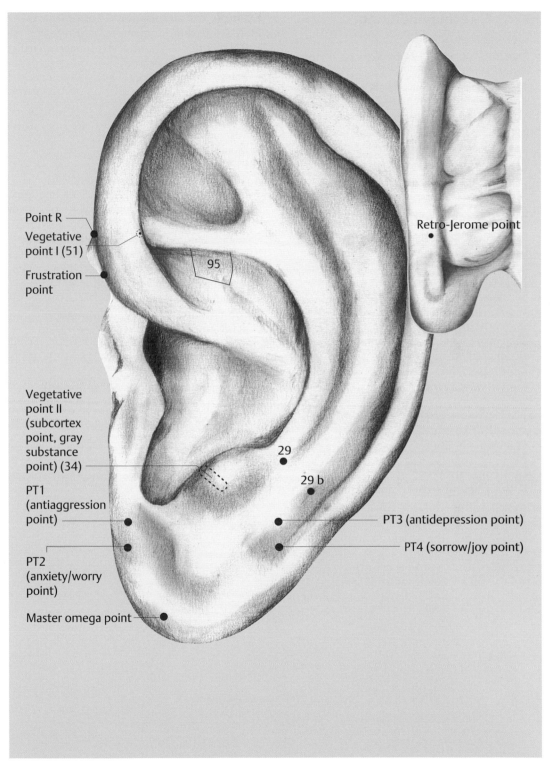

Fig. 10.37 Pool for depressive episodes.

10.11.5 Nicotine Addiction

> **Practical Tip**
>
> Prior to treatment, a 24-hour period of abstinence is indicated. In severe cases, a schematic set of points does not provide sufficient support. One should, therefore, aim for an individual set of points, depending on the patient's history and the sensitivity of points, and should also include body acupuncture (e.g., GV-20, HT-7).

Pool of Feasible Points (Fig. 10.38)

- ACTH point.
- Craving point (29 c).
- Psychotropic points: PT1 (antiaggression point), frustration point.
- Sensitive points in the lung zone (101).
- Vegetative point I (51), or heart zone (100), or vegetative point II (34).
- *Shen men* point (55).
- Occiput point (29).
- Mouth zone (84).
- Master omega point.

Example for Schematic Treatment (According to Nogier):

- Craving point (29 c).
- PT1.
- Lung zone (101).
- If warranted, also frustration point.

Example for an Individual Set of Points

Indicated in difficult cases, such as repeated recidivism, or in cases of severe underlying diseases and emotional stress.

- Master omega point (if warranted, omega I point).
- Craving point (29 c).
- Occiput point (29).
- Vegetative point II (34).
- Mouth zone (84).

A single treatment is often sufficient.

In principle, treatment is feasible on both ears. However, when considering laterality, treatment should start on the contralateral auricle with respect to right- or left-handedness. Hence, in a right-handed person, the left auricle is examined and needled first; it is then possible that only a few sensitive points will be detected on the right auricle.

Combination with Body Acupuncture

LI-4, GB-20, ST-36, LU-7, HT-7, PC-6, GV-20.

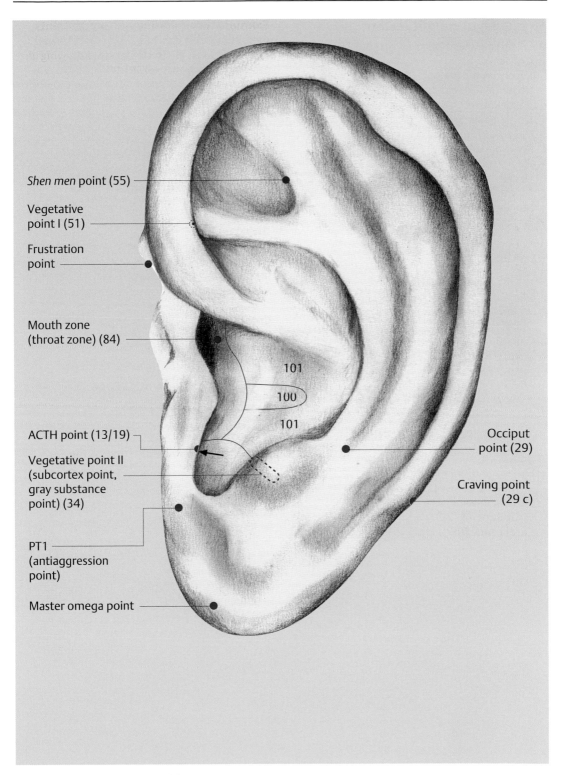

Shen men point (55)

Vegetative point I (51)

Frustration point

Mouth zone (throat zone) (84)

101

100

101

ACTH point (13/19)

Vegetative point II (subcortex point, gray substance point) (34)

PT1 (antiaggression point)

Master omega point

Occiput point (29)

Craving point (29 c)

Fig. 10.38 Pool for nicotine addiction.

10.11.6 **Overweight, Bulimia**

Pool of Feasible Points (Fig. 10.39)
- Craving point (29 c).
- Psychotropic points: PT1 to PT4, frustration point.
- Point R.
- Omega points.
- Vegetative points I (51) and II (34).
- Solar plexus point.
- *Shen men* point (55).
- Occiput point (29).
- Mouth zone (84).
- Stomach zone (84).
- Food craving point (level C7/T1, transition of stomach to liver area).
- Cardia zone (86).

Primary Point Selection
- Stomach zone (87) (sieving technique).
- Food craving point.
- Mouth zone (84).
- Point R.
- Vegetative point II (34).
- Solar plexus point.
- Master omega point.
- Craving point (29 c).

Supplementary Points
- Psychotropic points: PT1 to PT4, frustration point.
- Omega points I and II.
- Vegetative point I (51).
- *Shen men* point (55).
- Occiput point (29).
- Cardia zone (86).

Combination with Body Acupuncture
LI-4, LI-10, GV-20, ST-25, ST-36, SP-6, LR-3.

A series of 10 to 15 treatments is recommended. If there are no positive results (appetite reduction) after the second session, it is pointless to continue treatment. Treatment is carried out at intervals of 6 to 7 days as appetite reduction usually lasts for that long. A series of 10 to 15 treatments is sufficient to induce physiological weight reduction. In order to achieve long-term results, series of five sessions may be repeated at intervals of 3 to 6 months.

Example
First Session
- Craving point (29 c).
- Master omega point.
- Vegetative point II (34).
- Mouth zone (84).
- Cardia zone (86).
- PT1.

Second Session
- Stomach zone (87) (sieving technique).
- Solar plexus point.
- Point R.
- Food craving point (level C7/T1, transition from stomach to liver area).
- *Shen men* point (55).
- Psychotropic points: PT1 to PT4, depending on sensitivity.

Third Session
- Mouth zone (84).
- Cardia zone (86).
- Psychotropic points: PT1 to PT4, depending on sensitivity.
- Craving point (84).
- Vegetative point I (51).
- Occiput point (29).

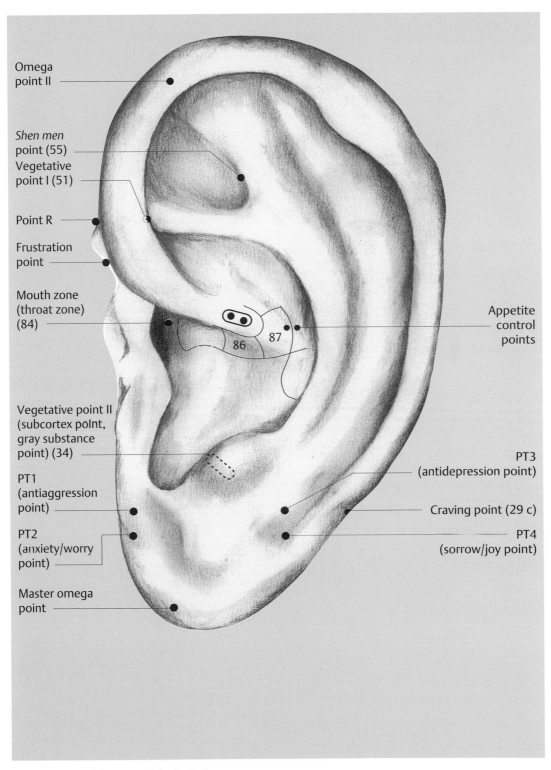

Omega
point II

Shen men
point (55)
Vegetative
point I (51)

Point R

Frustration
point

Mouth zone
(throat zone)
(84)

86 87

Appetite
control
points

Vegetative point II
(subcortex polnt,
gray substance
point) (34)

PT1
(antiaggression
point)

PT2
(anxiety/worry
point)

Master omega
point

PT3
(antidepression point)

Craving point (29 c)

PT4
(sorrow/joy point)

Fig. 10.39 Pool for overweight, bulimia.

Appendix

11 Numerical Index of Points and Zones (Page, Figure, Location)

Front – lateral surface of auricle
Back – medial surface of auricle
m – medial

1	Tooth point (dental analgesia point I), p. 32, **Fig. 3.8** ⟶ Front, lobule
2	Upper palate point, p. 33, **Fig. 3.8** ⟶ Front, lobule
3	Lower palate point, p. 33, **Fig. 3.8** ⟶ Front, lobule
4	Tongue Point, p. 33, **Fig. 3.8** ⟶ Front, lobule
5	Upper jaw point (Chinese), p. 33, **Fig. 3.9** ⟶ Front, lobule
6	Lower jaw point (Chinese), p. 33, **Fig. 3.9** ⟶ Front, lobule
7	Tooth point (dental analgesia point II), p. 33, **Fig. 3.9** ⟶ Front, lobule
8	Eye point, p. 34, **Fig. 3.9** ⟶ Front, lobule
9	Inner ear point, p. 34, **Fig. 3.9** ⟶ Front, lobule
10	Tonsil point (Chinese), p. 34, **Fig. 3.11** ⟶ Front, lobule
11	Cheek zone, p. 35, **Fig. 3.11** ⟶ Front, lobule
12	Apex of tragus point, p. 26, **Fig. 3.3** ⟶ Front, tragus
13	ACTH point (Nogier; adrenal gland point), p. 24, **Figs. 3.3 and 3.4** ⟶ Front, tragus
14	External nose point, p. 24, not shown ⟶ Front, tragus
15	Larynx/pharynx point (Chinese), p. 26, **Fig. 3.3** ⟶ Front, tragus
16	Inner nose point, p. 26, **Fig. 3.3** ⟶ Front, tragus
17	Thirst point, p. 26, **Fig. 3.3** ⟶ Front, tragus
18	Hunger point (appetite control point), p. 26, **Fig. 3.3** ⟶ Front, tragus
19	Antihypertension point (high blood pressure point), p. 26, **Fig. 3.3** ⟶ Front, tragus
20	External ear point, p. 24, **Fig. 3.2** ⟶ Front, supratragic notch
21	Heart point, p. 24, **Fig. 3.2** ⟶ Front, supratragic notch
22	Endocrine zone, p. 26, **Figs. 3.3 and 3.4** ⟶ Front, intertragic notch
23	Ovary point (gonadotropin point), p. 27, **Fig. 3.4** ⟶ Front, intertragic notch
24 a, 24 b	Eye points, p. 27, **Fig. 3.4** ⟶ Front, intertragic notch
25	Brainstem point, p. 24, **Fig. 3.7** ⟶ Front, postantitragal fossa
26 a	Thalamus point, pp. 27, 65, **Figs. 3.5, 3.6, and 4.1** ⟶ Front, antitragus
29	Occiput point (pad point), pp. 30, 65, 68, **Figs. 3.7, 4.1, 4.3, and 4.4** ⟶ Front, postantitragal fossa
29 a	Kinetosis point (nausea point, antiemetica point), p. 30, **Fig. 3.7** ⟶ Front, post-antitragal fossa
29 b	Jerome point (Nogier; relaxation point, sexual suppression point, pp. 30, 69, **Figs. 3.7 and 4.4** ⟶ Front, postantitragal fossa
29 c	Craving point (desire point), p. 30, **Fig. 3.7** ⟶ Front, postantitragal fossa
30	Parotid gland point, p. 28, **Fig. 3.5** ⟶ Front, antitragus

12 Alphabetical Index of Points and Zones (Name, Page, Figure)

13 Figure Sources

Figs. 1.1, 1.2, 2.3–2.10, 6.1–6.3, 6.5, 6.6, 7.1, 7.8–7.12, Dr. Hans-Jürgen Weise, Rheinfelden, Germany.

Fig. 1.5 The cortical representation of different parts of the body in the primary somatosensory cortex of the postcentral gyrus (left) and the primary motor cortex of the precentral gyrus (right) in the human being (after Penfield W, Jasper H), from: Mumenthaler M, Mattle H. Fundamentals of Neurology. Stuttgart–New York: Thieme Publishers; 2006.

Fig. 3.17 from: Schiffter R, Harms E. Connective Tissue Massage. Bindegewebsmassage According to Dicke. Stuttgart: Thieme Publishers; 2014.

Fig. 6.1 With kind permission from schwamedico Medizintechnik, Ehringhausen, Germany.

Fig. 7.2 With kind permission from SEDATELEC Chemin des Mûriers, 69540 Irigny/France (www.sedatelec.com).

14 References

Alimi D, Rubino C, Pichard-Leandri E. Analgesic effect of auricular acupuncture for cancer pain: a randomized, blinded, controlled trial. J Clin Oncol 2003;21:4120–4126

Avants SK, Margolin A, Holford T, Kosten TR. A randomized controlled trial of auricular acupuncture for cocaine dependence. Arch Intern Med 2000;160:2305–2312

Bachmann G. Die Akupunktur—eine Ordnungstherapie. 3. Aufl. Heidelberg: Haug; 1980

Backmund M, Meyer K, Baeyens H, Eichenlaub D. Akupunktur und stationärer Drogenentzug—eine kontrollierte Pilotstudie. Dt Ztschr f Akup 1999;42(4):206–209

Bahn J, Küblböck J. Laserstrahlen in der Akupunktur. Wien: Wilhelm Maudrich Verlag; 1997

Bahn J. Laser und Infrarotstrahlen in der Akupunktur. 4. Aufl. Heidelberg: Haug; 1990

Becke H, Richter K. Akupunktur. 3. Aufl. Wiesbaden: Ullstein Medical; 1995

Berman AH, Lundberg U. Auricular acupuncture in prison psychiatric units: a pilot study. Acta Psychiatr Scand 2002;106:152–157

Bier IA, Wilson J, Studt P, Shakleton M. Auricular acupuncture, education and smoking cessation: a randomized, sham-controlled trial. Am J Public Health 2002;92:1642–1647

Birngruber, R. Gabel, V. P. Augengefährdung durch Lasereffekte in Diskotheken. Sozialpädiatrie Prax Klin 1984; 6(9):487–494

Bischko J. Handbuch der Akupunktur und Aurikulotherapie. Heidelberg: Haug; 1998

Bossy J. Formation réticulaire at acupuncture. Méridiens1981;55–56:73–93

Bossy J, Prat-Pradal D, Teullemolier J. Die Microsysteme der Akupunktur. Essen: VGM-Verlag; 1993

Bourdiol RJ. Elements of auriculotherapy. Moulins-les-Metz: Maisonneuve; 1982

Bucek R. Die Rolle der kombinierten Ohr- und Körperakupunktur bei der Raucherentwöhnung und Gewichtsabnahme. Dt Ztschr f Akup 1986;2:27–32

Buhk H, Busch W, Feldkamp J, Koch U. Ergebnisse einer Studie zur ambulanten Akupunkturbehandlung von alkohol- und medikamentenabhängigen Klienten in einer Beratungsstelle. Suchttherapie 2001;2:35–44

Bullock ML, Kiresuk TJ, Sherman RE, et al. A large randomized placebo controlled study of auricular acupuncture for alcohol dependence. J Subst Abuse Treat 2002;22:71–77

Caspers KH. Laser Reiztherapie. Physik Med Rehabil 1977;9:426–455

Chen G. Advances on ear acupoints research. Paper presented at: International Symposium on Diagnosis and Treatment with Auricular Points, October 16–19, 1989; Beijing, China

Cole B, Yarbery M. NADA training provides PTSD relief in Haiti. Dt Ztschr f Akup 2011;54(1):21–24

D'Alberto A. Auricular acupuncture in the treatment of cocaine/crack abuse: review of the efficacy, the use of the National Acupuncture Detoxification Association protocol, and the selection of sham points. J Altern Complement Med 2004;10:985–1000

Dinstl K, Fischer PL. Der Laser, Grundlagen und Klinische Anwendung. Heidelberg: Springer Verlag; 1981

Dung AC. Die Rolle des Vagus bei der Gewichtsreduktion durch Ohrakupunktur. J Trad Chin Med 1986;14(3):183

Durinjan RH. Physiological basis of auricular reflexes to viscera-endocrine functions, acupuncture and electrotherapy. Research International Journal 1983;8:9–80

Eichner H, Kampik G, Gleditsch J. Akupunkturbehandlung bei akuter Sinusitis bei Kindern und Erwachsenen. Akupunktur Theorie und Praxis 1987;15(1):6–15

Einstein A. Zur Quantentheorie der Strahlung. Theorie des thermodynamischen Gleichgewichts. Berlin: Springer; 1917

Gaponjuk VPJ, Scherkovina TJ, Leonova MV. Differenzierte aurikuläre Elektroakupunktur bei der Behandlung der Hypertension. Akupunktur 1993;21:265–268

Gates S, Smith LA, Foxcroft DR. Auricular acupuncture for cocaine dependence. Cochrane Database Syst Rev 2006 Jan 25;(1):CD005192

Gleditsch JM. Mikroakupunktsysteme: Maps; Grundlagen und Praxis der somatotopischen Therapie. Stuttgart: Hippokrates; 2002

Gleditsch JM. Mundakupunktur. 8. Aufl. München: Elsevier; 2004

Gleditsch JM. Reflexzonen und Somatotopien. 9. Aufl. München: Elsevier; 2005

Grüsser SM, Mörsen CP, Rau S, et al. Der Einfluss von Ohrakupunktur auf das Drogenverlangen und das emotionale Befinden bei Opiatabhängigen und nicht abhängigen Alkoholkonsumenten. Dt Ztschr f Akup 2005;48(2):20–27

Head H. On disturbances of sensations with especial reference to the pain of visceral disease. Brain 1893;1–133

Helms JM, Walkowski SA, Elkiss M, et al. HMI Auricular Trauma Protocol: an acupuncture approach for trauma spectrum symptoms (NADA-verwandte Methode). Dt Ztschr f Akup 2012;55(4):5–8

Kampik G. Zuverlässige Hilfe bei Singultus durch Ohrakupunktur. Akupunktur. Theorie und Praxis 1975;3:75

Kampik G. Propädeutik der Akupunktur. 4. Aufl. Stuttgart: Hippokrates; 1998

Klauser AG, Rubach A, Bertsche O, Müller-Lissner SA. Body acupuncture: effect on colonic function in chronic constipation. Z Gastroenterol 1993;31(10):605–608

König G, Wancura I (eEds). Praxis und Theorie der Neuen Chinesischen Akupunktur. Band III. 2. Aufl. Wien: Maudrich; 1998

König G, Wancura I. Einführung in die chinesische Ohrakupunktur. Heidelberg: Haug; 1999

Krivorutskii B. Attachment for electroacupuncture of the external ear in treating smoking. Vopr Kurortol Fizioter Lech Fiz Kult 1986;4:71–73

Kropej H. Systematik der Ohrakupunktur. 3. Aufl. Heidelberg: Haug; 1977

Kropej H. Systematik der Ohrakupunktur. 7. Aufl. Heidelberg: Haug; 1993

Krüger H, Krüger CP.Grundlagen der Auriculotherapie bei Hund und Pferd. Akupunkturarzt 1980;13:7

Lange G. Akupunktur der Ohrmuschel. Schorndorf: BMV-Verlag; 1985

Lapeer GL. Auriculotherapy in dentistry. Cranio 1986;4(3):266–275

Li L, Wang ZY. Clinical therapeutic effects of body acupuncture and ear acupuncture on juvenile simple obesity and effects on metabolism of blood lipids. Zhonegguo Zhen Jiu 2006;26:173–176

Li QS, Liu ZY, Ma HJ, et al. A preliminary study on the mechanism of ear-acupuncture for withdrawal of smoking. J Trad Chin Med 1987;7:243–247

Lian Y. TCM Methods of Obstetrical Care. Tinajin, China: TCM University of Tianjin, China, 1996

Maciocia G. Die Praxis der chinesischen Medizin. Kötzting: Verlag für Traditionelle Chinesische Medizin; 1997

Mainman T. Optical and microwave-optical experiments in ruby. Phys Rev Lett 1960;4:564

Margolin A, Chany P, Kelly S, Vosten R. Effects of sham and real auricular needling: implications for tricks of acupuncture for cocaine addiction. Am J Chin Med 1993;21:103–111

Margolin A, Kleber HD, Avants SK, et al. Acupuncture for the treatment of cocaine addiction: a randomized controlled trial. JAMA 2002;287:55–63

Markgraft A. Beitrag zur Ohrdiagnose. Naturheilpraxis 1982;10.

Marktl G, Payer K, Ots T, et al. PatientInnenzufriedenheit mit der NADA-Ohrakupunktur auf einer psychiatrischen Station. Dt Ztschr f Akup 2007;50(2):10–13

Marx HG. Medikamentenfreie Entgiftung von Suchtkranken. Bericht über den Einsatz von Akupunktur. Suchtgefahren 1984;30–34

Mastalier O. Reflextherapie in der Zahn-, Mund- und Kieferheilkunde. 2. Aufl. Berlin: Quintessenz Verlags; 1992

Melzack R, Wall PD. Pain mechanisms: a new theory. Science 1965:Nov 19;150(3699):971–979

Mester E. The biomedical effects of laser-application. Lasers Surg Med 1985;5:31–39

Niederecker M. Akupunktur nach dem NADA-Protokoll am Fachkrankenhaus für Psychiatrie und Psychotherapie Taufkirchen (Vils). Dt Ztschr f Akup 2004;47(2):14–17

Nogier PFM. Über die Akupunktur der Ohrmuschel. Übersetzung von G. Bachmann. Dt Ztschr f Akup 1957;3–8

Nogier PFM. Lehrbuch der Auriculotherapie. Sainte-Ruffine: Maisonneuve; 1969

Nogier PFM. Treatise of auriculotherapy. Moulinsles-Metz: Maisonneuve; 1972

Nogier PFM. Loki auriculo medicinae. Verlag: Moulins-les-Metz; 1976

Nogier PFM. Praktische Einführung in die Aurikulotherapie. Sainte-Ruffine: Maisonneuve; 1978

Nogier PFM. Lehrbuch der Auriculotherapie. Saint-Ruffine: Maisonneuve; 1981

Nogier PFM. From auriculotherapy to auriculomedicine. Moulins-les-Metz: Maisonneuve; 1983

Nogier PFM. Points réflexes auriculaires. Sainte-Ruffine: Maisonneuve; 1987

Nogier PFM. Complément des points réflexes auriculaires. Moulins-les-Metz: Maisonneuve; 1989

Nogier PFM, Nogier R. The man in the ear. Moulins-les-Metz: Maisonneuve; 1987

Nogier R. Introduction practique à l' auriculo medicine. Bruxelles: Haug; 1993

Nogier R. Auriculotherapy. Thieme, 2009

Ogaï BCh, Pashkova TL, Kolganova NA. [Effectiveness of acupuncture and berotec aerosol in bronchial asthma.] Sov Med 1986;9:98–100

Ogal H, Ogal M, Hafer J, Hennig J, Brockemeyer H, Kracht R. Beginn der Anxiolyse und Relaxation unter Ohrakupunktur. Dt Ztschr f Akup 2004;47(2):6–12

Oleson TD. Auriculo therapy manual: Chinese and Western systems of ear acupuncture. Los Angeles, CA: Health Care Alternatives; 1990

Ornstein RE. Die Psychologie des Bewusstseins. Frankfurt: Fischer Taschenb; 1982

Ots T. Leib und Empowerment. Dt Ztschr f Akup 2013;56(2):55–56

Ots T, Rubach A, Raben R. Gibt es eine soziale Kompetenz der Akupunktur? Impressionen einer Amerika-Reise. Dt Ztschr f Akup 2010;53(2):4–7

Pennala M, et al. Primary Effect of permanent ear acupuncture on appetite and ventricular feelings in 374 outpatients research. Nordic Acupuncture Society. Acupuncture seminar at: Joensuu 1983. Finnish Acupuncture Ass. Espoo; 1984

Pennala M, Pöntinen JP, Kalinowski J. Langzeitergebnisse in der Behandlung der Adipositas mit Ohrakupunktur (1200 Patienten). Akupunktur—Theorie und Praxis. 1986;4:69–77

Pert A, Dionne R, Ng L, Bragin E, Moody TW, Pert CB. Alterations in rat central nervous system: endorphins following transauricular electro-acupuncture. Brain Res 1981;224(1):83–93

Peuker ET. Wissenschaftliche Grundlagen der Ohrakupunktur. Dt Ztschr f Akup 2003;3:6–13

Pildner v. Steinburg R, Pildner v. Steinburg D. Die Behandlung der zentralen vestibulären Dysfunktion mittels Akupunktur (Reflextherapie), HNO Praxis Heute. 1983;3:161–167

Pimentel-Paredes J. Medical missions for the victims of Typhoon Ondoy. Dt Ztschr f Akup 2010;53(3):45–46

Porkert M. Die Entwicklung der Ohrakupunktur aus chinesischer Sicht. Vol. 10.1 Wiss. Akupunktur und Auriculomedizin. Heidelberg: VfM Dr. E. Fischer; 1987

Portnov FG. Aurikulotherapija i aurikuldiagnostika. Nauka i technika 1979;5:11

Raben R. Akupunktur in der Behandlung drogenabhängiger Schwangerer. Dt Ztschr f Akup 1998;41(2):38–42

Raben R. Akupunkturgestützte Sressbewältigung. Dt Ztschr f Akup 2004;47(2):18–20

Raben R. Akupunktur nach dem NADA-Protokoll. Dt Ztschr f Akup 2004;47(2):35–41

Raben R. Akupunktur nach dem NADA-Protokoll—eine Übersicht zur Sucht-Therapie. Dt Ztschr f Akup 2004;2:47

Raben R. Phasen der Stressbewältigung. Dt Ztschr f Akup 2011;54(4):13–17

Raben R, Carola S. Heroinabhängig—Akupunktur in einem Fall chronischer Drogenabhängigkeit. Dt Ztschr f Akup 2004;47(3):38–41

Romoli M. Auricular Acupuncture Diagnosis. Churchill Livingstone, 2009

Romoli M, Allais G, Airola G, Benedetto C. Ear acupuncture in the control of migraine pain: selecting the right acupoints by the "needle-contact test". Neurol Sci 2005;26: 158–161

Rubach A, Ots T. Auf in die USA—Berichte vom Besuch dreier Akupunktur-Konferenzen . Dt Ztschr f Akup 2010;53(2):78–81

Sator-Katzenschlager SM, Wölfler MM, Kozek-Langenecker SA, et al. Auricular electroacupuncture as an additional perioperative analgesic method during oocyte aspiration in IVF treatment. Hum Reprod 2006;21(8): 2114–2120

Schlehbusch KP. Der heutige Stand der Grundlagenforschung in der Akupunktur. Ärztezeitschrift Naturheilverfahren 1982;5:214

Schulte-Uebbing C. Gibt es verbotene Akupunkturpunkte in der Schwangerschaft? In: Römer A, Weigel M, Ziegler W, eds. Akupunkthurtherapie in Geburtshilfe und Frauenheilkunde. Stuttgart: Hippokrates Verlag; 1998:59–64

Schulte-Uebbing C. Aku-Tokolyse bei vorzeitigen Wehen In: Römer A, Weigel M, Ziegler W, eds. Akupunkthurtherapie in Geburtshilfe und Frauenheilkunde. Stuttgart: Hippokrates Verlag; 1998:75–82

Smith MO, Aponte J, Bonilla-Rodriguez R, et al. Acupuncture detoxification in a drug and alcohol abuse treatment setting. Am J Acupunct 1984;12(3):251–255

Smith MO. An acupuncture programme for the treatment of drug addicted persons. Bull Narc 1988;1:35–44

Sternlieb JJ, Gau GT, Davis GD, Rutherford BD, Frye RL. The ear crease sign in coronary artery disease (abstr). Circulation. 1974;50:152

Umlauf R. Zu den wissenschaftlichen Grundlagen der Aurikulotherapie. Dt Ztschr f Akup 1988;3:59–66

Usichenko TI, Dinse M, Hermsen M, et al. Auricular acupuncture for pain relief after total hip arthroplasty—a randomized controlled study. Pain 2005a;114:320–327

Usichenko TI, Hermsen M, Witstruck T, et al. Auricular acupuncture for pain relief after ambulatory knee arthroscopy—a pilot study. Evid Based Complement Alternat Med 2005b;2:185–189

Usichenko TI, Kuchling S, Witstruck T, et al. Auricular acupuncture for pain relief after ambulatory knee surgery: a randomized trial. CMAJ 2007;2:176–179

Velchover ES. O signalnoj funkcii usnoj rakoviny. [Über die Signalfunktion der Ohrmuschel.] Ezegodnik nauc. rabot Alma-Atinskogo IUV 1967;3:217

Vorobiev W, Dymnikov AA. The effectiveness of auricular microneedle acupuncture at the early postoperative period under conditions of the day surgical department. Vestn Khir im II Grek 2000;159:48–50

Wang SM, Peloquin C, Kain ZN. The use of auricular acupuncture to reduce preoperative anxiety. Anesth Analg 2001;93:1178–1180

Warnke U. Dosis-Wirkungskoordinaten der 904 nm Laserstrahlung auf Zellsuspensionen. In: Proceedings of the German Society of Laser Medicine, 1986. Munich: EBM Verlag; 1987:49–56

Weidig W. Erfahrungen mit Akupunktur beim Entzug von Jugendlichen in der Fachklinik Bokholt. Dt Ztschr f Akup 2004;47(3):24–31

Weidig W. Akupunktur in Sucht und Psyche—ein Update. Dt Ztschr f Akup 2012;55(3):12–15

Wimmer MU. Zur Akupunkturbehandlung der akuten Sinusitis bei Kindern und Erwachsenen [dissertation]. München: Ludwig-Maximilians-Unversität München; 1984

Witstruck T, Usichenko T, Dinse M, Hermsen M, Lehrmann C, Merk HR. Beeinflussung des Schmerzmittelverbrauchs durch Ohrakupunktur nach Hüft-TEP-Implantation—eine prospektive, randomisierte, kontrollierte Studie. Orthopädische Praxis 2004;40:110

Xu B, Fei J. Clinical observation of the weight-reducing effect of ear acupuncture in 350 cases of obesity. J Trad Chin Med 1985;5:87–88

Xu B, et al. Effective observation on 350 cases of reducing weight treated by emplanting earneedles. Chin Acup Mox 1984;4(6):167

Yarberry M. The use of the NADA-Protocol for PTSD in Kenya. Dt Ztschr f Akup 2010;53(4):6–11

Yuan S, et al. Comparison of Chinese and Nogier's ear point systems. Paper presented at: International Symposium on Diagnosis and Treatment with Auricular Points. October 16–19, 1989; Beijing, China

Zhang Zh: Weight reduction by auriculo-acupuncture—a report of 110 cases. J Trad Chin Med 1990;10(1):17–18

Zhao H. Auriculo-Acupuncture. Tianjin, China: TCM University of Tianjin; 1996

15 Subject Index

Notes

The numerical nomenclature is not used in the index, for details please refer to the appendix on
  pages 248-251
Page numbers in *italics* denote figures and tables

A

abdomen point 37, *37*
abdominal organs, reflex zones 22–23
abnormal placental detachment 132
abortion 128
achillodynia 208, *209*
acoustic meatus 15
acoustic state point 112
ACTH point 24, *26*, 27
– joint distortion/contusion 146
– nicotine addiction 159
acupressure 101
acute diseases 10
acute entcrocolitis 122
acute torticollis 142
addiction treatment 10, 156–162, *157*
– patient motivation 158
– during pregnancy 130
adrenal gland point (Chinese) *see* ACTH point
adrenal gland point (French) 39, *40*
adrenal plexus point 41, *42*
aggression 32
agitation, premature birth 129
alcohol addiction 161–162
allergens, migraine 150
allergic bronchial asthma 114–116, 184, *185*
allergic conjunctivitis 106–107
allergic eczema 153–155
allergic rhinitis 92–94, *93*
allergy, skin 153–155
allergy point 49–52, *51*
– allergic conjunctivitis 107
– allergy treatment 52
– chronic bronchitis 117
– eye diseases 105
– headache 147
– microphlebotomy 52, 88
– pollinosis 110
– skin allergy 153
– trigeminal neuralgia 151
amenorrhea 124

analgesia
– coxalgia 146
– delivery 132, *134*
– in labor 132, *134*
analgesia point 34, *34, 66,* 67, 143
analgesic points 65–67, *66*
– choice of 100
– neuralgia 151, 152
ankle point *45*
antiaggression point (PT1) *31,* 31–32, *70,* 71, *72*
antidepression point (PT3) *32,* 33, *33, 72,* 73
antiemetic point 30, *30*
antihelical crura 15, *19*
– locomotor system points/reflex zones 44–47
– points 47–49, *48*
antihelical sulcus 17
antihelix 15
– Chinese zones of representation 36–38, *37*
– French/Western zones of representation *38,* 38–39
– points *35,* 35–41, *37*
– relief changes 36, *36*
antihypertension groove 61, *62,* 117
antihypertension point(s) 26, *26,* 47, *48*
anti-inflammatory points 100
antitragus 15, *19*
– points localization 27–29, *28, 29*
– rotatory vertigo 112
anxiety 32, 71
– imminent premature birth 129
– pre-examination 95
anxiety syndromes 236, *237*
anxiety/worry point (PT2) *31,* 32, 71–73, *72*
apex of the helix 15
apex of tragus point 24, *26,* 112
apoplexy 228–230, *229, 231*
appendix point(s) 48, 49
appendix point I 48
appendix point II 48
appendix point III 48
appendix zone IV 57, *57, 58*
appetite control point (hunger point) 26, *26*

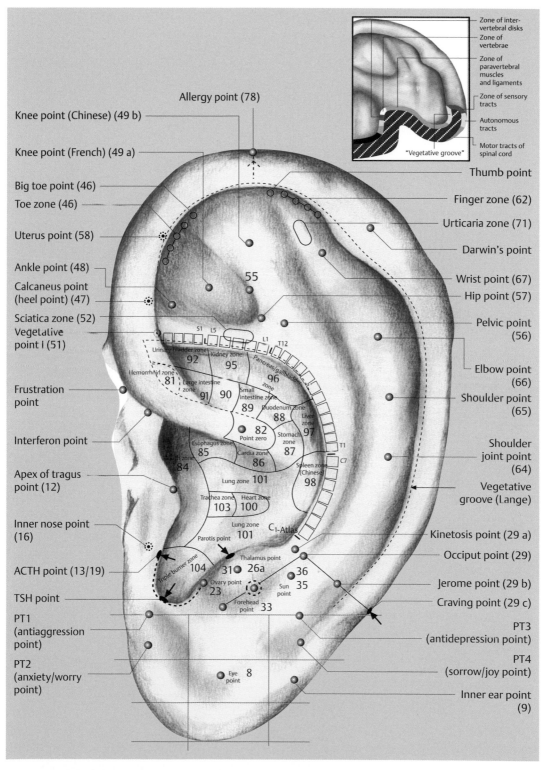

Allergy point (78)

Knee point (Chinese) (49 b)

Knee point (French) (49 a)

Big toe point (46)

Toe zone (46)

Uterus point (58)

Ankle point (48)

Calcaneus point
(heel point) (47)

Sciatica zone (52)

Vegetative
point I (51)

Frustration
point

Interferon point

Apex of tragus
point (12)

Inner nose point
(16)

ACTH point (13/19)

TSH point

PT1
(antiaggression
point)

PT2
(anxiety/worry
point)

Zone of inter-
vertebral disks
Zone of
vertebrae
Zone of
paravertebral
muscles
and ligaments
Zone of sensory
tracts
Autonomous
tracts
Motor tracts of
spinal cord
"Vegetative groove"

Thumb point

Finger zone (62)

Urticaria zone (71)

Darwin's point

Wrist point (67)

Hip point (57)

Pelvic point
(56)

Elbow point
(66)

Shoulder point
(65)

Shoulder
joint point
(64)

Vegetative
groove (Lange)

Kinetosis point (29 a)

Occiput point (29)

Jerome point (29 b)

Craving point (29 c)

PT3
(antidepression point)

PT4
(sorrow/joy point)

Inner ear point
(9)

55

S1   L5   L1   T12

Urinary bladder zone   Kidney zone

92   95

Pancreas/gallbladder
zone

96

Hemorrhoid zone

81   Large intestine
zone

91   90

Small
intestine zone

89

Duodenum zone

88

Liver
zone

97

T1

C7

Esophagus zone

85

82
Point zero

Stomach
zone

87

84

Cardia zone

86

Spleen zone
(Chinese)

98

Lung zone   101

Trachea zone   Heart zone

103   100

Lung zone
101

C1-Atlas

Parotis point

Thalamus point

104   31   26a   36

Triple burner zone

Ovary point

23

35

Sun
point

Forehead
point   33

Eye
point   8

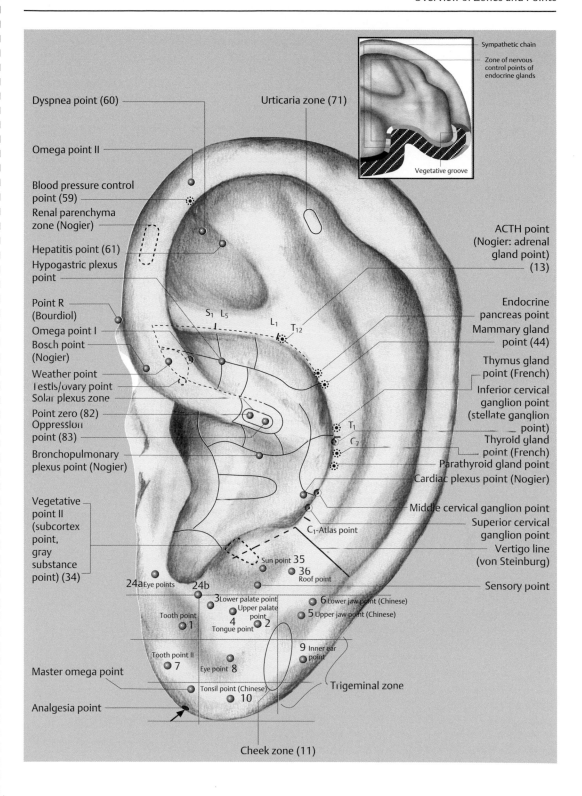

Dyspnea point (60)

Omega point II

Blood pressure control point (59)

Renal parenchyma zone (Nogier)

Hepatitis point (61)

Hypogastric plexus point

Point R (Bourdiol)

Omega point I

Bosch point (Nogier)

Weather point

Testis/ovary point

Solar plexus zone

Point zero (82)

Oppression point (83)

Bronchopulmonary plexus point (Nogier)

Vegetative point II (subcortex point, gray substance point) (34)

Master omega point

Analgesia point

Urticaria zone (71)

Sympathetic chain

Zone of nervous control points of endocrine glands

Vegetative groove

ACTH point (Nogier: adrenal gland point) (13)

Endocrine pancreas point

Mammary gland point (44)

Thymus gland point (French)

Inferior cervical ganglion point (stellate ganglion point)

Thyroid gland point (French)

Parathyroid gland point

Cardiac plexus point (Nogier)

Middle cervical ganglion point

Superior cervical ganglion point

Vertigo line (von Steinburg)

Sensory point

S_1 L_5

L_1 T_{12}

T_1

C_7

C_1-Atlas point

Sun point 35

36

Roof point

24a Eye points 24b

3 Lower palate point

Upper palate point

4 Tongue point 2

1 Tooth point

6 Lower jaw point (Chinese)

5 Upper jaw point (Chinese)

9 Inner ear point

Tooth point II 7

Eye point 8

Tonsil point (Chinese)

10

Trigeminal zone

Cheek zone (11)

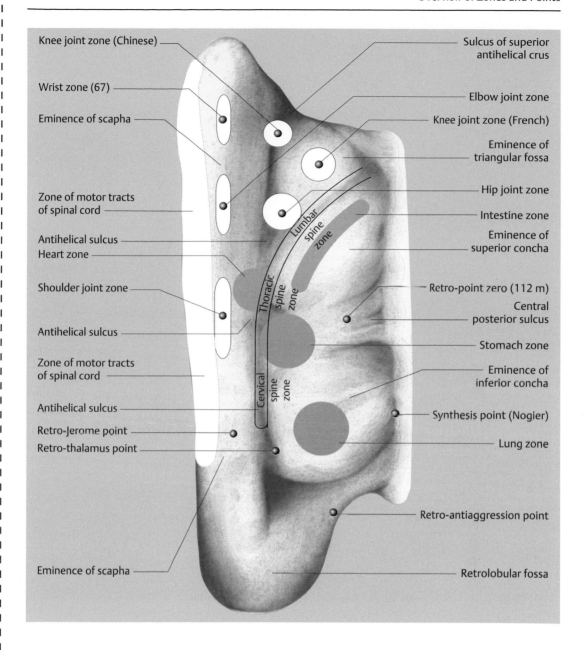

Knee joint zone (Chinese)

Wrist zone (67)

Eminence of scapha

Zone of motor tracts
of spinal cord

Antihelical sulcus

Heart zone

Shoulder joint zone

Antihelical sulcus

Zone of motor tracts
of spinal cord

Antihelical sulcus

Retro-Jerome point

Retro-thalamus point

Eminence of scapha

Sulcus of superior
antihelical crus

Elbow joint zone

Knee joint zone (French)

Eminence of
triangular fossa

Hip joint zone

Intestine zone

Eminence of
superior concha

Retro-point zero (112 m)

Central
posterior sulcus

Stomach zone

Eminence of
inferior concha

Synthesis point (Nogier)

Lung zone

Retro-antiaggression point

Retrolobular fossa

Lumbar spine zone

Thoracic spine zone

Cervical spine zone